FROM MEDICAL POLICE TO SOCIAL MEDICINE

Essays on the History of

Health Care

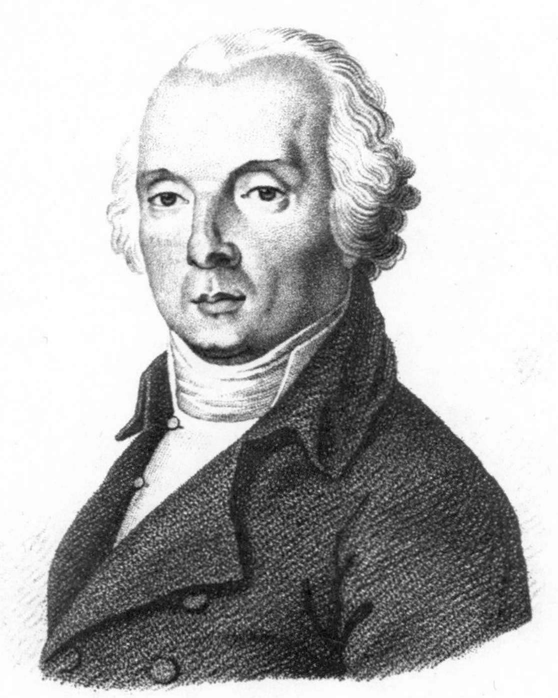

1 Johann Peter Frank (1745–1821), German physician, professor at Pavia and later at Vienna. The outstanding representative of community health action in the 18th century, he endeavored to systematize the health knowledge of his day and to show how it might be applied through government action for the benefit of the people. Frank's views, characteristic of public health thought and practice in an environment of enlightened despotism, are contained in his *System einer vollständigen medicinischen Polizey*, 1779 – 1827. COURTESY HISTORICAL LIBRARY, YALE UNIVERSITY MEDICAL SCHOOL.

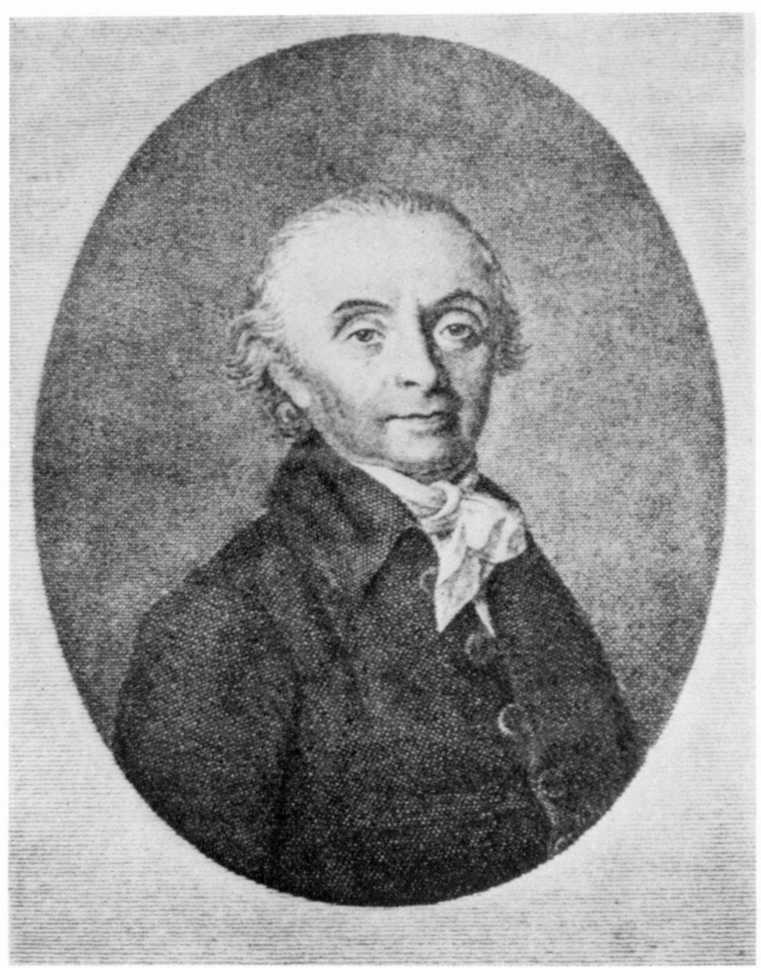

2 Franz Anton Mai (1742 – 1814), German physician and humanitarian who endeavored to put into practice the proposals made by Johann Peter Frank. In 1800 he submitted to the government of the Palatinate a draft of a health code as broad in scope as Frank's treatise. Though approved by the Elector, the medical officials of Mannheim, and the medical faculty of Heidelberg, his proposal was not realized due to political and administrative conditions.

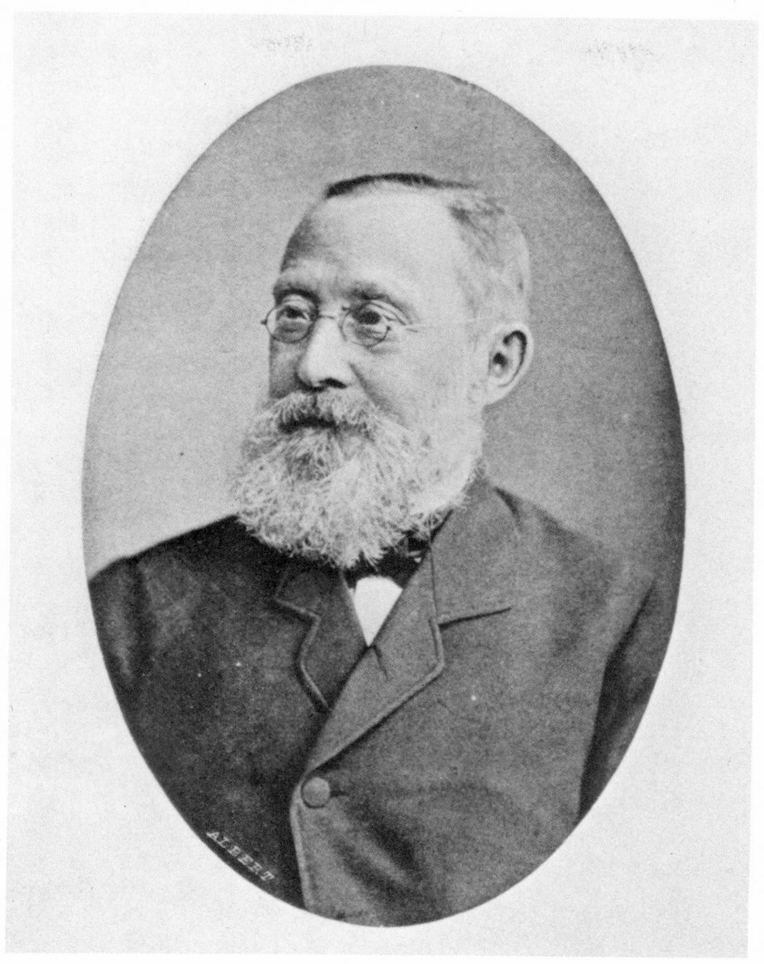

3 Rudolf Virchow (1821–1902), German pathologist, anthropologist and politician. Early in his career, he developed a concept of social epidemiology, and later helped to improve sanitary conditions and community health in Berlin. COURTESY THE JOHNS HOPKINS UNIVERSITY INSTITUTE OF THE HISTORY OF MEDICINE.

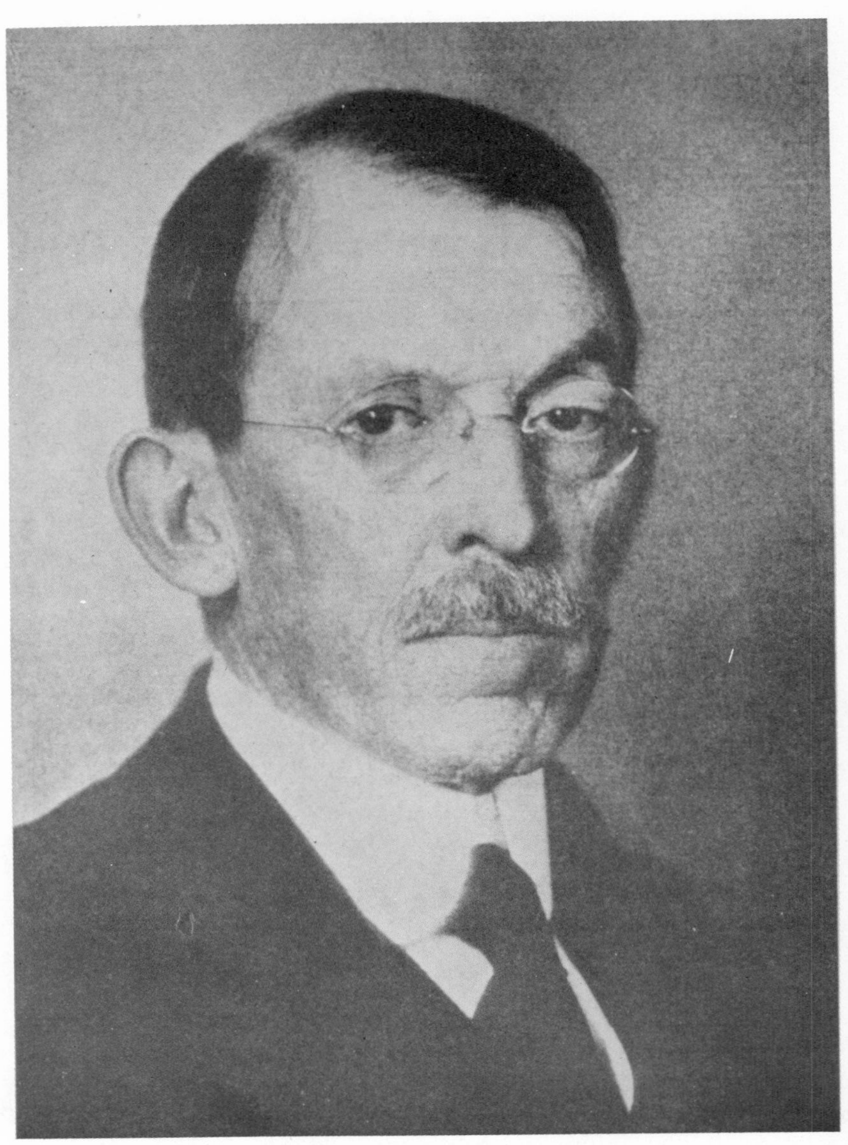

4 Hermann M. Biggs (1859 – 1923), a pioneer in tuberculosis control, the provisions of medical care, and in health education. He gave the public health laboratory a significant place in community health action, and was fully aware of the need for government to deal with social problems at the root of sickness and disease.

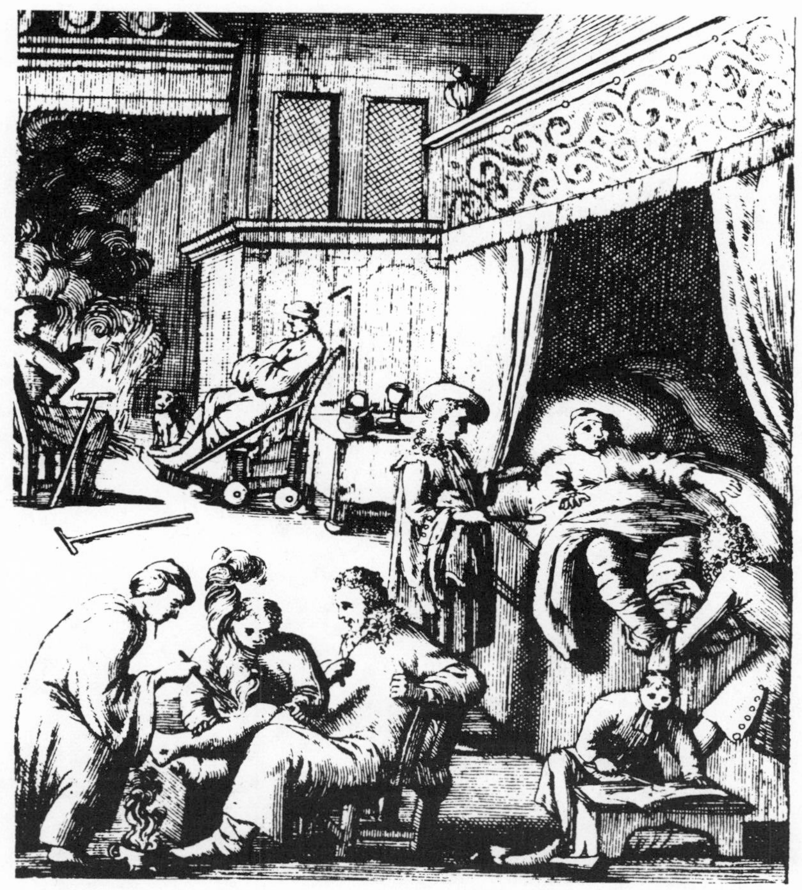

5 Medical care at the end of the 17th century in a more affluent household, as portrayed on the title-page of Stephen Blankaart's treatise on gout and its treatment, originally published at Amsterdam in 1684. Several different forms and aspects of treatment are represented. Near the fireplace in the background the gouty patient is seated in a wheelchair, his bandaged foot resting on a platform. At the right the patient is in bed; his foot is being bandaged, while a physician drops a medicinal fluid onto a spoon. At the lower left the patient is being treated by moxibustion, which had recently been introduced from the Orient. The bearded healer, presumably a Chinese, is igniting the moxa with an incense stick. The physician's assistant in the right foreground is preparing an ointment. OWEN H. WAGENSTEIN HISTORICAL LIBRARY OF BIOLOGY AND MEDICINE, UNIVERSITY OF MINNESOTA, MINNEAPOLIS, MINNESOTA.

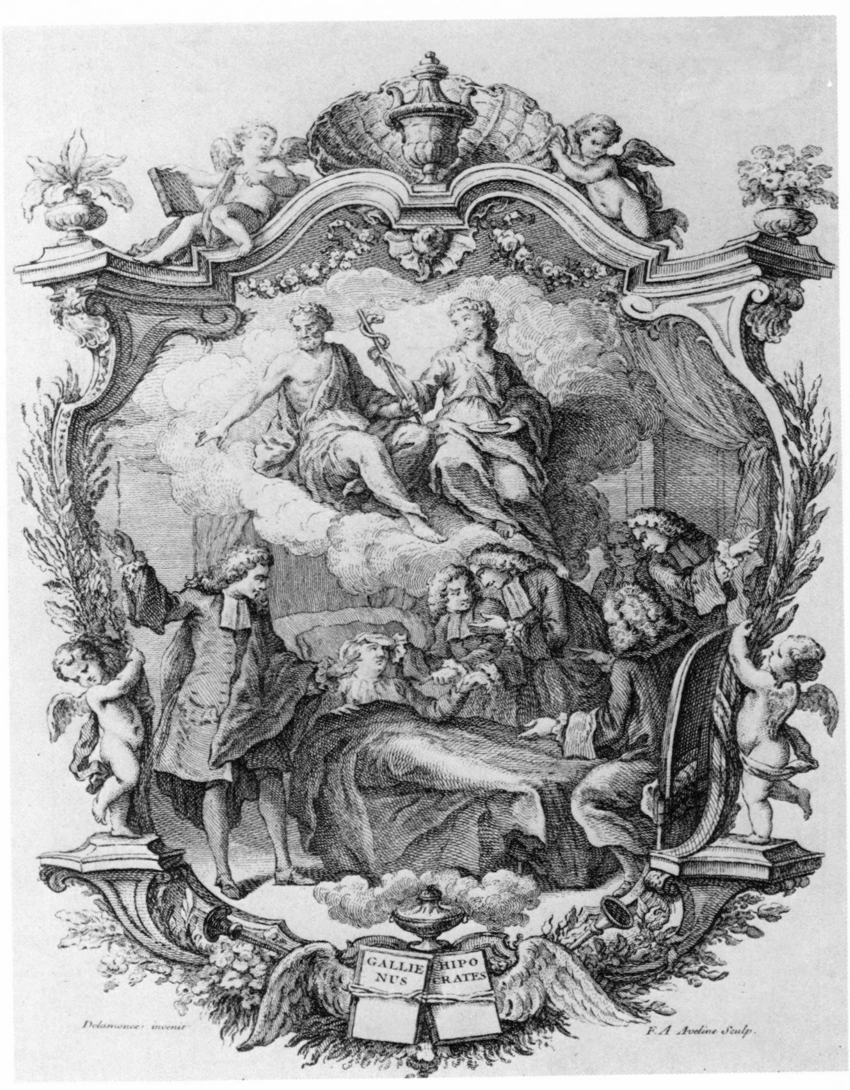

6 Medical care in the middle of the 18th century. A medical consultation at the bedside, under the aegis of Asclepius and Hygeia and based on Hippocrates and Galen. The rococo frame is typical of such illustrations in books of the period. Frontispiece, *Historia morborum que annis MDCXIX. MDCC. MDCCI. MDCCII. Vratislaviae grassati sunt . . .* LAUSANNE & GENEVA, MARC-MICHAEL BOUSQUET, 1746.

7 An 18th century hospital. View of the St.-Hubertus Hospital in Düsseldorf, founded 1709. From 1772 on, it was a military hospital for the garrison stationed in the city. The Holy Trinity is represented above the hospital which includes a church, wings for male and female patients, for foreigners, a school for pauper children, a flower garden, and herb garden and a fruit orchard.

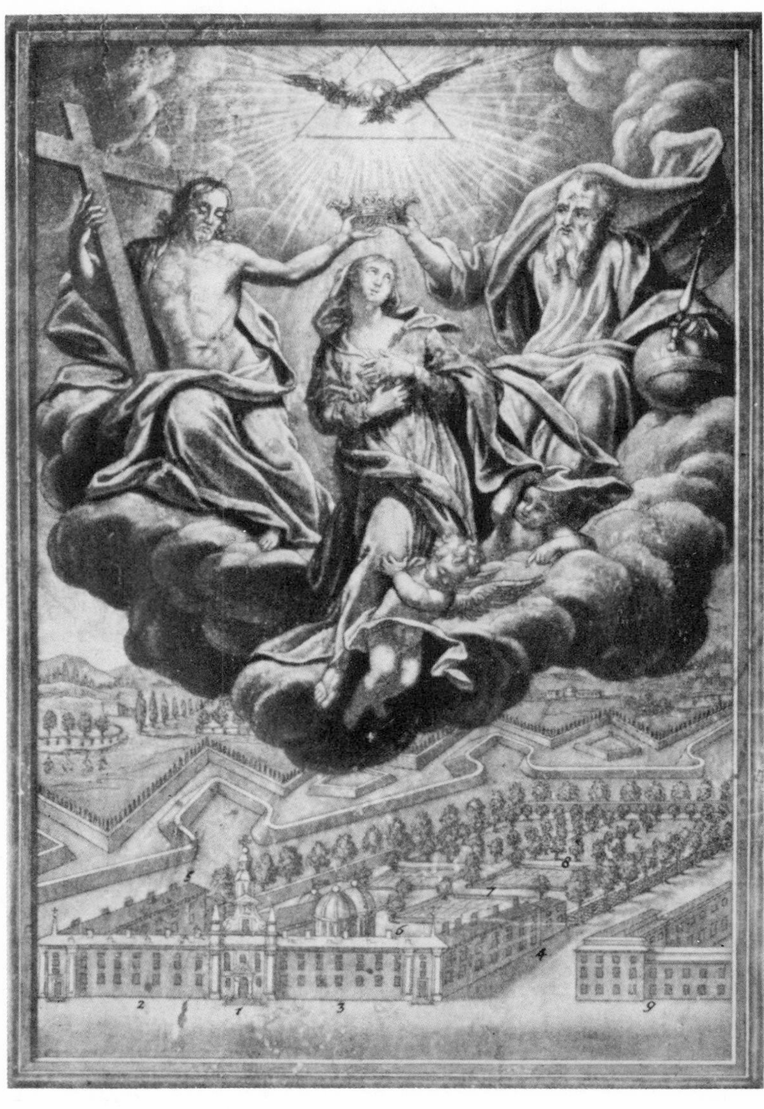

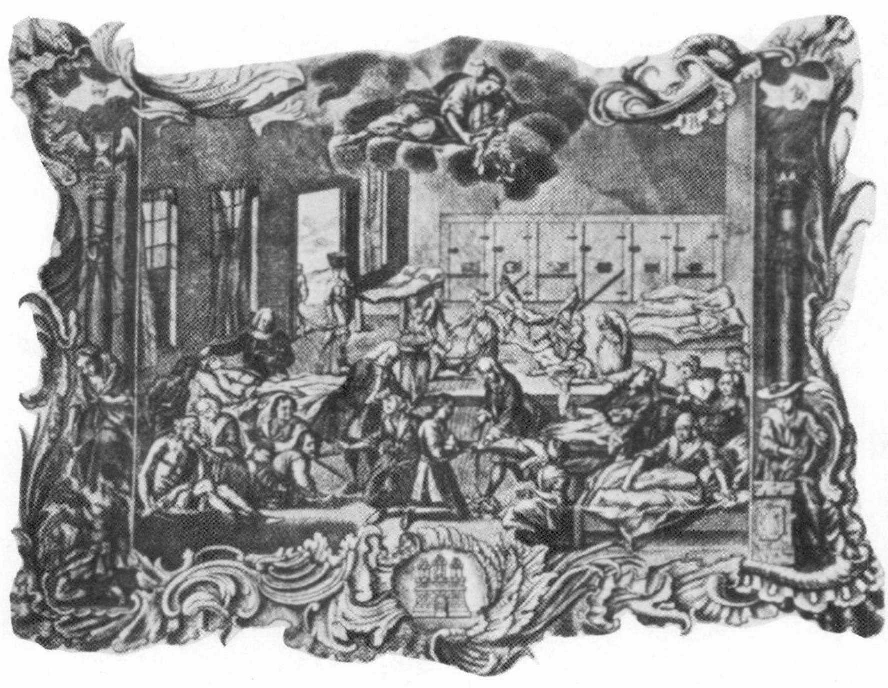

8 Medical care in a Hamburg hospital in 1746. Cells for lunatics are depicted in the background. In the center foreground a surgeon is amputating a man's leg. Patients with various conditions are all together in one room. STAATSARCHIV HAMBURG.

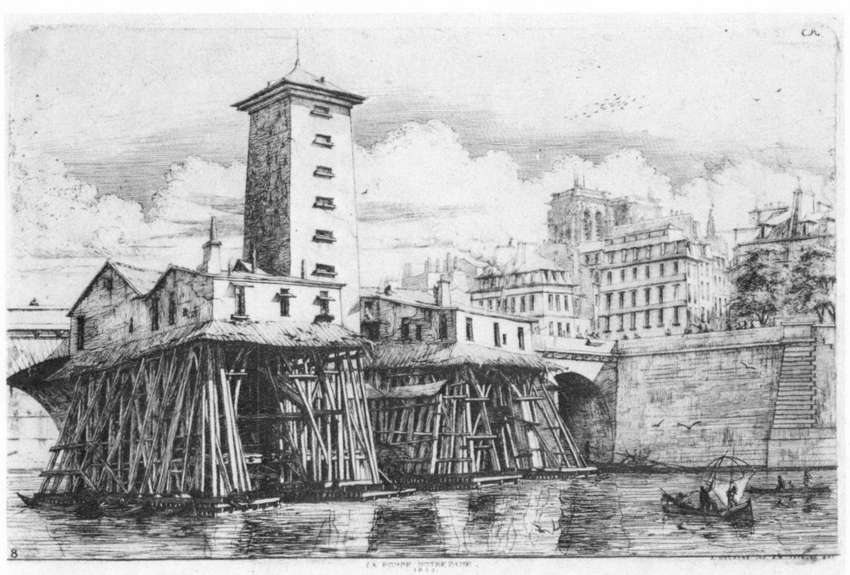

9 Charles Meryon (1821–1868). Le Pompe Notre Dame (1852). The use of polluted water pumped from the Seine was an important cause of ill health in Paris, producing various gastrointestinal infections. Foreigners unaccustomed to the local bacterial flora frequently experienced the equivalent of *la turista*. COURTESY YALE UNIVERSITY ART GALLERY.

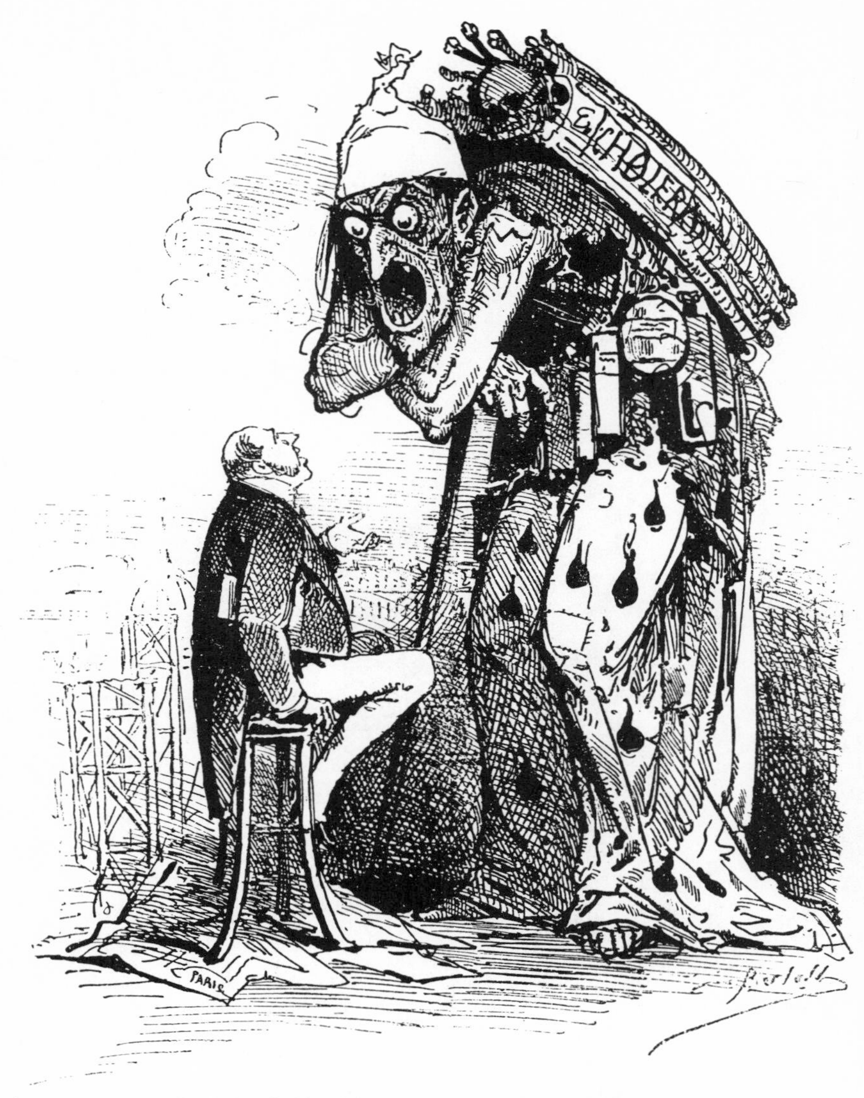

S. A. le Choléra fait aussi ses petites réclamations.

Les maisons où je me plaisais si bien, vous vous êtes plu à jeter tout par terre.
Eh bien! et moi! où vais-je me loger maintenant?

10 Cholera protests to Baron Haussmann that the destruction of old houses involved in the urban renewal of Paris has left him homeless, reflecting the view that the disease erupted where filth and poor housing existed. *L'Illustration,* PARIS, MARCH 13, 1869.

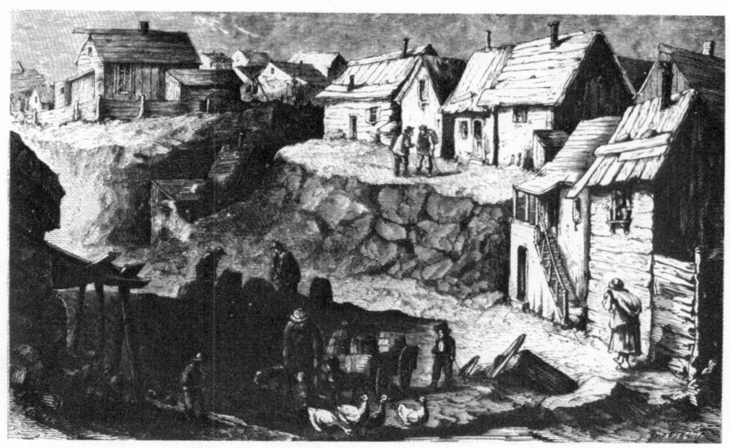

11 A shanty town on the outskirts of New York City in 1871, where the very poor lived. APPLETONS JOURNAL OF LITERATURE, SCIENCE AND ART, 5: 573, 1871.

12 How the Alms-House Children are Reared. Investigators find three half-starved Alms-House children in the room of a hired nurse, 152 E. 34th St., New York City. Infant mortality was a major health problem during the 18th and 19th centuries, resulting from social conditions plus defective medical knowledge. The infant poor, frequently placed in alms houses or with hired women were in the worst situation and died from malnutrition, gastro-intestinal infections, and dosing with opium or alcohol. HARPER'S WEEKLY, FEBRUARY 19, 1859.

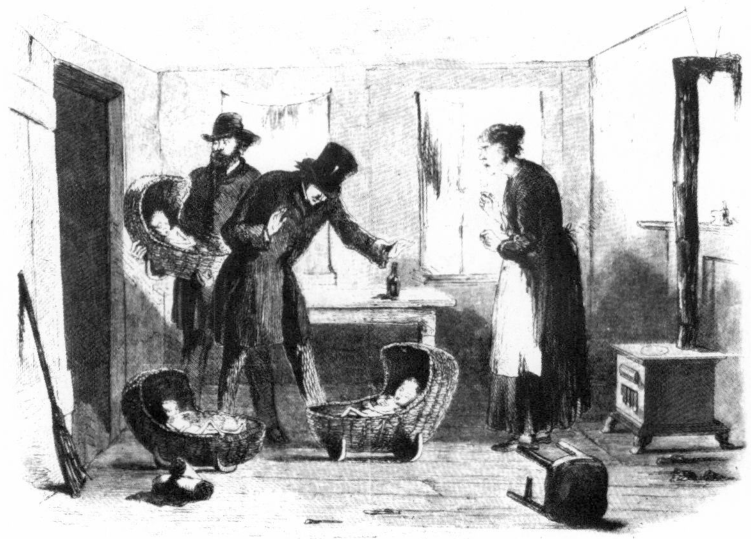

13 Scavengers at a New York City garbage dump in 1871. These people like similar groups in London described by Henry Mayhew about the same time lived from their findings which they sold or used in other ways. APPLETONS JOURNAL OF LITERATURE SCIENCE AND ART, 5: 41, 1871.

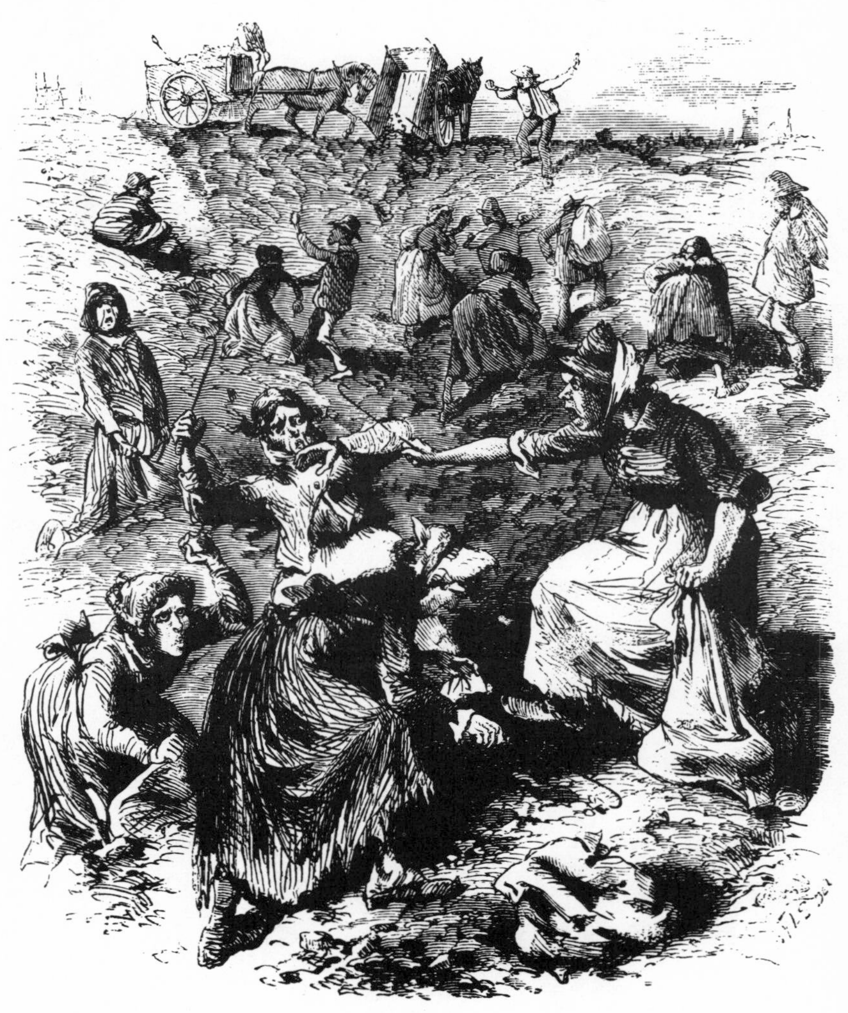

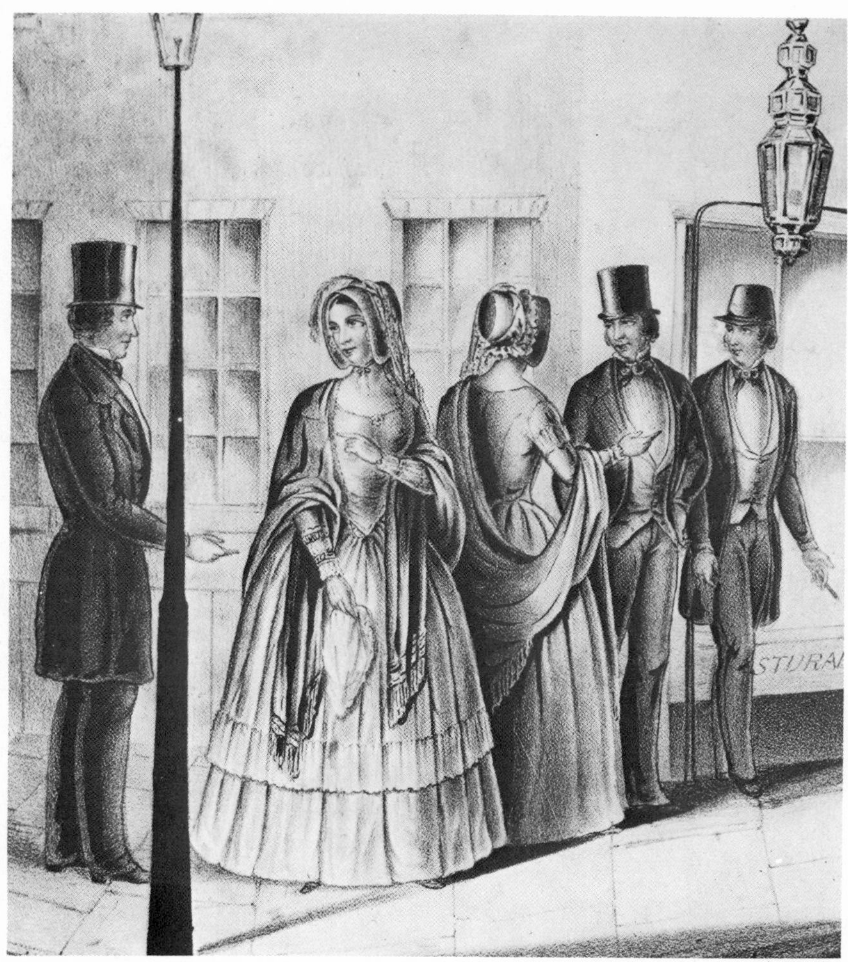

14 Hooking a Victim. New York by gas-light, circa 1850. Lithograph, Serrell and Perkins. Prostitution, a significant socio-medical problem, in cities during the 19th century, as it had been in earlier periods, was due to the precarious economic situation of women workers, overcrowded dwellings and lodging houses, and exploitation by employers and members of families where young women were employed as domestics. Public opinion in the later 19th century was greatly concerned about the extent of prostitution and its consequences, particularly venereal disease. PHOTO LIBRARY DEPARTMENT, MUSEUM OF THE CITY OF NEW YORK.

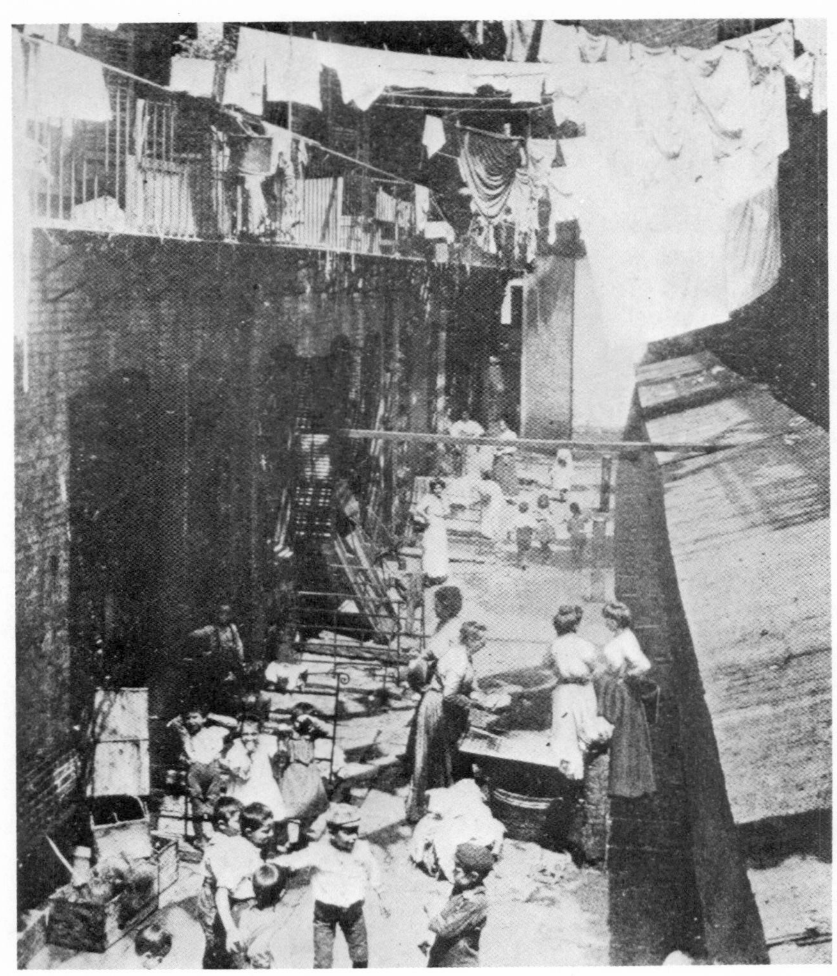

15 A typical backyard scene in the lower East Side of New York City around the turn of the century. Although housing conditions had improved somewhat toward the end of the 19th century, older tenements where poor immigrants lived had many defects. Buildings erected before 1881 generally had no indoor toilets, only outdoor privies, the row of sheds at the right. These were frequently fouled and the seats covered with fecal matter. Outside in the yard, women did their washing and children played. FROM ROBERT W. DeFOREST AND LAWRENCE VEILLER: *The Tenement House Problem,* 1903, VOL. 1, PAGE 304.

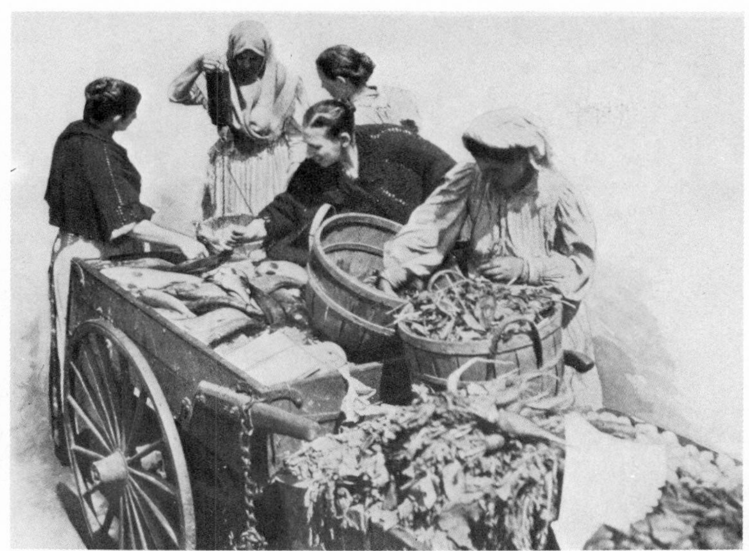

16 Another health problem involved with social conditions of the urban poor was the sanitation of food. The sale of food by pushcart vendors was common in cities such as New York and London, and added to the toll of ill health. The New York street scene shown here is from E. J. ZEISLOFT: *The New Metropolis,* NEW YORK, 1899.

17 An ambulance delivering a patient to Bellevue Hospital in New York, circa 1890. FROM E. J. ZEISLOFT: *The New Metropolis:* NEW YORK, 1899.

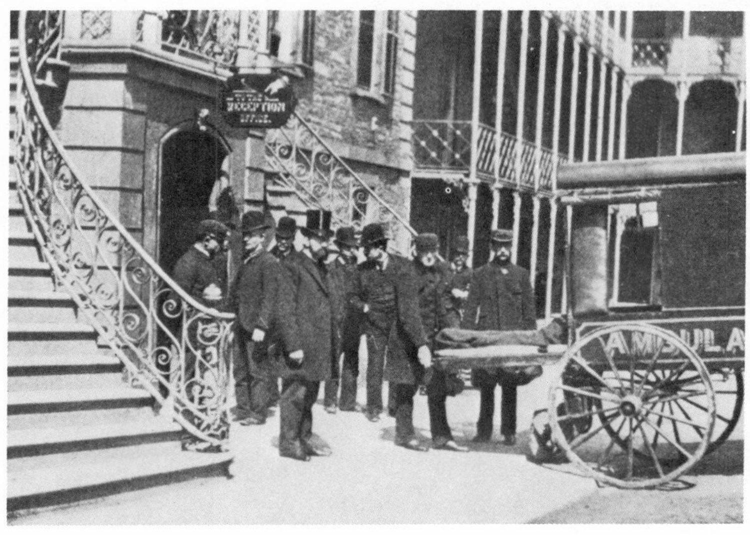

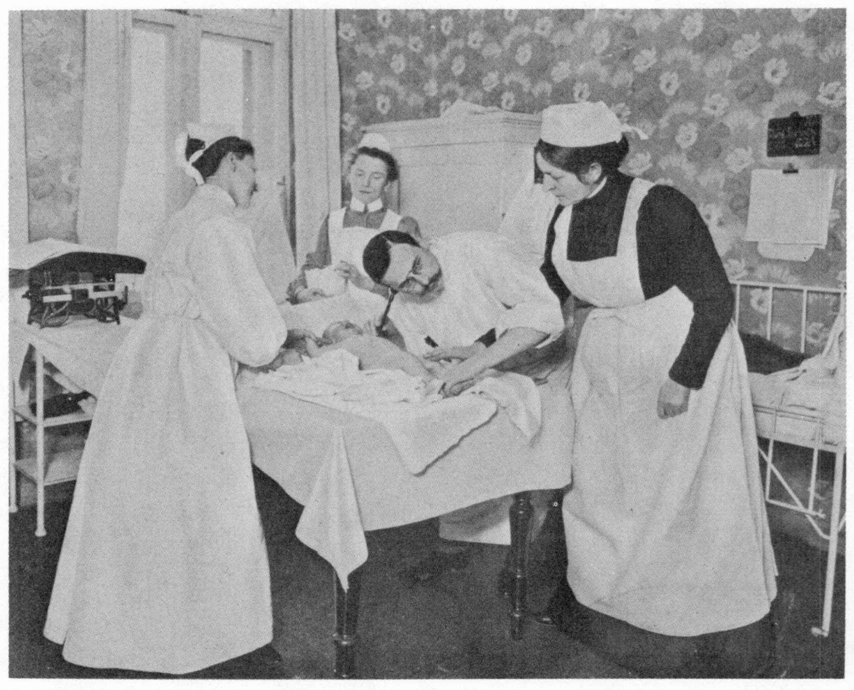

18 A pediatrician examining a baby by means of a monaural stethoscope at the Children's Refuge (Kinderasyl), a hospital in Berlin in 1906. The hospital was beginning to assume its important role in the provision of health care. FROM THE *Illustrirte Zeitung*, BERLIN, 1906.

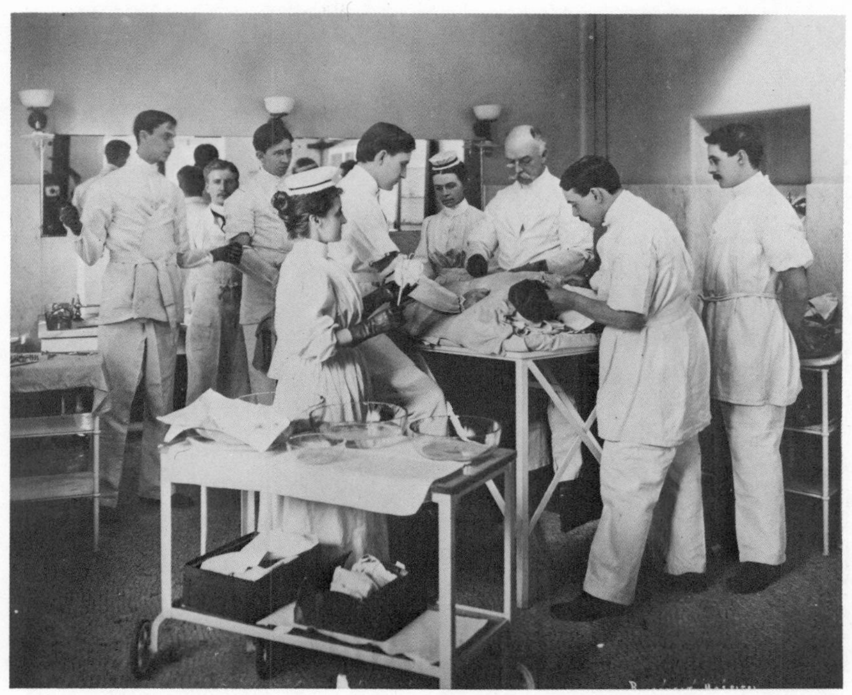

19 The New York surgeon, Charles McBurney (1845–1914) operating in 1900 at the Roosevelt Hospital. In 1889, he described one painful spot in the lower right quadrant of the abdomen indicative of appendicitis which is known as McBurney's point. At this time surgery led the way toward the development of the hospital as a center for medical care. Note that none of those participating in the operating room is wearing a face mask or cap covering the head. FROM THE BYRON COLLECTION, MUSEUM OF THE CITY OF NEW YORK.

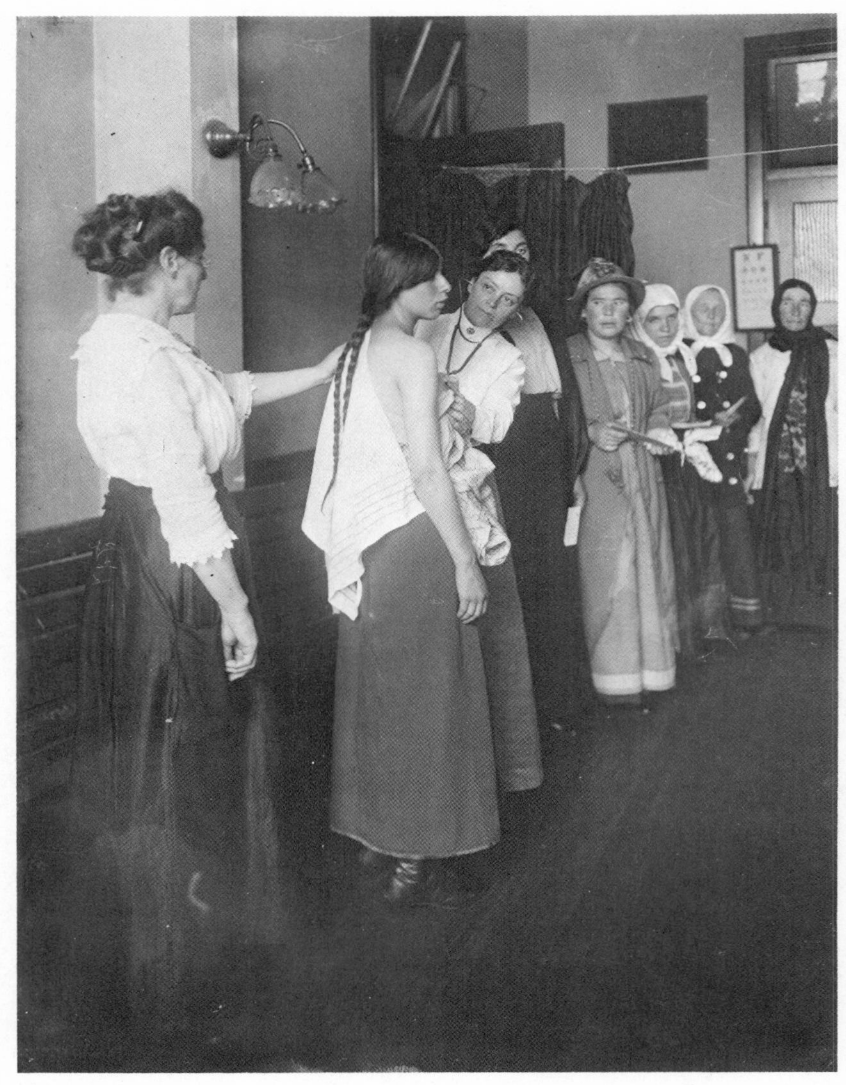

20 A woman physician of the U.S. Public Health Service examining an immigrant girl about the time of the First World War. PHOTO BY BROWN BROTHERS, STERLING, PA: NATIONAL ARCHIVES, PUBLIC HEALTH SERVICE FILE, PHOTO 90–G–22D–8.

GEORGE ROSEN

From Medical Police to Social Medicine:

Essays on the History of Health Care

SHP

1974 SCIENCE HISTORY PUBLICATIONS NEW YORK

First published in the United States by
Science History Publications
a division of
Neale Watson Academic Publications, Inc.
156 Fifth Avenue, New York 10010

Science History Publications 1974

First Edition 1974

(CIP Data on final page)

Designed and manufactured
in the U.S.A.

CONTENTS

ACKNOWLEDGMENTS We should like to express our sincere appreciation to a number of scholarly publications for granting us permission to reprint articles in this current volume. They are as follows: Bulletin of the History of Medicine, The Johns Hopkins University Press, "The Place of History in Medical Education", 22:594–627, 1948; "What is Social Medicine?", 21:674–733, 1947; "Cameralism and the Concept of Medical Police", 27: 21–42, 1952; "Hospitals, Medical Care and Social Policy in the French Revolution", 30:124–129, 1956; "Political Order and Human Health in Jeffersonian Thought", 26:32–44, 1952; "The Medical Aspects of the Controversy Over Factory Conditions in New England", 15:483–497, 1944; American Journal of Public Health, "The First Neighborhood Health Center Movement: Its Rise and Fall", 61:1620 – 1637, 1971; Bulletin of the New York Academy of Medicine, "Medical Care and Social Policy in Seventeenth Century England", 29 (2nd series):420–437, 1953; Journal of the History of Medicine, "Economic and Social Policy in the Development of Public Health", 8:406–430, 1953; Centaurus, "The Fate of the Concept of Medical Police, 1700–1890", 5:97–113, 1957; Medical History, "Mercantilism and Health Policy in Eighteenth Century French Thought", 3:259–275, 1959; Social Science and Medicine, "Health, History and the Social Sciences", 7:233–248, Pergamon Press, 1973; The Hospital in Modern Society, edited by E. Freidson, "The Hospital: Historical Sociology of a Community Institution", 1–36, Macmillan, 1963. If the publishers have unwillingly infringed the copyright in any illustration reproduced, they will gladly pay an appropriate fee on being satisfied as to the owner's title.

INTRODUCTION

The history of social medicine is to a very large extent the history of social policy and action in relation to health problems. In this sense, social medicine is an applied discipline. To a considerable degree, social medicine has been pragmatic, using whatever knowledge and methods were available and seemed to suit the purpose of its practitioners. As an example, the availability of statistical data and survey methods led to their use and further development. Basically, social medicine has been oriented to health problems and their social roots or causes so that action might be taken to deal with them. At the same time, proponents and practitioners of social medicine have also emphasized its basis in social science. Obviously those concerned with such problems of health and disease in the past have had to use the social science of their time, such as it was, just as we do today.

Long before social medicine was identified as a special field of study and action, men concerned with affairs of state and matters of policy—politicians, administrators, economists, physicians and social reformers — were aware of sociomedical problems and acted to deal with them. Health concerns have always been intimately related to the political, economic and social conditions of particular groups of people, but in earlier periods these relationships were not the subject of systematic investigation. In particular, the influence of social structure, and especially of socioeconomic status, on the provision of health care was plainly recognized by ancient authors, but this point was not pursued and developed. Nonetheless, sporadic observations linking social and cultural factors or situations with the health of the members of a community were recorded in antiquity and in medieval times. During the Renaissance, and later, in the seventeenth and eighteenth centuries, the need to provide medical care and the wish to foster population growth produced other observations about the relationships between social factors and health.

By the end of the seventeenth century and the beginning of the eighteenth, some of the basic elements of a concept of social medicine had been brought together. These included the need to study the relation between the health of a given population and the living conditions determined by its social position, the noxious factors that act in a particular way or with special intensity on a group because of its social situation, and the elements that exert a deleterious influence on health and which impede the improvement of general well-being.

The development of social medicine from the seventeenth century to the present reflects the problems perceived by communities and states at any given time, the contemporary status of the health and social sciences, and the way in which a society is organized structurally and ideologically to deal with them. Whether and how scientific and medical knowledge is brought to bear on health problems not infrequently depends more on the interests and ideology of politically and economically powerful groups than on medical or scientific validity. Thus, for example, the arrangements for health care in the United States are an expression of "free" enterprise, the product of a medical market system, which like other markets of our society is being modified in various ways, but which despite these modifications still depends on the manner in which payment is made for medical service.

Over the past thirty-odd years I have studied the evolution of social medicine with respect to both theory and application in Europe and America. The results of these investigations have appeared in several books and in a series of papers. From among these publications the present collection has been chosen as representing major themes within the general framework sketched above. To understand our society, the times in which we live, to be capable of playing an intelligent role in shaping our civilization toward the future, we must have a knowledge, not only of the actions of the past, but of the mental struggles, the ideological and philosophical conflicts that preceded action, and of the groups and interests they represented. In this way insight can be gained into the problems of the present, and that is the purpose of this volume.

ADDITIONAL READINGS

Papers on other aspects of social medicine which I have published but which could not be included and may be of interest to the reader are listed here:

1. An Eighteenth Century Plan for a National Health Service, *Bull. Hist. Med.* 16: 429–436, 1944.
2. Biography of Dr. Johann Peter Frank . . . . Written by Himself. Translated from the German . . . by George Rosen, *Journal of the History of Medicine* 3: 11–46, 279–314, 1948.
3. The Idea of Social Medicine in America, *Canadian Med. Assn. J.* 61: 316–323, 1949.
4. Charles Turner Thackrah in the Agitation for Factory Reform. *Brit. J. Ind. Med.* 10: 285–287, 1953.
5. The Impact of the Hospital on the Physician, the Patient and the Community, *Hospital Administration* 9: 15–33, 1964.
6. Social Variables and Health in an Urban Environment: The Case of the Victorian City, *Clio Medica* 8: 1–17, 1973.
7. Disease, Debility and Death, in *The Victorian City: Images and Realities*, eds. H. Dyos and Michael Wolff, 2 vols., London, Routledge & Kegan Paul, 1973, vol. 2, pp. 625–667.
8. Emotion and Sensibility in Ages of Anxiety: A Comparative Historical Review, *Amer. J. Psychiat.* 124: 771–784, 1967.

THE PLACE OF HISTORY IN MEDICAL EDUCATION

Ours is an age of crisis and social upheaval, a transitional period characteristically marked by revaluation of all values. Reflecting these conditions and affected by them, medical education is slowly but inevitably undergoing transformation and adapting itself to changing conditions. Medical education will be something very different tomorrow, and the historian may well raise the question: What part has history in the training of tomorrow's physicians? To answer this question he must raise another: Is the study of medical history only a fad; is it simply "a delightful hobby for retired practitioners," [1] and a mark of culture and intellectual refinement; or is it sufficiently important to be considered an essential element in medical education? No definite place in the scheme of modern medical education has yet been assigned to history. Apart from a few outstanding exceptions, opportunism has characterized the attitude of medical education toward the history of medicine. Nevertheless, it is possible to obtain an unequivocal answer to our question. Historical analysis, by explaining how it came into existence, will throw into clear-cut relief the prevailing relation between medical education and history.

The historical element in medical teaching is not new. For example, *Anonymus Londinensis*, the earliest history of medicine, is extant in a version that W. H. S. Jones believes to be "a copy, made by a medical student, of lecture notes also made by a student." [2] It is in the late eighteenth century and the early nineteenth century, however, that the beginnings of the modern teaching of medical history are to be sought.

Pragmatism was the dominant mode of thought in the medical history of the later eighteenth century. The pragmatic trend in medical historiography first showed itself in England, but it was in Germany under the influence of Albrecht von Haller that it achieved its fullest development. Guided by the idea of progress, pragmatic history was practical in intention. It endeavored to learn from the medicine of the past, in order to instruct the medical reader and to teach him a useful lesson.[3] Haeser

[1] H. E. Sigerist: *The University at the Crossroads*, New York, Henry Schuman, 1946, p. 19.

[2] W. H. S. Jones: *The Medical Writings of Anonymus Londinensis*, Cambridge, At the University Press, 1947, p. 8.

[3] G. von Selle: *Die Georg-August Universität zu Göttingen 1737-1937*, Göttingen, Vandenhoeck and Ruprecht, 1937, pp. 69-70; Edith Heischkel: Die Medizinhistoriographie

called attention to the historical spirit that prevailed in Göttingen in the eighteenth century, and attributed its origin and development to Haller. The inclusion of medical history in the curriculum at Göttingen may be taken as indicative. From 1750 on the professor of medical theory was also obligated to give lectures on medical history.[4] It should be noted however, that in 1743 the Statute of the University of Würzburg already required that a *Collegium privatum* on the history of medicine, be given, " so that nothing might be lacking which could serve to provide a more complete knowledge of the art of medicine." Furthermore, in 1749, the professor of medical theory was charged with the teaching of medical history.[4a] In other schools, however, the history of medicine was, for the most part, summarily disposed of in the professor's introductory lecture to his course. That the teaching of medical history was becoming more widespread in Germany toward the end of the eighteenth century is suggested by the publication in 1786 of Blumenbach's *Introductio in historiam medicinae litterariam* and in 1792 of Ackermann's *Institutiones historiae medicinae*, which were intended as textbooks, as well as by the announcement of lectures on the subject in 1798 at Heidelberg.[5]

The teaching of medical history on pragmatic grounds first made its appearance in France following the Revolution. The Convention abolished the medical faculties in 1793, but the exigencies of war and the need for a regulation of medical training led to the establishment of three medical schools (*écoles de santé*). These schools were created by the decree of the 14 primaire, Year III (December 4, 1794).[6] This decree also established at Paris a joint chair for legal medicine and medical history.

im XVIII. Jahrhundert, *Janus* 35:91-95, 1931; Stephen d'Irsay: *Albrecht von Haller. Eine Studie zur Geistesgeschichte der Aufklärung*, Leipzig, Georg Thieme Verlag, 1930, pp. 70-79.

[4] H. Haeser: *Lehrbuch der Geschichte der Medizin und der epidemischen Krankheiten*, 3. Bearbeitung, Jena, Gustav Fischer, 1881, II, pp. 565 ff., 1089.

[4a] Alfons Fischer: *Geschichte des deutschen Gesundheitswesens*, Berlin, F. A. Herbig, 1933, vol. II, pp. 31-32.

[5] J. C. G. Ackermann: *Institutiones historiae medicinae*, Nürnberg, 1792; *Medizinische Bibliothek*, 1785-1787, p. 724; August Hirsch: *Geschichte der medicinischen Wissenschaften in Deutschland*, München und Leipzig, R. Oldenbourg, 1893, p. 365; H. von Seemen: *Zur Kenntnis der Medizinhistorie in der deutschen Romantik*, [Beiträge zur Geschichte der Medizin, III], Zürich, Leipzig, Berlin, Orell Füssli, 1926, p. 61.

[6] Stephen d'Irsay: *Histoire des universités françaises et étrangères* (2 vols.) Paris, Editions Auguste Picard, 1933-35, vol. II, pp. 142-143, 149; A. Prévost: *La Faculté de médecine de Paris, ses chaires, ses annexes, et son personnel enseignant de 1794 à 1900*, Paris, A. Maloine, Editeur, 1900, *passim*; A. Prévost: *L'Ecole de santé de Paris (1794-1809)*, [Paris], 1901, *passim*.

Shortly thereafter, in 1795, two other courses with historical implications were added to the curriculum.[7] Pierre Sue, librarian of the school, was charged with the teaching of medical bibliography, and M. A. Thouret, its director, undertook to give a course on the " Doctrine of Hippocrates."

Underlying these acts was an essentially pragmatic motivation. On October 14, 1799, at the reopening of the school, Thouret pointed out that medical history is " so commendable for the useful examples that it offers us, and even more instructive, perhaps, because of the errors that it teaches us to avoid than for the precepts that it transmits. . . ."[8] Furthermore, the philosophy of Ideology was strongly represented in the Paris school (Cabanis, Chaussier, Pinel, Sue, Thouret).[9] Ideology tended to reinforce and to foster the trend toward empirical investigation in medicine, and in this endeavor medical history, with special emphasis on Hippocrates, was employed to strengthen the Ideologic position. The function of Hippocratism in Ideologic thinking on medical problems was to support its realistic approach.[10]

Undertaken in the first flush of enthusiasm two of these courses remained only expressions of good intentions. Thouret died in 1810 without ever having given a single lecture on Hippocratic doctrine.[11] It is of interest to note that Laennec endeavored to obtain this chair, but it was finally suppressed at the end of August or early in September 1811.[12] Similarly, Sue does not seem to have given his course on medical bibliography. The subject was removed from the curriculum in 1808, but was restored in 1815 as a position for Moreau de la Sarthe. In 1819, the chair of bibliography was combined with that of medical history.

[7] Ch. Daremberg: *Histoire des sciences médicales* (2 vols.), Paris, J.-B. Baillière et Fils, 1870, vol. I, pp. 3-4; R. Blanchard: L'Enseignement de l'histoire de la médecine à la Faculté de Paris, *Janus* 8: 583, 1903.

[8] Daremberg, *op. cit.*, pp. 3-4.

[9] G. Rosen, The Philosophy of Ideology and the Emergence of Modern Medicine in France, *Bull. Hist. Med.* 20: 328-339, 1946.

[10] See for example P. J. G. Cabanis: *Du degré de certitude de la médecine*, nouvelle édition, Paris, 1803; P. J. G. Cabanis: *Rapports du physique et du moral de l'homme*, 3rd edition (2 vols.), Paris 1815, vol. I, p. 23; also J. A. Chaptal: *Memoires personnels rédigés par lui-même de 1756 à 1804* . . . in, *Mes Souvenirs sur Napoleon*, par le Cte Chaptal, Paris, E. Plon, Nourrit et Cie, 1893, p. 19.

[11] Alfred Rouxeau: *Laennec après 1806, 1806-1826,* Paris, J.-B. Baillière et Fils, 1920, pp. 112-113.

[12] *Ibid.*, p. 115. On Sept. 15, 1811 Laennec wrote to his father: " The professorship of Hippocratic doctrine vacated by the death of M. Thouret, has finally been abolished because M. Thouret, who at the same time was director of the school, never gave a single lecture. Together with the hope of competing for this position, I lose my hope of becoming a professor at the school, at least for a long time and perhaps for ever."

On the other hand, the professorship of medical history created in 1794 was filled, and courses were given from 1795 to 1822, when the position was abolished.[13] The number of students attending the lectures on medical history varied considerably, from as few as 24 in 1797-1798 to as many as 142 during 1800-1801.[14] Nevertheless, this venture in the teaching of medical history left only few and rather minor achievements when it was terminated. Of the men who held the chair of medical history, only the name of Cabanis is still remembered, and his contributions lie rather in the fields of philosophy and psychology than in that of history.[15] In 1830, the medical faculty requested the reestablishment of a chair of medical history, but without success; and it was not until 1870 that this was realized.[16]

The status of medical history in the German universities throughout most of the nineteenth century offers a marked contrast to the situation in France. Courses of lectures on the general history of medicine and on special medico-historical subjects are common in the university catalogues.[17] In addition to the strictly historical lectures, there was also a course for entering medical students which was generally offered as " Encyclopedia and Methodology of Medicine." [18] Under this imposing title, the student was given a survey of medicine.[19] In 1825, for instance,

[13] A. Prévost: *La Faculté de médecine de Paris, ses chaires, ses annexes et son personnel enseignant de 1794 à 1900*, Paris, A. Maloine, Editeur, 1900, pp. 29-31, 203-204; Daremberg, *op. cit.*, p. 5 (Daremberg's chronology does not agree with that of Prévost, but since the latter's statements are based on archival study, I have given them preference.)

[14] A. Prévost: *Les études médicales sous le Directoire et le Consulat*, Paris, H. Champion, 1907, pp. 21-22.

[15] The occupants of the chair of medical history were: Lassus, full professor (14 frimaire to 2 messidor an III); Mahon, associate professor (14 frimaire to 2 messidor an III); Goulin, associate professor (2 messidor an III to 9 prairial an VII); Mahon, full professor (2 messidor an III to 1 pluviôse an IX); Cabanis, associate professor (9 prairial an VII to May 6, 1808); Le Clerc, full professor (9 pluviôse an IX to January 23, 1808); Sue, full professor (January 30, 1808 to March 28, 1816); A.-A. Royer-Collard, full professor (May 12, 1816 to February 23, 1819); J.-L. Moreau de la Sarthe (February 23, 1819 to November 21, 1822). See A. Prévost: *La Faculté de médecine de Paris* . . . pp. 30-31.

[16] Prévost, *op. cit.*, pp. 47-48.

[17] Von Seemen, *op. cit.*, pp. 51-69.

[18] H. E. Sigerist: Enzyklopädie und Methodologie der Medizin, *Internationale Beiträge zur Geschichte der Medizin. Festschrift zur Feier seines 60. Geburtstages am 8. December 1928 Max Neuburger gewidmet von Freunden, Kollegen und Schülern*, Wien, 1928, pp. 273-277.

[19] See, for instance, August Förster: *Grundriss der Encyclopaedie und Methodologie der Medicin*, Jena, Friedrich Mauke, 1857, p. VII (" Historische Uebersicht der Ansichten über die Aufgaben und die Bedeutung der Medicin ").

during the summer semester, Johannes Müller gave such a course in Bonn.[20]

Of the influences which contributed to this result, several are particularly significant. The pragmatic approach was carried over from the eighteenth century. The knowledge and experience of the ancients were to help in solving the problems of the present. Even more influential, however, was the tremendous increase of interest in history and the rise in the importance assigned to it. This development dates from the end of the eighteenth century and is to be attributed to the movement known as romanticism.

It is generally recognized that the romantic movement had an important share in the rise of modern historiography.[21] Romanticism was an ideology of cultural crisis, having developed in opposition to the Enlightenment and its culminating achievement, the French Revolution. Romanticism emphasized the principles of organicism, continuity and development. In the dialectic of romantic philosophy, reality developed according to certain simple ideas. Carl Becker pointed out that "If we would discover the little backstairs door that for any age serves as the secret entranceway to knowledge, we will do well to look for certain unobtrusive words with uncertain meanings that are permitted to slip off the tongue or the pen without fear and without research. . . ."[22] In the romantic vocabulary three terms are particularly characteristic in this respect—*das Ganze* (the whole), [23] *das Streben* (striving, or aspiration), and *Einmaligkeit* or *Eigentümlichkeit* (uniqueness). Indicative of the influence of romantic thought on medical history is the frequent occurrence of these concepts in historical writing.[24] Dietrich Georg Kieser, professor at Jena, and one of the chief representatives of *Naturphilosophie*

[20] Wilhelm Haberling: *Johannes Müller. Das Leben des rheinischen Naturforschers,* Leipzig, Akademische Verlagsgesellschaft, 1924, p. 59.

[21] G. von Below: *Die deutsche Geschichtschreibung von den Befreiungskriegen bis zu unseren Tagen,* Leipzig, Quelle and Meyer, 1916, pp. 8-15; Georg Mehlis: *Die Deutsche Romantik,* München, Rösl and Cie., 1922, pp. 64, 130, 131-138; Jacques Barzun: Romantic Historiography as a Political Force in France, *Journal of the History of Ideas* 2: 318-329, 1941.

[22] Carl L. Becker: *The Heavenly City of the Eighteenth Century Philosophers,* New Haven, Yale University Press, 1946, p. 47.

[23] The ideas of holism and organicism were not discovered by the Romantic philosophers. See, for instance, Immanuel Kant's *Kritik der Urtheilskraft,* herausgegeben von Benno Erdmann, zweite Stereotypausgabe, Hamburg and Leipzig, Leopold Voss, 1884, pp. 219-223 (¶ 65. "Dinge als Naturzwecke sind organisirte Wesen").

[24] Von Seemen, *op. cit.,* pp. 33-49; [A. W. E. T. Henschel]: Ein Blick auf das Ganze der Geschichte der Medizin, *Janus,* 3: 1-28, 1848. Over Henschel's article there still falls the long shadow of Romantic idealism.

in medicine, in 1817, stated his point of view on the study of medical history. "Not enough attention," he wrote, "has been devoted to the description of Life, the essential idea of history, as an organic whole in a constant process of development; or to the demonstration of this progressive tendency, which is its purpose, in the life of nations, as well as in the life of the sciences. Even though this has been vaguely recognized by some, still we feel that it has been worth the trouble to demonstrate this also for the history of medicine." Furthermore, Kieser pointed out, "History is the portrayal of the origin, development and cultivation of an organic whole, and the knowledge of this history is knowledge of the object itself. . . . All life consists only in progressive development, and this is true also of science." [25] In 1829, Heinrich Damerow, profoundly influenced by Hegel, published a history of medicine in which he defines his subject as "a living organ in the great organism of history. . . ." [26] Finally, it is noteworthy that even those who overtly renounced the philosophical history of the Romantics were not yet entirely free of their philosophical bias. When Henschel, the editor of *Janus*, asserts that history manifests itself through an eternal triad which is the organic soul of history, one cannot fail to see the categories of the Hegelian system.[27]

A third significant influence may be seen in the humanism best represented perhaps by Wilhelm von Humboldt. The great majority of university students, he saw, were impelled by utilitarian motives of study to prepare for the professions of law, medicine, or theology. While accepting the existence of professional education in the university, he warned against the accumulation of unintegrated information and believed that history might exercise a unifying function.[28]

These influences are reflected in the wide variety of historical courses offered by the medical faculties. Among the special subjects dealt with were the history of anatomy and physiology; ancient medicine with particular reference to Aristotle, Hippocrates, Celsus, Pliny, Galen, Aretaeus and Caelius Aurelianus; medical systems from Hippocrates to Hahnemann; the lives and achievements of great doctors; the history of pathology and therapy; the literature of surgery; on the surgical instruments

[25] Dietrich Georg Kieser: *System der Medicin*, Bd. I, Halle, 1817-19, cited by von Seemen, *op. cit.*, p. 42.

[26] Werner Leibbrand: *Romantische Medizin*, Hamburg-Leipzig, H. Goverts Verlag, 1937, p. 173.

[27] Henschel, *op. cit.*, p. 23.

[28] Wilhelm von Humboldt: *Ausgewählte Schriften*, Berlin, Wilhelm Borngräber, n. d., pp. 19-43, 443-455.

of ancient and recent times; the history and literature of obstetrics; the history of psychiatry. Several courses on the history of cholera given in 1831, reflect the epidemic prevalent at that time. Finally, further evidence of the romantic influence may be seen in the numerous presentations of the history of animal magnetism, mesmerism, and Gall's phrenology.[29]

It is useful in taking the full measure of this historical movement to look at the ideas held by the teachers of medical history on its function and value as a desirable feature in medical education. The teaching of medical history was an effort to impart a broader culture to the medical student, as well as a deeper knowledge of the development of medicine and its aims. From a broader point of view the physician would be made aware of his place in the scheme of things, and at the same time historical instruction would serve the practical purpose of training the doctor to learn from the experience of the past. According to Karl Friedrich Burdach, in 1800, the history of medicine is " the history of the different methods that have been used at various periods to cure diseases. Thus it is also the history of the changes experienced by all the separate sciences on which medicine is based." At the same time, however, " It presents the causes and effects of these different forms of treatment and thus becomes our teacher, by showing us by what paths the highest aim of the [medical] art has been approached most closely, and by warning us against the various ways in which others have been led astray by improper methods." [30] Burdach conceived medical history broadly, indicating as sources for its study medical literature, coins and medals, laws, linguistics, political and cultural history, and the history of philosophy.

These characteristic themes appear again and again. In 1826, J. F. Hofacker asserted that " The history of medicine investigates and teaches how medicine, including its individual branches, developed from its beginnings and gradually became what it is today; and it does this in relation to the general history of mankind of which the history of medicine is only a part." Emphasizing the educational influence of the historical approach, Hofacker points out that it stimulates the student to critical observation. The history of medicine is the " best teacher to protect us against bias and pride, and to maintain that humility which an experiential science should never lose. It does this by acquainting us with a series of theories which have prevailed and have been repudiated in

[29] Von Seemen, *op. cit.*, pp. 51-69.

[30] Karl Friedrich Burdach: *Propädeutik zum Studium der gesamten Heilkunst*, Leipzig, 1800, cited by von Seemen, *op. cit.*, p. 15.

medicine in the course of its history. Much that is praised as new and infallible, history proves to be old, and it accepts no credo but that of experience and sound reason." [31] Similarly, J. W. Arnold, who taught anatomy in Heidelberg and Zürich, insisted that the study of medical history belongs to general education; and that without history the physician remains "ignorant forever of the origin, the successive development, and the interrelations of many medical experiences." The ultimate aim of teaching medical history is "to give physicians a clear insight into the present state of medicine, and the relations of the branches of medicine to each other and with other sciences." [32]

Consideration was also given to the time at which the student should be made acquainted with the history of medicine. In general, it was felt that medical history should be presented at the end of the medical course. Burdach recommended that the student attend a course on medical bibliography in the eighth semester and hear the history of medicine in the ninth semester. Hofacker believed that medical history should be dealt with briefly in the first semester within the framework of the lectures on "Encyclopedia of Medicine," and again in greater detail in the last semester of medical study.[33] Friedrich Trendelenburg, the surgeon, who attended the lectures of August Hirsch in 1863, during his first semester at the University of Berlin, commented in his autobiography: "I should naturally have left the history of medicine for later semester, since one can understand the history of a science only when one is familiar with the science itself." [34]

By the middle of the century, however, it was becoming evident that the very elements which had helped to bring this widespread historical movement into being were adding less to the strength than to the vulnerability of history's place in medical education. The theoretical underpinning by which medical history justified its place in the curriculum was sapped by the growth and progress of experimental science. When it became painfully obvious that more useful and sounder knowledge could be garnered faster by looking through a microscope than by studying older medical literature, the pragmatic argument lost its force.[35] Of

[31] J. F. Hofacker: *Anleitung zum Studium der Medicin oder äussere Encyclopädie und Methodologie derselben,* Tübingen 1826, cited by von Seemen, *op. cit.*, pp. 24-25.

[32] J. W. Arnold: *Hodegetik für Medicin-Studierende oder Anleitung zum Studium der Medizin* . . . Heidelberg and Leipzig, 1832, cited by von Seemen, *op. cit.*, pp. 26-27.

[33] Von Seemen, *op. cit.*, pp. 16-24.

[34] Friedrich Trendelenburg: *Aus heiteren Jugendtagen*, Berlin, Julius Springer, 1924, p. 118.

[35] A. W. E. T. Henschel; Ist die Geschichte der Medicin an der Zeit? *Janus*, 1851, pp. 6-7, 10-11.

equal, if not greater, significance for the further development of the teaching of medical history in the German universities was the conflict of romantic idealism with experimental science. This conflict assumed a form most injurious to the place of history in medical education.[36] Indicative is the situation in 1863 at Berlin. Friedrich Trendelenburg, then a student, later recalled that "August Hirsch, the excellent scholar who only recently had been called to Berlin from Elbing, . . . lectured to very few auditors." [37] It had taken a struggle of several decades to eliminate *Naturphilosophie* from medicine, so that the earlier generations of scientifically trained physicians in Germany were in no mood to traffic with anything having the slightest relation to romantic thought. In essence, this attitude was shared by medicine with science in general; and the fate of the teaching of medical history is actually one aspect of the crisis in educational and cultural values that Germany experienced during the latter half of the nineteenth century. This climate of opinion was to exercise a profound influence on the further development of the teaching of medical history, an influence still to be felt at present. Before tracing this development, however, let us glance at the place of history in the medical schools of other countries during the nineteenth century.

The teaching of medical history in Vienna dates from the beginning of the century. Separate lectures for the history of medicine were first given in 1808 by Heinrich Attenhofer. A year later, Joseph Eyerel, a pupil of Maximilian Stoll, also received permission to teach this subject. In 1811, Andreas Wawruch began to give a course devoted particularly to the history of epidemics.[38] Voices were not lacking, however, to deny the need for independent instruction in medical history. Without denying the importance of knowledge of history for medical men, Johann Peter Frank felt that special courses on this subject were unnecessary. It would suffice if each teacher presented a brief historical sketch of his field.[39] Not until 1833, when Romeo Seligmann obtained the *venia legendi*, was the teaching of medical history at Vienna firmly established. Seligmann initiated a tradition which continued without interruption

[36] Hermann von Helmholtz: *Vorträge und Reden* (2 vols.), Fünfte Auflage, Braunschweig, Friedrich Vieweg und Sohn, 1903, vol. 1, pp. 163-165.

[37] Trendelenburg, *op. cit.*, p. 118.

[38] Max Neuburger: Ueber den Unterricht in der Geschichte der Medizin in Oesterreich-Ungarn, *Janus* 8: 583, 1903; Max Neuburger: Die Geschichte der Medizin als akademischer Lehrgegenstand, *Wiener klinische Wochenschrift*, 1904, p. 1217.

[39] J. P. Frank: *System einer vollständigen medicinischen Polizey.* Band 6, Teil 2, Vienna, 1817, p. 15.

for a century. He became associate professor in 1848, and full professor in 1869. Upon his retirement in 1879, Seligmann was succeeded by Theodor Puschmann, who occupied the chair of medical history for two decades until 1899. Max Neuburger followed him as professor in 1904 and remained active until forced out by the Nazis.

At Budapest, instruction in medical history was given by August Schöpf from 1835 to 1844, by Stockinger from 1844 to 1849, and later by Sigmund Purjesz and T. von Györy.[40]

As in Austria, the teaching of medical history in Italy is already to be found early in the century.[41] It began at Florence in 1806, with Giovanni Bertini as the occupant of the first chair. Transferred to Pisa at the close of the Napoleonic period, this position was held until 1845 by C. Pigli. In 1846, upon the death of the incumbent, the Grand Duke of Tuscany appointed Francesco Puccinotti to the chair which he held until his death in 1872.

At Naples, the medical faculty was constituted in 1811 with nine professorships, of which one was devoted to the history of medicine and medical bibliography. In 1816, this position was divided, and instruction was given in two courses, one dealing with the history of medicine, the other with the text of Hippocrates and Greek medicine. The two divisions were reunited in 1848 into a chair of the history of medicine and the text of Hippocrates. In 1860, Salvatore de Renzi, the outstanding historian of the Salernitan school, was appointed to this position which now became a professorship of medical history. It may be noted that De Renzi combined the teaching of history with that of medical geography.

At the time of the unification of Italy, in 1861, the history of medicine was taught at Bologna, Florence, Modena, Naples, Palermo and Turin. At Modena the subject was obligatory for third-year medical students. But as in other countries, the last third of the century saw a decline of interest in the subject, and a slow but unmistakeable disappearance of instruction in medical history from the curriculum. This development went hand in hand with the rise of scientific medicine. It was a result of the conflict between the new experimental and the older speculative medicine. The physiologist Salvatore Tommasi was an ardent exponent of the experimental standpoint in medicine, and in his zeal to dissociate

[40] Max Neuburger: Ueber den Unterricht in der Geschichte der Medizin in Oesterreich-Ungarn, *Janus*, 8: 583, 1903.

[41] Modestino del Gaizo: L'Enseignement de l'histoire de la médecine aux universités italiennes pendant la seconde moitié du dixneuvième siècle, *Janus*, 6: 351-357, 1901; Arturo Castiglioni: *A History of Medicine*, New York, Alfred A. Knopf, 1941, p. 754.

himself completely from the past wrote a series of letters on the uselessness of medical history and its inability to contribute to scientific progress.[42] Not until the end of the century was there a revival of history in the medical faculties.

Medical history was also taught in Spain during the nineteenth century.[43] A course on " Bibliography and History of the Medical Sciences " was listed in 1845 in the curriculum of the Medical Faculty of Madrid. Similar courses were given in 1847, 1850, 1852 and 1857. From 1875 on instruction in the history of medicine was given regularly. In Spain, the doctorate in medicine was not required for admission to practice. For those students who wished to acquire the academic degree of Doctor of Medicine, attendance at a course in medical history was obligatory.

The first course in medical history in Denmark was given about 1803-1804 by J. C. Tode at Copenhagen.[44] Two decades later, from 1823 to 1826, J. D. Herholdt again took up the history of medicine paying particular attention to the medical history of Denmark. During the second third of the century, from 1839 to1859, courses on the history and literature of anatomy and physiology were given frequently by D. F. Eschricht, professor of physiology. In 1845-46, A. G. Sommer, professor of pathological anatomy, gave a series of lectures surveying the history of medicine. After 1859, the teaching of medical history lapsed until 1870-71 when T. S. Warncke, professor of pharmacology at Copenhagen, again covered the history of medicine in a series of lectures. Finally, in the spring of 1874, medical history struck root in Copenhagen when Julius Petersen began the lectures upon which he later based his book, *Hovedmomenter i den medicinske Laegekunsts historiske Udvikling* (1876).[45] Not until 1889, however, was he appointed professor of medical history.

In Sweden, there was no professorship for medical history during the nineteenth century. Such instruction as was imparted to the students appears to have been given very irregularly, and toward the end of the century became more and more sporadic.[46] Yet medical history was a

[42] A. De Martini: *Di Salvatore Tommasi e dell' indirizzo moderno della medicina,* Naples, 1888; L. Galassi: *Discorso intorno alla dottrina d'Ippocrate ed allo spirito della medicina moderna,* Milan, 1861.

[43] R. Ulecia: L'Enseignement de la médecine en Espagne, *Janus* 8: 33, 1903.

[44] K. Caröe: Histoire de la médecine en Danemark, *Janus* 4: 299-303, 1899.

[45] The German translation, *Hauptmomente in der geschichtlichen Entwicklung der medicinischen Therapie,* appeared in 1877.

[46] Ernst Nachmanson: Anteckningar om studiet av medicinens historia, förnämligast i Tyskland, *Svenska Läkaresällskapets Handlingar* 49: 1-25, 1923.

required subject for medical students in their final examination, and its importance was officially recognized. In 1859, a Commission studying medical education in Sweden, expressed the opinion that the inclusion of history as an examination subject " does not need justification, since every physician must have knowledge of the history of his science and his art." [47] The University Statute of November 13, 1874 required medical history in the final examination, and indicated the scope of the subject as comprising "the general outlines of the history of medical theories, medical literature, and of the most important epidemic diseases." [48]

In the medical faculties of the Russian universities during the nineteenth century, the teaching of medical history in many respects followed the pattern established in Germany and Austria.[49]

Only a few sporadic ventures in the teaching of medical history characterize the United States during this period. Dunglison's lectures held at the University of Virginia from 1824 to 1833 are noteworthy only in being the first American project of its kind, and in having been stimulated by Thomas Jefferson.[50] No further effort in this direction was attempted until 1877 when John Shaw Billings, who had been appointed Lecturer in the History of Medicine at the Johns Hopkins a year earlier, gave a course of twenty lectures on medical history, medical legislation and medical education. In 1891, while holding the post of Lecturer in Municipal Hygiene, Billings gave another series of lectures on the history of medicine. With the opening of the Medical School in 1893, he received an appointment as Lecturer in the History and Literature of Medicine, a position which he held until 1905 when he resigned.[51] The third American venture in the teaching of medical history was made in 1897 by Roswell Park at the University of Buffalo.[52]

It should not be overlooked, however, that there was probably also a considerable amount of informal teaching of medical history. Dr. Winslow Lewis, a teacher of Oliver Wendell Holmes, is described as having

[47] *Ibid.*, p. 21.

[48] *Ibid.*, pp. 21-22.

[49] The following account is based upon D. M. Rossiski: The Study of the History of Medicine in Russia, *Bull. Hist. Med.* 21 : 959-965, 1947. See also *Janus* 8 : 654, 1903 for review of a book by L. S. Morochovetz.

[50] R. Dunglison: *History of Medicine*, 1872, pp. III-IV.

[51] John Shaw Billings Memorial Number, *Bull. Inst. Hist. Med.* 6 : 223-386, 1938. (See in particular Alan M. Chesney: "John Shaw Billings and the Johns Hopkins Medical School," pp. 271-284; and Sanford V. Larkey: "John Shaw Billings and the History of Medicine," pp. 360-376.)

[52] Roswell Park: *An Epitome of the History of Medicine*, Philadelphia, New York, Chicago, F. A. Davis Company, 1897, pp. V ff.

" mixed medical history and talk of old books with anatomical puzzles." [53] Indicative also is Dr. Ordronaux's account of how he came to translate the *Regimen Sanitatis*.

> Somewhere in the early days of our Civil War I happened to be passing an evening with the late Dr. John W. Francis, of New York, a personal friend and in many senses my preceptor. . . .
>
> On the occasion of my visit, I found him discussing with an English colonial bishop the merits of the *Regimen Sanitatis Salerni* as a repository of ancient medical wisdom. At the conclusion of some quotation which he made from the Latin text, the bishop made some remarks about the quantity of its verse and the difficulty of any symmetrical translation. To this criticism the Doctor assented, and turning to me, said:
>
> " Here is a book that needs a new English version. The last translation is still in somewhat ancient English. It ought to be made anew and by an American physician, as a classical contribution to our medical literature, which, as yet, contains no translation of the Salernian masters. Why don't you undertake it as a duty to the Profession? You must do it."
>
> This request he repeated on several subsequent occasions, until I finally promised to take up the task.[54]

In France, during the second third of the century, there were signs of a revival of interest in the teaching of medical history.[55] In 1837, Dezeimeris, then librarian in the medical faculty, energetically urged the usefulness of medical history and the consequent necessity of reestablishing a chair for the teaching of this subject. The surgeon Malgaigne, in 1841, gave a series of lectures on the history of surgery. In 1845, a French medical congress urged the need for reorganizing the teaching of history in the medical faculties, but nothing came of this. Two years later, Daremberg persuaded the authorities of the Collège de France to announce a course on the history of medicine. Several years after this, from 1852 to 1854, Andral gave a course on the history of medical theories. In 1859, the Faculty of Medicine, on being consulted by the Minister of Public Instruction regarding any existing gaps in the teaching program, urged the creation of a chair of medical history. This proposal was rejected, and it was not until March 9, 1870 that a new chair of medical history was established, to which Daremberg received the appointment.

[53] Eleanor Tilton: *Amiable Autocrat. A Biography of Dr. Oliver Wendell Holmes*, New York, Henry Schuman, 1947, p. 71.

[54] Transactions of The Johns Hopkins Hospital Historical Club, *Medical Library and Historical Club* 2: 49, 1904.

[55] Ch. Daremberg: *Histoire des sciences médicales* (2 vols.), Paris, J.-B. Baillière et Fils, 1870, vol. i, pp. VII-IX, 6-7; *Janus* 2: 399, 1847; Förderung des medicinischen Geschichtsstudiums in Paris, *Janus* 3: 833-834, 1848.

Daremberg's approach to the teaching of medical history derived from his aim of carrying out the intentions of his master, Emile Littré. In 1829, Littré had pointed out that "If the science of medicine did not wish to drop to the rank of a craft, it must occupy itself with its history and care for the old monuments inherited from the past."[56] Moreover, Littré was not alone a medical historian, but also a social philosopher; a disciple and friend of Auguste Comte, the philosopher of positivism. As such, Littré believed that the task of the historian was to follow the development of the human spirit through time, and to show the relation between past and present. Analysis of this kind would provide the laws underlying the variegated phenomena with which the historian dealt. As the major emphases in his lectures, Daremberg mentioned their concern with the general development of medicine, the determination of the laws underlying this development, the circumstances that have advanced or retarded it, and finally, the consideration of the reciprocal influences that the diverse branches of medicine have exercised on each other and on the advance of science.[57]

Nevertheless, despite the promising start made by Daremberg, the renaissance of the teaching of medical history was not to come from France. Several circumstances contributed to this end. In the first place, Daremberg died in 1872, after having occupied his chair for only two years, and was thus unable to develop anything resembling a school. Secondly, none of his successors were men of outstanding achievement either in the teaching or the writing of medical history. His immediate follower was Lorain, who died in 1875, thus also occupying the chair for some two years.[58] The position was then held by Parrot, Laboulbène, Brissaud, Déjerine and Ménetrier, none of whom were distinguished in the history of medicine, however excellent they may have been in the branches of medicine which were their primary interest. The third factor which militated against a significant development of instruction in medical history was the unfavorable intellectual climate, dominated as it was by the religion of science,[59] or better perhaps by the idolatry of science.

This third factor was not specifically characteristic of France. In

[56] Daremberg, *op. cit.*, Dedication to Émile Littré.

[57] Daremberg, *op. cit.*, p. 15.

[58] *American Medical Weekly* 3:273, 1875; Blanchard, *op. cit.*, p. 583.

[59] I have borrowed the phrase "religion of science" from a paper by Edwin H. Ackerknecht: Paul Bert's Triumph, *Essays in the History of Medicine presented to Professor Arturo Castiglioni on the occasion of his seventieth birthday April 10, 1944* [Supplements to the Bulletin of the History of Medicine, No. 3], Baltimore, The Johns Hopkins Press, 1944, p. 17.

fact, it was a marked feature of European culture after the middle of the century; but nowhere was this bias in favor of omnipotent science more evident, and its meaning for the teaching of medical history more clearly and more radically expressed in terms of practical consequences than in Germany. Under the pressure of specialized experimental work the older tradition of the *universitas litterarum* was rapidly undermined, and the university threatened to dissolve into a conglomeration of narrowly specialized professional and technical schools.[60] The methods and aims of university teaching were reinterpreted in terms of the assumption that the purposes of a university and of research in natural science were identical. As medicine became more and more scientific, it was content to accept these attitudes. Helmholtz, in 1877, undoubtedly expressed the consensus of the majority of physicians when he concluded a discussion of the state of medicine with the comment, ". . . I believe we have every reason to be satisfied with the success of the treatment which the natural scientific school has applied, and to the younger generation we can only recommend that they continue the same therapy." [61]

Medicine and the humanities had come to a parting of the ways, and the consequences of this unfortunate development for the teaching of medical history soon made themselves manifest. One by one the lights of medical history went out in Germany. Several isolated teachers of medical history remained in a few universities, but the situation around the turn of the century is probably most clearly illuminated by Richard Koch's statement that in 1907, when he attended the lectures of Julius Pagel at Berlin, he was the only auditor.[62]

Yet it was in this very period that the seeds were sown which would give rise to a renaissance of medical history. Some of the leading scientists soon realized that historical studies could not be jettisoned without the loss of certain elements necessary for a liberal education. Du Bois-Reymond, in 1872, pointed out the advantages of the historical approach to the teaching of natural science; and he emphasized that no matter whether one studies an organism, a political organization, a language, or a scientific theory, the significance and the relations of the object of study are best revealed by the history of its development.[63]

[60] Hermann von Helmholtz: Ueber das Verhältniss der Naturwissenschaften zur Gesammtheit der Wissenschaften, in: *Vorträge und Reden* (2 vols.), Fünfte Auflage, Braunschweig, Friedrich Vieweg und Sohn, 1903, vol. 1, pp. 157-185.

[61] Helmholtz; Das Denken in der Medicin, *op. cit.*, vol. 2, p. 190.

[62] R. Koch: Die Bedeutung der Geschichte der Medizin für den Arzt, *Fortschritte der Medizin* 38:217-225, 1921, (p. 217).

[63] Emil Du Bois-Reymond: Ueber Geschichte der Wissenschaft, in: *Reden* (2 vols.), Leipzig, Veit and Comp., 1886-87, vol. 2, p. 350.

An equally important, although more indirect influence was exerted by the critical approach to academic positivism represented by Wilhelm Dilthey, the philosopher of historicism, and by Wilhelm Windelband and Heinrich Rickert, the South German value theoreticians, all of whom were concerned with reestablishing the study of history as an essential element of liberal education. Suggestive of this influence are Sudhoff's use, in 1906, of the concept of nomothetic and idiographic sciences, and Diepgen's attempt, in 1913, to apply to the history of medicine Rickert's differentiation between natural sciences and cultural sciences, or the humanities.[64]

Most significant, however, from an immediate point of view, was the circumstance, during the last quarter of the nineteenth century, that in Theodor Puschmann medical history had not only a very able representative and a most eloquent spokesman, but also a man who laid the foundation for a renaissance of medical history.

It was just ten years before his death, at the Heidelberg meeting of German scientists and physicians in 1889, that Puschmann presented his well-known address on the significance of history for medicine and the natural sciences.[65] This was not the first time that he had dealt with the subject. Upon the assumption of his professorship in 1879, Puschmann had delivered an inaugural address on medical history as an object of academic instruction.[66] Taken together, these addresses present in clear and cogent form the ideas upon which Puschmann believed the teaching of medical history should be based, and which justify its inclusion in the medical curriculum.

Historical knowledge, he pointed out, is not indispensable for the practice of medicine in a strictly technical sense. A physician can treat a wound successfully without knowing anything about the methods used by Hippocrates and Galen. But having said this, Puschmann felt that medicine as a learned profession had interests that transcended the purely utilitarian. As a part of his education the physician must be imbued with a sense of the evolution and gradual refinement of what he comes to know as scientific truth. In the same spirit in which Dilthey wrote, " What man

[64] Karl Sudhoff: Theodor Puschmann und die Aufgaben der Geschichte der Medizin, *Münchener Medizinische Wochenschrift, 1906*, p. 1672; Paul Diepgen: Ueber das Verhaeltnis der Geschichte der Medizin zur modernen Heilkunde und den Wert medizinhistorischer Forschung für diese, *Die Naturwissenschaften*, 1913, p. 1290.

[65] Th. Puschmann: Die Bedeutung der Geschichte für die Medicin und die Naturwissenschaften, *Deutsche medizinische Wochenschrift* 15: 817-820, 1889.

[66] Th. Puschmann: Die Geschichte der Medizin als akademischer Lehrgegenstand, *Wiener medizinische Blätter*, 1879, pp. 1069-1072, 1093-1096.

is, he can learn only from history,"[67] Puschmann emphasized that "Anyone who wants to have a complete and thorough understanding of scientific facts must study the history of their origin."[68]

The values of the genetic viewpoint are threefold—pragmatic, cultural, and ethical. In a very real sense, the teaching of medical history has a practical side. For anyone who wants to contribute to the extension of knowledge in a particular field of science the study of its history is an imperative duty. In order to avoid the reproach of superficiality and to achieve true success, such a person, when he approaches the investigation of his problem, must already have mastered completely everything on it in the literature. Furthermore, a sound historical basis gives the physician a more secure vantage point from which to judge newer developments as they appear. It enables him to understand that medical ideas have their source not only in technique, but to a much greater extent in human imagination and judgment. Indeed, once this point has been grasped broad vistas open up for the physician. Our understanding of ourselves is enhanced as we learn to enter into the experience and thought of others. The broad relations of medicine to politics, social conditions, philosophy, and religion become apparent, and the physician learns that the history of medicine is a part of the general history of culture. In this way, the history of medicine expands its horizon and becomes a history of the human spirit.[69]

To accomplish this, Puschmann urged that chairs for the history of medicine and science be established in the German universities. This would also encourage young physicians to devote time and energy to a field from which they turned away because it offered no openings.

The immediate response to Puschmann's plea was meager. At the Czech University in Prague, A. Schrutz became *dozent* for medical history in 1897, and in 1900 was appointed professor.[70] At Graz, in 1898, Viktor Fossel became professor for the history of medicine, yet, as he pointed out in his introductory lecture, the situation had changed but little in the course of a decade. The history of medicine was still taught at only a few of the German language universities. "Of these," said Fossel, "the University of Vienna is at present the only one with a full professorship for medical history, while several German faculties have

[67] Wilhelm Dilthey, *Gesammelte Schriften*, vol. VIII, p. 224.

[68] Puschmann, *Wiener med. Blätter*, 1879, p. 1070.

[69] Puschmann, *Deutsche med. Wochenschrift*, 1889, p. 818.

[70] Max Neuburger: Ueber den Unterricht in der Geschichte der Medizin in Oesterreich-Ungarn, *Janus*, 8: 583, 1903.

tried to remedy the situation by charging the teacher of pharmacology hygiene or ophthalmology with the task of lecturing on the history of our science." [71]

The year 1905 marks a turning point in the teaching of medical history. The widow of Theodor Puschmann in 1901 bequeathed her fortune to the University of Leipzig for the promotion of scientific work in the field of medical history. In 1905, Karl Sudhoff accepted the newly created chair of medical history at Leipzig on condition that a department be established.[72] It is noteworthy that in 1904 an anonymous writer in the *Münchner medizinische Wochenschrift* proposed that the Puschmann bequest be used for the establishment of a special institute for the history of medicine, citing in this connection Sudhoff's suggestion in 1901 for a museum of medical history, and Baas's proposal to organize a medico-historical research seminar.[73] For the staff of such an institute the writer proposed a full professor, who would also be the director, and an associate professor, whose chief task besides sharing the teaching load with the director would be to guide the medico-historical seminar. To fill these posts the names of Sudhoff and von Oefele were suggested.

Puschmann had recognized that interest in medical history could be furthered by organizing sections on the history of medicine at scientific congresses. Following this suggestion, a section was organized in 1896 at the Braunschweig meeting of German scientists and physicans, but it was only a small beginning.[74] Not until 1898, when the *Gesellschaft deutscher Naturforscher und Aerzte* held its annual meeting at Düsseldorf, where Sudhoff organized a brilliant exhibition illustrating the history of medicine, was the place of the section firmly established. This activity was followed in 1901 by the organization of the German Society for the History of Medicine and Science, with Sudhoff as president.

Thus, when Sudhoff began his academic career at the age of fifty-two, he had already had considerable experience as an organizer, and this he applied to the development of medical history within the University. Under his aegis, the Institute developed from year to year. It would not

[71] V. Fossel: Die Geschichte der Medicin und ihr Studium, *Wiener klinische Wochenschrift*, 1898, p. 1028.

[72] Henry E. Sigerist: Karl Sudhoff, the Man and the Historian, *Bull. Inst. Hist. Med.* 2: 3-6, 1934.

[73] Die Puschmann-Stiftung für Geschichte der Medicin, *Muenchener medizinische Wochenschrift*, 1904, pp. 884-885.

[74] Theodor Meyer-Steineg: Die Entwicklung der medizinischen Geschichts-Wissenschaft in den letzten Dezennien, *Reichs-Medizinal Anzeiger*, 35: 321-325, 1910.

be exaggerated to say that the establishment of the Leipzig Institute and the appointment of Karl Sudoff as director to a very considerable degree determined the objectives and directions for the investigation and teaching of medical history during the first half of the twentieth century.

Indicative of the influence exerted by the example which Sudhoff set at Leipzig is the fact that in 1910 medical history was being taught at Berlin, Bonn, Budapest, Edinburgh, Erlangen, Geneva, Jena, Lemberg, Leyden, Vienna and Würzburg.[75] At these schools there were professors or instructors specifically charged with the teaching of this subject. In addition, occasional instruction was given at Basel, Breslau, Freiburg, Göttingen, Graz, Halle, Heidelberg, Munich, and Tübingen. Furthermore, medico-historical collections were started in Vienna and Jena.

The work of Karl Sudhoff was not an isolated phenomenon. It was only the culmination of a movement which at the end of the nineteenth century and during the first two decades of the twentieth century brought about a renaissance of medical history.[76] This movement manifested itself in various ways both in Europe and America. In 1896, *Janus*, an international journal for the history of medicine, was founded by H. F. A. Peypers. Medical history in Great Britain, despite outstanding achievements by such men as Greenhill, Adams, Creighton and Payne, was largely neglected. In 1899, E. T. Withington remarked that "in Britain the introduction of history as a definite portion of the medical curriculum has not yet reached the stage of serious suggestion." [77] Yet by 1903 proposals were being made to establish professorships or lectureships in medical history, and the Royal College of Physicians of London accepted a gift of £2000 given by Mrs. Fitz Patrick to establish a lectureship on the history of medicine.[78] In Germany, the *Bundesrat* received a draft for a law to reintroduce medical history into the university curriculum.[79] The significance of medical history for the physician and its place in medical education were also under discussion in Sweden and Denmark at this time. In 1903, Julius Wiberg made a strong plea for the teaching of medical history in Denmark.[80] At the same time societies for medical

[75] *Ibid.*, p. 324.

[76] H. F. A. Peypers: L'Avancement de l'histoire de la médecine, *Janus*, 6: 490-493, 1901.

[77] E. T. Wittington: Medical History in England, *Janus* 4: 22-25, 1899.

[78] The Study of Medical History, *Janus* 8: 53-54, 1903; James Finlayson: Library Demonstrations in the Teaching of the History of Medicine, *Janus* 8: 190, 1903.

[79] *Janus* 6: 59, 1901.

[80] J. Wiberg: Om Studiet af Medicinens Historie og den historiske Medicin, *Bibliotek for Laeger* 4: 113-124, 1903; see also Nachmanson, *op. cit.*, pp. 22-23.

history were founded. Mention has been made of the organization of the German society in 1901. About this time the *Société française d'histoire de la médecine* was established. Similar organizations were founded in Holland in 1903 and in Italy in 1908.[81] Impressive was the medical history movement in the United States. In many instances American activities were held up to Europeans as examples to follow.[82]

The original impetus to the medical history movement in the United States came from John Shaw Billings, whose lectures at Johns Hopkins have already been mentioned. It is not surprising therefore to find Baltimore playing a distinguished part in this movement. Nevertheless, there is evidence that active interest in medical history was widespread. In 1901, the following were mentioned as teachers of medical history: C. W. Dulles in Philadelphia, Thomas Gray at Minneapolis, C. L. Nichols in Boston, Roswell Park at Buffalo, Burnside Foster in St. Paul, and Sarah Hackett Stevenson at the Women's Medical School in Chicago. Commenting on this information, a writer in *Janus* said that it showed how much more seriously the teaching of medical history was taken in American schools.[83] It is quite likely that sporadic instruction was given in various medical institutions, usually by some member of the faculty interested in the subject. Alfred E. Cohn remarks that when he went to medical school, at the turn of the century, the professor of physiology "gave a few lectures on the history of the discovery of the circulation of the blood." [84] The survey which Eugene F. Cordell made in 1904 probably gives the best picture of the place of medical history in the American medical school in the first decade of the century.[85] He investigated conditions in 14 leading medical schools (Harvard, Yale, Cornell, Buffalo, Columbia, New York, Pennsylvania, Johns Hopkins, Maryland, Virginia, Tulane, Chicago, Michigan and Minnesota) and found that only three (Pennsylvania, Maryland and Minnesota) were giving full courses of 14 to 16 lectures. As for the others, "there are four 'lectureships,' one just established and still without an incumbent, and another held jointly with a 'Clinical Professorship of Dermatology.' One of the 'courses' consists of three lectures! There is but one professorship, and that an 'honorary' one. In two institutions 'some' instruction is given by the

[81] Meyer-Steineg, *op. cit.*, p. 324.

[82] See for instance *Janus* 8: 53, 504, 537, 1903; *Janus* 2: 601-603, 1897-98.

[83] Peypers, *op. cit.*, p. 492.

[84] Alfred E. Cohn: *No Retreat From Reason*, New York, Harcourt, Brace and Company, 1948, p. 252.

[85] Eugene F. Cordell: The Importance of the Study of the History of Medicine, *Medical Library and Historical Journal* 2: 268-282, 1904.

Professor of Therapeutics and the Assistants of Surgery, respectively; in the latter case only in surgery. In one, and that one, strange to say, Harvard, lectures were attempted, but 'no great interest was shown' and they were discontinued. There is no uniformity in those receiving instruction; sometimes it is the sophomores, sometimes the juniors or seniors, and sometimes any that *choose* to attend. In but one is the claim made that the course is compulsory. In none is there any examination. One can readily imagine what the attendance must be under such circumstances, and the experience of Harvard is instructive." [86] It must be added that Cordell did not overlook the important rôle of the Johns Hopkins Hospital Historical Club, commenting that since its founding it "has exercised a profound influence not only locally, but throughout the entire country."

As to the values to be derived from the teaching of medical history, there was general agreement. These were summed up by Cordell in the following statement:

1. It teaches what and how to investigate.
2. It is the best antidote we know against egotism, error and despondency.
3. It increases knowledge, gratifies natural and laudable curiosity, broadens the view and strengthens the judgment.
4. It is a rich mine from which may be brought to light many neglected or overlooked discoveries of value.
5. It furnishes the stimulus of high ideals which we poor, weak mortals need to have ever before us; it teaches our students to venerate what is good, to cherish our best traditions, and strengthens the common bond of the profession.
6. It is the fulfillment of a duty—that of cherishing the memories, the virtues, the achievements, of a class which has benefited the world as no other has, and of which we may feel proud that we are members.[87]

Opinions differed, however, on the way in which the history of medicine should be taught in order to achieve these values. In 1902, William Osler, writing in the *British Medical Journal* gave a brief statement of the methods adopted in the Johns Hopkins Medical School.[88] After mention-

[86] *Ibid.*, p. 270.

[87] *Ibid.*, p. 281. For earlier statements of these points see John S. Billings: Medical Bibliography, *Transactions of the Medical and Chirurgical Faculty of the State of Maryland*, 1883, pp. 58-80; Two Letters by John Shaw Billings on the History of Medicine. With a Foreword by Sanford V. Larkey, *Bull. Inst. Hist. Med.* 6: 394-398, 1938; Roswell Park: *An Epitome of the History of Medicine*, Philadelphia, New York, Chicago, F. A. Davis Company, 1897, pp. V-VII; The Teaching of Medical History, *Medical Library and Historical Journal* 2: 57-58, 1904.

[88] William Osler: A Note on the Teaching of the History of Medicine, *British Medical Journal*, 1902, vol. 2, p. 93.

ing Billings's lectures, and the Historical Club, Osler went on to discuss his own method of instruction.

In the everyday work of the wards, and of the out-patient department, the student may be helped to get into the habit of looking at a subject from an historical standpoint. In my outpatient class this is made a special feature of the teaching. A case of exophthalmic goitre comes in and the question at once is put, Who was Graves? Who was Parry? Who was Basedow? Of course the student does not know; he is told to bring, on another day, the original article, and he is given five or ten minutes in which to read a brief historical note. . . .

Once a week, over a little "Beer and baccy," I meet my clinical clerks in an informal conference upon the events of the week. For half an hour I give a short talk on one of the "Masters of Medicine," in which, as far as possible, the original editions of the works are shown. In the present crowded state of the curriculum it does not seem desirable, to add "The History of Medicine" as a compulsory subject. An attractive course will catch the good men and do them good, but much more valuable is it to train insensibly the mind of the student into the habit of looking at things from the historical standpoint. . . .

There is no doubt that a method of this kind has definite advantages. Above all it is flexible, and, as James Finlayson, of Glasgow, pointed out, can be adjusted to the requirements of one's audience. Moreover, it can be combined with instruction by other and more usual methods.[89] On the other hand, it is equally clear that this type of instruction is dependent upon local opportunities both as to the availability of a teacher and a demand from students. Nor should one forget that Osler, in addition to being available himself, had another advantage in favor of his approach. He was one of a group of medico-historical collectors who greatly influenced the development of medical history in the United States during the first three decades of the present century. Dr. Viets has characterized the members of this group as "men of scholarship, charm, book collecting instincts and the long purse.[90]

Eugene Cordell, on the other hand, drew very different conclusions from his study of 1904.

Having now shown the value—nay, I should rather say the necessity—of the study of medical history, I shall conclude with a few words regarding its teaching. So important a branch should receive the highest consideration. It should be taught in no desultory fashion, but as thoroughly as any other. There should be a full chair of the history of medicine in every university. A systematic course of reading should be required in addition to the lectures, which should be not less

[89] See above footnote 78.

[90] Henry R. Viets: Edward Clark Street (1874-1947), *Bull. Hist. Med.* 21:843-845, 1947.

than sixteen to twenty in number. It should be made a subject of examination, for all experience proves that in no way can the attendance of the students be enforced. The time is near at hand when the standing of universities will be judged by their attitude to this branch, and when it will be assigned a front rank in the curriculum.

Ten years after this forceful recommendation, Arnold Klebs again looked at the place of history in the medical school and concluded " that the study of the history of medicine has [not] made very decided progress as a feature in medical education."[91] He did point out, however, that the number of academic courses on the subject was not an exact measure of the interest manifested in the subject itself. Even where academic instruction is given in medical history, " It cannot be said that it enjoys a very great popularity, here or abroad." Klebs attributed this state of affairs more to an inadequate approach to the problem than to lack of interest. " I believe," he said, ". . . that we have a fertile soil, which, properly tilled and sown, will some day bring forth a bountiful harvest." Emphasizing that the lukewarm interest hitherto shown in history as an element in medical education should not discourage further efforts, he asserted that " If a distinct place were assigned to it in the medical curriculum, it could, by its achievements, by the influence it would exert on students and teachers of all departments, form one of the most useful and inspiring features in the whole of medical education." As to the method by which this could be accomplished Klebs recommended that pursued at the University of Leipzig. " Didactic lectures alone," he concluded, " are insufficient and time-consuming. Whatever direct teaching is given students would be based best on objective demonstration and practical work in bibliographical and historical methods rather than on systematic historical lectures. Such instruction will be given in separate premises easily accessible to all departments, where the objects for demonstration should be collected and classified and where special research can be carried on." Nevertheless, fifteen years were yet to elapse before this program would be implemented.

Clearly underlying these American developments is a pragmatic trend. Through an understanding of the evolution of medicine the physician can participate in general culture, thereby enhancing the prestige of the profession and his own education. In 1916, Robert E. Schlueter reiterated that history is an essential study for the physician. " The history of science," he states, " like general history is an instrument of culture. . . .

[91] Arnold C. Klebs: The History of Medicine as a Subject of Teaching and Research, *Bull. Johns Hopkins Hosp.* 25: 1-10, 1914.

She contributes to form citizens who are not only scientists but who are also men and citizens. History rounds off and completes an education. . . ." [92] Like Puschmann, he insisted that medical history is necessary for "the completion of a general education, for the fixation of technical knowledge, the prevention of professional narrowness and the ennobling of character."

Lewis S. Pilcher, in 1924, forcefully stated the same point. The physician "cannot respond adequately to his duties, either to himself, his patients, his community, or to his profession, without acquiring a knowledge that must extend far beyond familiarity with tools of daily use. He must become a man of culture as well as a man of skill; and just to the degree that he answers to such higher professional ideals will not only his own enjoyment and success in his work be increased, but the estimation and influence in which he will be held by all men will be magnified." [93] To achieve this aim medical history should be systematically taught in every medical school. "How early in the medical curriculum should subjects of medical history, medical ideals and ethics be introduced? My answer," said Pilcher, "would be, as early as possible. They should be a part of the ABC of medical studies. The atmosphere of the great names of the past and the ideals by which they were animated should surround the medical student from the beginning of his career."

Meanwhile, medical history in Europe, particularly in Germany, had developed in another direction. Non-medical scholars gradually began to cultivate various fields of medical history. The increasing significance of this trend may be grasped from the fact that it was the Academies of Berlin and Copenhagen which in 1905-1906 initiated the *Corpus medicorum graecorum*. The help of the philologists was welcomed,[94] but it was not long before their point of view began to dominate the history of medicine. These scholars had no need to relate their studies to the problems of contemporary medicine, and medical history tended more and more to become an independent discipline. The pragmatic element in the history of medicine was relegated to the background.[95] It was recognized, however, that this development harbored the danger that medical history

[92] Robert E. Schlueter: The Necessity for Studying Medical History, *Journal Missouri State Medical Association,* 13: 385-390, 1916.

[93] Lewis S. Pilcher: Medical History in Medical Education, *Long Island Medical Journal* 18: 400-407, 1924.

[94] Meyer-Steineg, *op. cit.*, p. 323.

[95] Owsei Temkin: An Essay on the Usefulness of Medical History for Medicine, *Bull. Hist. Med.* 19: 9-47, 1946 (See particularly the changes undergone by Pagel's *Einführung in die Geschichte der Medicin* from 1898 to 1922, on page 37).

might become an ivory tower for a few specialists. Voices were raised in sharp criticism. In 1904, a year before Sudhoff came to Leipzig, a *privatdozent* at that university commented as follows: [96]

> I have no desire to represent the philological-antiquarian study of the older history of medicine as useless or superfluous. Indeed, I recognize its value and justification. Nevertheless, such researches are of value only to a relatively narrow group of physicians who are interested in literary and cultural history, and consequently, can expect only a limited reception. . . .
>
> If the history of medicine is to have any value for the further development of medical science and for the general education of future medical generations, something which can justifiably be demanded, then it cannot consist solely . . . in a study of sources, or in the discovery, criticism and annotation of literary remains of greater or lesser age.

Similarly, Hellpach in 1919, contemptuously referred to the existing medical history as "pathophilology," and characterized it as much too interested in archival material to be of any use in giving medical students a cultural point of view.[97] Instead, he suggested that the student would be provided with a better cultural background if he were led to discover for himself such materials as the chapter on physicians in Theodor Gomperz's *Greek Thinkers*, Burckhardt's *Civilization of the Renaissance in Italy*, or Ricarda Huch's study of the Romantic Movement. The reference to Burckhardt is worth commenting on, for as early as 1870 he had written to a friend: "A rather remarkable phenomenon has become clear to me as a teacher of history, that is, the sudden devaluation of all mere 'events' of the past." [98] In the study of history, Burckhardt laid emphasis not on erudition and research but on interpretation of selected historical periods, and this point of view Hellpach wished to have applied to medical history.

And in 1921 Richard Koch attributed the wide gap that still existed between medicine and medical history to the spirit that had motivated the medical historians of the preceding generations.[99] Just as in the natural sciences, he pointed out, historical research attempted to arrive at historical truth by collecting *all* the facts so as to arrive at a picture of the past as complete as possible. As a result, the history of medicine became the domain

[96] M. Seiffert: Aufgabe und Stellung der Geschichte im medizinischen Unterricht, *Münchener medizinische Wochenschrift*, 1904, pp. 1159-1161.

[97] Willy Hellpach: *Die Neugestaltung des medizinischen Unterrichts*, Berlin, 1919, p. 59.

[98] Jacob Burckhardt: *Briefe zur Erkenntnis seiner geistigen Gestalt* Mit einem Lebensabriss herausgegeben von Fritz Kaphahn, Leipzig, Alfred Kröner Verlag, 1935, p. 337.

[99] R. Koch: Die Bedeutung der Geschichte der Medizin für den Arzt, *Fortschritte der Medizin* 38:217-225, 1921.

of scholarly philologists, bibliographers, and lexicographers, such as Littré, Daremberg, Hirsch, Pagel, Sudhoff and many others. Yet with all their zeal and diligence the aim they set themselves was not achieved. What did happen was that enormous masses of facts were collected which are not yet synthesized or interpreted. It was a scientific labor of love performed by a small group, and for this reason could have little influence on medical education in general.

In 1918, Germany had collapsed, and yet, in the midst of chaos, there were soon signs of recovery. A reorganization of the educational system was undertaken as a part of the attempted restructuring of German society. The question of having medical history taught in the medical faculties was raised again in this connection.[100] The demand of the German Society for Medical History in 1913 that medical students be required to attend a course in the history of medicine had passed unnoticed. But now when preparations were being made to abolish all the old injustices and absurdities, it appeared urgent to demand that chairs for medical history be established in all the universities. Haberling pointed out that in seven Prussian universities there were no teachers for medical history, and in three there were only *dozenten* to offer the subject. In the non-Prussian schools, four had chairs for medical history while five did not. To support this demand, emphasis was placed on the usefulness of medical history.

A medical student wrote to the *Deutsche medizinische Wochenschrift* supporting this demand, and urged that the history of medicine be made a required subject in the final examination.[101]

Meyer-Steineg emphasized the need for instruction in the history of medicine on several grounds.[102] Gone was the unified structure that medicine had once been. Now it was simply a conglomeration of many specialties. Some element was needed to counterbalance this condition, and this element was history. Not only would it make possible for the student a synthesis of the various branches of medicine, but it would provide him also with a cultural point of view and thus strengthen the place of the humanities in medicine. Finally, said Meyer-Steineg, it would illuminate the social relations of the medical profession.

[100] W. Haberling: Zur Frage des Unterrichts in der Geschichte der Medizin an den Universitäten, *Deutsche medizinische Wochenschrift* 45: 1420-1421, 1919.

[101] Hubert Beisele: Die Frage des Geschichtsstudiums; Zu dem Artikel von Oberstabsarzt Haberling in Nr. 51, *Deutsche medizinische Wochenschrift* 46: 102, 1920.

[102] Theodor Meyer-Steineg: Geschichte der Medizin als Lehrgegenstand, *Berliner klinische Wochenschrift*, 1920, p. 158.

Pointing out that a good deal of the current discussion on the means whereby a broader cultural background could be provided for the medical student was too diffuse to be of value, Karl Sudhoff went on to analyze how this might be accomplished through the teaching of medical history.[103] On the basis of his long experience, he felt that students would most easily be introduced to such matters through a course resembling the old " Encyclopedia and Methodology of Medicine." The actual teaching of medical history Sudhoff wished to have at the end of the medical course, because the student would then be in a better position to appreciate the development of medical knowledge.

Despite the urging of these leading German medical historians, the medical faculties remained lukewarm to all proposals for the systematic teaching of medical history. In 1921, representatives of the faculties and of the medical societies presented to the German government a memorial in which the wish was expressed that in reorganizing the medical curriculum an opportunity be provided for the student to become acquainted with the history of medicine.[104]

The first World War had temporarily interrupted the renaissance of medical history that we previously noted as having begun at the turn of the century, but with the cessation of hostilities medico-historical activities increased both in Europe and America. An international society of the history of medicine was organized in 1921, and the American Association of the History of Medicine in 1924. International congresses were held at intervals. Evidence of this ongoing development is also to be found in the increased attention given to the teaching of the history of medicine.

Great Britain had had almost no provision for the teaching of medical history. The subject was ignored by all the universities, except Edinburgh, where John D. Comrie had held a part-time lectureship since the early part of the century. In 1919, Charles Singer urged that more attention be given to the teaching of medical history.[105] Two things, he maintained, were necessary to develop a " generalized interest in history and effective work along historical lines." The first of these was the establishment of

[103] Karl Sudhoff: Neuordnung des Studiums und medizingeschichtlicher Hochschulunterricht, *Jahreskurse für aerztliche Fortbildung* 11: 31-39, 1920; see also Paul Diepgen: Ueber Wert, Aufgabe und Methode des medizin-historischen Unterrichtes, *Fortschritte der Medizin* 37: 517-520, 1920.

[104] Vorschläge der Kommissionsberatung der Abgeordneten medizinischer deutscher Fakultäten und Vertreter des deutschen Aerztevereinsbundes zur Neuordnung des medizinischen Studiums und der Prüfungen, *Fortschritte der Medizin* 38: 26, 1921.

[105] Charles Singer: The Teaching of Medical History, *British Medical Journal*, 1919, pp. 141-142.

two or three chairs " to be held by men who would devote their lives to the task of setting forth the history of medicine as a continuous whole." The second need for an adequate study of medical history was the establishment of a special institute, preferably situated in London. The chief advantage to be derived from such a program was that the student in learning how medicine had come to be what it is, would also learn to see all the branches of medicine as parts of an organic unity. Finally, concluded Singer, " Those who are best acquainted with the work done in other countries for the history of medicine will have no doubts that the introduction into the country of a systematic treatment of the subject will do much to raise the educational standing and with it the self-respect, happiness and efficiency of the medical profession as a whole." Not long after, Charles Singer himself held positions, such as he had suggested, at Oxford and at University College in London.

At the same time medical history in Italy had an eloquent spokesman in Arturo Castiglioni. In word and in deed he demonstrated the significance of history in medical education, and insisted that a proper place be accorded to it in the curriculum.[106]

In 1922, Henry E. Sigerist, entering upon a brilliant career, devoted his inaugural lecture as *privat dozent* to a discussion of the tasks and the aims of medical history.[107] Surveying the events of the preceding fifty years, he showed that there was reason to be optimistic about the future of medical history. Sigerist felt that a major function of the history of medicine was to bridge the gap between the natural sciences and the humanities. In this way the medical student would be enabled to acquire a broad cultural background. The growing interest in medical history and its increasing significance in medical teaching were also emphasized in 1923 by Isidor Fischer of Vienna.[108]

At Leipzig, Karl Sudhoff was succeeded in 1925 by Henry Sigerist. Early in 1927, to determine the state of medico-historical instruction, Sigerist undertook a survey covering Europe and the New World.[109] The survey revealed that in six European countries (Bulgaria, Esthonia,

[106] A. Castiglioni: Sul riordinamente dell' insegnamento universitario della storia medicina, *Rivista di storia critica delle scienze mediche e naturali* 11 : 97, 1920.

[107] Henry E. Sigerist: Aufgaben und Ziele der Medizingeschichte, *Schweizerische medizinische Wochenschrift*, 1922, pp. 318-322.

[108] I. Fischer: Der historische Fachunterricht, *Wiener klinische Wochenschrift* 36: 888-890, 1923.

[109] Henry E. Sigerist: Die Geschichte der Medizin im akademischen Unterricht. Ergebnisse einer Rundfrage des Institutes, *Kyklos*, Leipzig, 1928, vol. i, pp. 147-156.

Finland, Latvia, Sweden and Yugoslavia) there was no teaching of medical history. Poland had created institutes for the history and philosophy of medicine in its five universities. In addition, full professorships were reported as established in Athens, Baltimore, Copenhagen, Leipzig, Lisbon, Madrid, Montreal, Moscow, Paris, Toronto, Vienna and Würzburg. At Prague and Coimbra, the chair of medical history was combined with another subject. Institutes or seminars in medical history were noted in Athens, Baltimore, Cluj, Frankfurt a.M., Freiburg i. Br. Jena, Leipzig, Naples, Vienna and Würzburg. The history of medicine was reported to be a required subject in Greece, Poland and Rumania, as well as at the universities of Modena, Padua and Madrid. It was a required examination subject for the doctorate in medicine at the universities of Madrid, Modena, Greece, Poland and Rumania and was optional at the universities of Bari, Padua, and Naples.

An event of major importance for the teaching of medical history in the United States was the creation in 1929 of the Institute of the History of Medicine at The Johns Hopkins University. During the decade of the 'twenties interest in medical history had been growing. In 1920, Victor Robinson founded and edited *Medical Life*, at that time the only monthly magazine in English devoted to the history of medicine. The founding, a few years later, of the American Association of the History of Medicine has already been mentioned. By 1929, Garrison's *History of Medicine* had achieved its fourth edition. The teaching of medical history, however, continued on a desultory and sporadic basis. Some men followed the informal Osler tradition. For example, in 1921, Edward C. Streeter was appointed Lecturer on the History of Medicine at the Harvard Medical School. No formal lectures were given at the school, but according to Dr. Viets, "he gave a few discerning students delightful evenings at his home on Beacon Street. . . ."[110] Temple University in 1929, created a professorship of medical history for Victor Robinson. While a required course of lectures was given to freshmen, the position was unsalaried and not full-time, and there was no department. Again, at the University of Chicago Medical School, medical history was taught by the professor of anatomy.

Meanwhile, forces had been set in motion to create a powerful center for the study of medical history. In 1925, William H. Welch agreed to do something to advance the history of medicine in America. As he wrote to his niece, he felt that "The time is ripe and the opportunity

[110] Viets, *op. cit.*, p. 844.

splendid for getting the subject of medical history well established and properly recognized both on the research and the teaching sides in our medical schools. . . ." [111] Welch's interest in the history of medicine was of long standing, extending back to his student days; and this despite the fact that when he attended Heinrich Haeser's lectures at Breslau, he found them "deadly dull." In 1888, for instance, in a speech at Yale, he had advocated the study of medical history and deplored its neglect, on the ground that there is nothing "more liberalizing and conducive to medical culture than to follow the evolution of medical knowledge." [112] Throughout his career at Hopkins, Welch continued to manifest a keen interest in history.

In 1926, funds were secured for the endowment of a chair of medical history, and a decision was reached to establish a library. In November of that year Welch became professor of the history of medicine, but he was fully aware that more than just a professorship was needed. In 1927, he noted in his diary, "A mere 'Lehrstuhl' of medical history is like a chair of anatomy, physiology, pathology, etc., without laboratory, assistants, staff, and budget." The logical consequence had already been decided on earlier that year. "I want to get launched as soon as possible," he wrote, "a genuine Institute of Medical History connected with the professorship and the library—altogether a good-sized job." [113]

After a visit at Leipzig with Sudhoff and Sigerist, where he "obtained some idea of what a real Institute for the History of Medicine should be," and was confirmed in his belief that a mere professorship for medical history was inadequate, Welch set out on his travels through Europe as a book buyer. Finally, on October 17 and 18, 1929, the department of the history of medicine and the library were officially dedicated, with Harvey Cushing, Karl Sudhoff and Abraham Flexner as the principal speakers.

Cushing related the functions of the department and the library to the increasing specialization of medicine, pointing out that medical history had much of great value to give to the physician, but that it would also have to remain vigilant to avoid the creation of an ivory tower for another specialist.

> What possible relation . . . does this rapidly moving account of the cleavages in medicine, past and apparently on the way, have to the dedication of this library

---

[111] Simon Flexner and James Thomas Flexner: *William Henry Welch and the Heroic Age of American Medicine*, New York, Viking Press, 1941, pp. 418-419.

[112] *Ibid.* p. 421.

[113] *Ibid.*, p. 425.

and its inseparable association with the establishment of a chair of the History of Medicine? Will this foundation merely mean still another group of specialists having their own societies, organs of publication, separate places of meeting, separate congresses, national and international, and who will also incline to hold aloof from the army of doctors made and in the making? Without lessening the opportunity and encouragement for historical and bibliographical research, on the part of those rare and highly gifted persons capable of it, is there not something far more important for Medicine that can radiate from here?

In the modern development of the physician into a scientist, have we not lost something precious that may without risk of pedantry be brought back to medicine? [114]

Sudhoff reiterated this point, and went on to show that the study of history brings our own experience into organic relation with the past, and teaches us to see our own work in relation to the whole. It teaches the medical man to look beyond the horizon of his own special field of activity "into the great wide world of mental activity around and beyond him, to see into the neighboring regions of mental science, of psychology, general philosophy, sociology, and into the general cultural life, the art and literature, of his own time. The physician cannot stand alone within his scientific specialty: as a creature of his time, he must remain in close relation with the general culture of his time. . . . The growing tendency to specialization, unavoidable in itself, is inimical to true professional development. The necessary corrective of its dissolving, dissociating effect is the unifying rôle of history." [115]

The Institute of the History of Medicine was launched, but Welch was aware that he would not be able to carry the burden of this venture. As a result the Institute did not really get under way until after Henry Sigerist had taken over in 1932. Welch wrote that Sigerist's "coming to Johns Hopkins is one of the most important events in the history of the University for years." [116]

Henry Sigerist brought home to his American auditors the meaning and potentialities of scholarship in relation to medical history. But the potentialities that he sees in history involve an organic linking of the past, not alone with the present, but equally so with the future. He has

[114] Harvey Cushing: The Binding Influence of a Library on a Subdividing Profession, *Bull. Johns Hopkins Hosp.* 46: 38, 1930.

[115] Karl Sudhoff: Address Delivered at the Inauguration of the Department of the History of Medicine at The Johns Hopkins University, Baltimore, October 18, 1929, *Bull. John Hopkins Hosp.* 46: 101-116, 1930.

[116] Flexner and Flexner, *op. cit.*, p. 443. See Henry E. Sigerist Valedictory Number, *Bull. Hist. of Med.*, Jan.-Feb., 1948.

added to the other values of medical history that of promoting a sociological comprehension of medicine. Or, stated differently, a medical history which approaches medicine with an understanding that it has always been involved in a matrix that is at once social, economic, political and cultural can be developed into a method that can contribute to the solution of urgent social problems of medicine.

My task has been to trace the historical evolution of the place of history in medical education; and the story of this development may be brought to a fitting close by glancing briefly at the situation in American medical schools shortly before the recent war. In 1937, Sigerist undertook to survey the status of medical history as a subject of instruction.[117] The results revealed that 54 of the 77 medical schools surveyed, or 7 percent, provided instruction of some kind. The courses were required in 28 schools, and in 22 of these there was a required examination in the subject, in six schools the final examination was optional. The courses in all the other schools were elective.

When compared with Cordell's survey of 1904, the results obtained by Sigerist showed that there had been a very considerable increase in interest in medical history, and that the majority of medical schools recognized that the subject had a place in the curriculum. Nevertheless, while the quantitative aspect of the survey was impressive, the qualitative aspect was much less so. Except at one school, history was taught by part-time instructors, that is, faculty members who happened to be interested in the subject, but whose main work was in some other branch of medicine. From the reported data it is clear that many of the courses were of inferior quality. Yet, taken as a whole, there is no doubt that progress had been made.

The coming of the recent war indubitably exerted a negative influence on the progress of medical history. Nevertheless, one significant positive achievement deserves mention, the creation of a full chair of the history of medicine at the University of Wisconsin, and the appointment to it of Erwin H. Ackerknecht. Much, however, still remains to be done to assure for the history of medicine a place in the scheme of medical education which accords with its intrinsic significance. Plans have recently been proposed for the creation of new centers of medical education, as well as for expansion of certain existing centers. It is noteworthy that at least one of these plans, that of the New York University Medical School,

[117] Henry E. Sigerist: Medical History in the Medical Schools of the United States, *Bull. Hist. Med.* 7: 627-662, 1939.

envisages a Department of Medical Humanities which would include the history of medicine. On the other hand, it is equally interesting that the proposed plan for the educational expansion of the Columbia-Presbyterian Medical Center contains no reference whatever to the subject of medical history.

What is the place of history in medical education? In our endeavor to answer this question, we have called on the past to shed light on the present and possibly to dispel a few of the shades that shroud the future. In view of the evidence presented to say that history has had a place in medical education for the past two and a half centuries is to be both correct and trite. Once said, this seems so obvious as to be embarrassing. Rather the problem is to indicate what that place is in the scheme of medical education. What are its significant characteristics? How does it articulate with the other elements of a medical education?

I shall not examine these questions. My task has been to show, what has been achieved so far, and where we stand at present, thus providing a point of departure for discussion of what the next tasks will be. I shall conclude, however, by summarizing what I conceive to be the advantages of medical history for practitioners and students of medicine.

We are aware that medicine involves the study and application of biological knowledge, and that this activity is linked in various ways with social, economic, political and ideological factors. In relation to the technical content of medicine, history shows this knowledge in proper perspective. It points up the way in which knowledge has evolved, and indicates how inquiry can be made to go forward into the unknown. Furthermore, the student of medical history soon discovers that the state of knowledge in one branch of medicine is of significance in understanding apparently unconnected developments in other branches. When properly presented, medical history counterbalances the divisive effects of specialization, and helps the medical man to synthesize for himself an organic conception of medicine.

But medicine is also a social activity. The student should acquire an understanding of the place of the medical profession in society. History as a social science facilitates this, and makes it possible for the student to understand the position of medicine in our complex social structure, and how the present has evolved from the past. Moreover, the health of our people is our most precious national asset. We are aware that the responsibilities of the physician today are more extensive than ever before. In the complex business of living, both theory and practice are necessary conditions of survival, and to both the history of medicine can make important contributions. In the words of the British historian, F. W. Maitland, "Today we study the day before yesterday, in order that yesterday may not paralyse today, and today may not paralyse tomorrow."

HEALTH, HISTORY AND THE SOCIAL SCIENCES

The term health, whether good or ill, designates a dynamic state of an organism resulting from the interaction of internal and environmental factors operating in a time-space setting. This generalization applies to all biological organisms and places health in an ecological context. A few examples will illustrate the point. Recently attention has been centered on the pathological effects of high levels of population density. Studies of animal groups suggest that overcrowding may have such adverse effects as lowered fertility rates, increased mortality particularly among the very young, and extremely aggressive behavior.[1] From a study of wild monkeys, Susiyama concluded that high density was followed by a breakdown of their social order, producing very aggressive behavior, killing of young monkeys, and the like.[2]

Aggressiveness as well as other deleterious consequences may also be produced by limited food supplies. Singh suggests that urban monkeys in India are much more aggressive than forest monkeys because of "the restrictive urban environment, particularly the limited availability of food, which forces the monkeys to compete among themselves and with human beings for survival. The urban monkeys are highly aggressive toward people as well as toward members of their own species".[3]

Another consequence of a limited or altered food supply was noted by Lack.[4] He observed that when birds such as the red grouse are in good condition they can carry a considerable burden of internal parasites without apparent deleterious effects. However, an adverse change in the quantity or quality of their staple plant food leads to an increased mortality due to parasitic infestation.

Analogous situations can also be found among human beings, and interest in the effects of differing levels of population density or of nutritional states has been active for a long time. A review of recent literature on housing led Alvin A. Schorr to conclude that poor, overcrowded housing produced such effects as "a perception of one's self that leads to pessimism and passivity, stress to which the individual cannot adapt, poor health, and a state of dissatisfaction; pleasure in company, but not in solitude, cynicism about people and organizations, a high degree of sexual stimulation without legitimate outlet, and difficulty in household management and child rearing".[5] In another connection, Leon Eisenberg, earlier this year, underscored "that the rapidly growing brain of fetus and infant is excruciatingly dependent on the adequacy of its nutrition", and "what has become equally evident is that the nutriment the growing brain requires is affective and cognitive as well as alimentary. The extraordinary dependence of the human young upon adult care and caring provides both an unparalleled opportunity for mental and emotional development and a period of vulnerability to profound distortion by neglect".[6]

The circumstance that the interactions of various animal organisms, including man, result in analogous phenomena does not necessarily mean that the factors and processes involved are the same, or even if they are similar that they operate in the same way for each group. This is particularly the case with human beings. The biological equipment of human beings is obviously related to other primates and can be studied comparatively. But men and women are more than just primates. human beings are creators and transmitters of culture. Though present in other animals, particularly the primates in rudimentary forms, the capacity to produce cultural systems and to transmit them through language and other forms of social communication is essentially human. Thus in the course of his evolution, man has become increasingly adaptable and capable of modifying not only his environment but himself as well. As Hugh M'Diarmid phrased it with poetic exaggeration, "Man's the reality that mak's A'things possible even himself".

One aspect of this capacity is evident in the various ways in which human beings living in larger or smaller groups have tried to deal with the health problems of their sick fellows. The essentially social nature of health care was recognized very early. describing the origins of medicine, the author of the Hippocratic treatise on *Ancient Medicine* wrote, "for the art of medicine would never have been discovered to begin with, nor would any medical research have been conducted—for there would have been no need for medicine—if sick men had profited by the same mode of living and regimen as the food, drink and mode of living of men in health, and if there had been no other things for the sick better than these. But the fact is that sheer necessity has caused men to seek and to find medicine because sick men did not, and do not, profit by the same regimen as do men in health."

As long as there has been life on earth, disease has been associated with it. Sickness has plagued man as long as he has existed, and everywhere he tried to deal with it as best he could. Studies in paleopathology have shown not only the antiquity of disease, but also its occurrence in the same basic biological forms, such as infection and infestation, disturbances of development and metabolism, neoplasia and traumatism.[7] Schistosomiasis, for example, is prevalent in Egypt today, but the disease is ancient there. Schistosomes, the infesting organisms, have been found in the kidneys of Egyptians who lived some 3000 years ago. Similarly, tuberculosis of the spine with collapse of several vertebrae leading to the characteristic hunchback, known as Pott's disease, has been found among ancient Egyptians, as well as among pre-Columbian Indians. But while these basic types and conditions have not altered, the incidence and prevalence of illnesses involving such processes have varied from time to time and place to place.

Our illnesses and accidents in various ways reflect the world in which we live, what we do in it and with it. Dermatitis due to make-up, nylon dermatitis, and bunions are related to fashions in cosmetics and dress. Tennis elbow is a hazard in a society where the game is played. Welder's conjunctivitis, hatters' shakes, or caisson disease occur as a result of occupational activity, and of the conditions under which workers earn a living. Diseases due to dietary deficiencies such as rickets and scurvy tell us a good deal about diet, living conditions, aspects of social class and other facets of a society. Moreover, this is true of the present and the past. In short, the occurrence of disease in a given population at a particular time is not just a matter of chance. It exhibits a characteristic pattern defined by etiology, incidence, prevalence and mortality as related to age, sex, social class, occupation, mode of life, or other factors connected in one way or another with the structure, culture and psychology of a society. In so far, then, as disease arises from, or affects, the social conditions or relations within which human beings live, it is a social phenomenon to be studied as such and completely comprehensible only within a biosocial context. This point can be illustrated by several examples.

Mental and emotional disorders have occurred among all peoples from the earliest times to the present. One of the most striking features of mental disorder is aberrant behavior, and every society designates certain forms of such behavior as mental derangement or insanity. In other words, along a spectrum of human behavior ranging from that considered normal to that regarded as abnormal, there is some point at which a judgment is made and an individual is designated as mad. In practice, the dividing line between normality and abnormality, between sanity and insanity, is not always easily established. People in a given community or social group tend to evaluate the behavior of those with whom they come in contact and interact in daily life in terms of some concept of the normal based upon cultural criteria. This applies not only to the patently psychotic but also to individuals whose behavior is not as extremely aberrant. Assessment of such behavior depends on a number of factors. One group includes the style and consistency of the behavior, its orientation to reality, its motivation and its consequences. A second set of factors involves the boundaries within which a society will accept, or at least tolerate, aberrant behavior, as well as the social institutions and cultural values which enable deviant individuals to function in some socially acceptable manner.

The Talmud, for example, contains several attempts to define mental disorder in behavioral terms. It was proposed that a person who wandered about alone at night, who spent the night in a cemetery, or who tore his garments and destroyed what was given to him might be considered deranged if such behavior appeared irrational. However, it was pointed out that otherwise normal persons could also behave in such ways—for example, one who spent the night in a cemetery might have done so to practice magic, or another who tore his clothes may have acted in a fit of anger or because he was a cynic philosopher exhibiting his contempt for material things.[8]

Among the Greeks and Romans, mental derangement was similarly defined in terms of appropriateness of behavior in a given context. Thus, some persons might be considered mentally disordered not merely because their behavior was perplexing or perverse, but because their actions, beliefs, and thought, and inferentially their orientation to reality, were considered excessively divergent from socially accepted norms. Socrates declared that most men "do not call those mad who err in matters that lie outside the knowledge of ordinary people; madness is the name they give to errors in matters of common knowledge. For instance, if a man imagines himself to be so tall as to stoop when he goes through the gateway in the Wall, or so strong as to try to lift houses or to perform any other feat that everybody knows to be impossible they say he's mad. They don't think a slight error implies madness, but just as they call strong desire love, so they name a great delusion madness".[9]

Indeed, from antiquity to the present, medical and nonmedical observers have noted and commented on the relationship between aberrant behavior and cultural context. In 1728, Voltaire wrote about England, "Reason is free here and walks her own way, hippocondriaks especially are wellcome. No manner of living appears strange; we have men who walk six miles a day for their health, feed upon roots, never taste flesh, wear a coat in winter thinner than your ladies do in the hottest days. All that is accounted a particular reason, but taxed with folly by no body".[10]

M. J. Field, an anthropologist and psychiatrist, has made the point even more specifically. She pointed out that in a country such as Ghana, where no one takes a second look at a truck announcing in large letters "Enemies all about me" or "Be afraid of people", the universality of the "normal" paranoid attitude requires the exercise of considerable caution in diagnosing paranoid schizophrenia.[11]

Clearly, the need to consider aberrant behavior with respect to socio-cultural factors has long been recognized in some degree. Furthermore, the views expressed in the cited comments point to a specific problem, namely, the relationship between socio-cultural deviance and psychological abnormality, a problem which the historian of mental disorder shares with the clinician, the epidemiologist, and the behavioral scientist—each of whom in his way must ask himself what is meant by *deviance, abnormality* and *mental illness*.

The importance of social situation and context in elucidating the occurrence of disease resides not only in the area of psychological judgment. For certain conditions socio-economic factors may be crucial. Pellagra is a case in point. How pellagra could be prevented or cured was known by 1920, yet in 1934 the disease caused 3602 deaths in the United States with about 20 reported cases for each death. The reason lay not primarily in a lack of knowledge, but rather in the economic factors that affected the dietary of the cotton-raising tenant farmers of the South. Joseph Goldberger, who elucidated the etiology of pellagra, studied the role of economic and social factors in its causation.[12,13] With Edgar Sydenstricker he carried out a series of classic studies in the social epidemiology of pellagra in cotton-mill villages and among tenant farmers. An unmistakable inverse correlation between family income and pellagra incidence was demonstrated. As income increased, the pellagra rate declined. However, income was not the only factor involved. Food supply and dietary habits played important roles as well. Given the restricted food pattern of the poorer people in the South, when families in mill villages were restricted to the mill store or commissary during the late winter or spring because of the absence of other sources of supply, pellagra was almost inevitable. Goldberger could recommend keeping cows and chickens, and planting gardens, but he could not change the economics of the situation. As he wrote in 1927 referring to the rural population: "It is necessary to keep in mind two considerations of essential importance. The first is that the economic status of this population is bound up in the tenant system, which, in turn, is involved in single-crop agricultural production and the speculative character of agricultural finance as practiced in this area, the seasonal fluctuation in income of the tenant . . . and other factors of an economic nature."

In the past 40 years, however, the pellagra problem has practically disappeared, in part through the application of scientific knowledge, but much more importantly as a result of social and economic developments. Among these have been the broad processes of industrialization and urbanization, and more specifically a decrease in the isolation of various areas as a result of better communication and travel facilities, the improved economic condition of the poorer classes of the population, an increased availability of a wide variety of nutritious processed foods, and some improvement in education. Indeed, the pressure by business interests to develop a profitable market for consumer goods in the South probably contributed significantly to the decline of pellagra.

Not only is disease related causally to the social and economic situation of the members of a given population, but the health care received also reflects the structure of a society, particularly its stratification and class divisions. Rank has its privileges in illness as in health. From antiquity to the present, the social class of patient has in various ways affected the medical transactions related to his illness. Members of the upper classes were supposed to differ from ordinary people even in their ailments, and did so even if only in the names applied to them. Thus, at the end of the 17th century, in imitation of the French fashion, *vapors* appeared at the court of William and Mary, and became almost *de rigueur* for aristocratic ladies after Queen Anne came to the throne. In consequence, terms such as the *spleen* and *vapors* were used to differentiate medically between persons of condition and the common run, a distinction upon which George Farquhar based a situation in *The Beaux Stratagem.* Archer, a gentleman of broken fortune, disguised as a valet, remarks inadvertently, "my constant drink is tea . . . 'Tis prescribed me by the physician for a remedy against the spleen." Thereupon a fellow servant bursts out, "O la! O la! a footman have the spleen!" and Mrs. Sullen to whom Archer is talking says, "I thought that distemper had been only proper to people of quality?" Whereupon Archer retorts, "Madam, like all other fashions it wears out, and so descends to their servants".[14]

As Farquhar indicates, such distinctions were not absolute. The *spleen* in a person of quality could become lowness of spirits in a patient of lower social status, but not infrequently these terms were used synonymously for the same person. When David Hume as a young man was incapacitated with melancholy, hypochondria, and various psychosomatic complaints, he was treated for the vapors, the spleen, lowness of spirits, melancholia or hypochondria. The names changed but the condition for which he was treated persisted until his recovery several years later. Noteworthy too is Hume's initial reaction that he could not be suffering from the vapors since this was a disease of the idle rich.[15]

The relation of social position to ill health and its consequences was also illustrated in 1677 by Sir William Temple in his essay on gout. Noting that the disease usually affected the wealthy, the lazy and those who lived high, he also pointed out that the poor and those who have to work for a living are not immune to the disease. If working men are attacked by gout, "either they mind it not al all, having no leisure to be sick; or they use it like a Dog, they walk on, or they toil and work as they did before, they keep it wet and cold; or they are laid up, they are perhaps forced by that to fast more than before; and if it lasts, they grow impatient, and fall to beat it, or whip it, or cut it, or burn it, and all this while perhaps never know the very name of the Gout".[16]

A pertinent comment in the same vein was made in 1713 by the Italian physician Bernardino Ramazzini. Concerning medical care for brickmakers he remarked, "Workers of this sort are mostly of the peasant class; so, when they are attacked by fever they betake themselves to their huts and leave the affair entirely to nature; or else they are carried off to hospitals and there are treated, like everybody else, with the usual remedies, purging and venesection. For the doctors know nothing of the mode of life of these workers, who are exhausted and prostrated by increasing toil".[17]

That the differential definition and provision of medical care by social class is still a fact of life can easily be confirmed. Hollingshead and Redlich in their study of *Social Class and Mental Illness* (1958) produced evidence that psychiatric diagnoses and the kinds of therapy administered to patients were significantly related to socio-economic position. Those who were relatively poor or uneducated were treated in ways that did not require as much of the doctor's time, while the more affluent and better educated tended to be treated by talk therapy (psychotherapy) which requires more time and a more personal relationship. Nor has much changed in this respect in the intervening 14 years. A more recent study by Duff and Hollingshead, entitled *Sickness and Society*, only adds more evidence to support the general proposition that medical care is not provided strictly in terms of need, and that it is governed to a considerable degree by other factors of a social nature.

This point applies as well to age categories. Before the nineteenth century, for example, when a high infant mortality prevailed, the attitude toward childhood differed from that generally prevalent in technically advanced societies. "I lost two or three children as nurslings" wrote Montaigne, "not without regret but without great grief". Even if Montaigne's attitude is viewed as determined in part by his philosophy, there is other evidence that children hardly counted until they had reached an age of probable survival. Certain *consilia,* i.e. written consultations, of physicians at the end of the medieval period seem to reflect this attitude and situation. Thus, among 309 *consilia* of Bartolomeo da Montagnana (d. 1466), 19 concern adolescents, 5 boys, 2 young children, and only one an infant. Similarly, among over 100 *consilia* of Ugo Benzi (1376-1439), one concerns a boy of ten, another a child of two and a half. Obviously such evidence is only suggestive, but it does point to the relevance of social values and demographic conditions in the provision of health care.[18]

To put the problem more generally, whether a given society emphasizes a particular stage of biological development in relation to health depends on social and cultural factors acting over a period of time. In medieval Europe, infancy ended at about the age of six or seven, and the individual was then considered an adult. The concept of childhood emerged gradually during the seventeenth and eighteenth centuries. Even more recent in origin is the concept of adolescence, which dates from the nineteenth and twentieth centuries. In other words, the stages of the life cycle depend not only on physiological maturation, but even more on the way in which a society recognizes, defines and structures such stages in terms of social attitudes and roles. Such changing concepts are reflected in various social institutions and have an impact on them, for example, in the organization and provision of medical care. Instances in point are the various institutional arrangements for the health care of mothers and children, and also old people, among them such medical specialties as pediatrics and geriatrics.

Other examples can be cited, but what I am emphasizing is that medicine, or, more broadly speaking, health care, is a functional aspect of society. Attention to the maintenance of good health, and care of the sick and disabled, have been an element of group life throughout recorded history and in all likelihood long before. As a social activity such care is interlocked in various ways and in differing degree with the structure of group living of which it is a part—with the family, religion, the economy, government, the value system and other elements. Furthermore, not only is the structure of health care inseparable from the general organization of society, but its reality cannot be fully discovered from static, cross-sectional analysis. Like any other social institution, medicine experiences both continuity and change, so that its past differs from its present, and it will be something different in the future, and yet for good or for ill what happened in the past influences the present and the future.

This dynamic aspect is the history of health care. History derives from challenges experienced by various groups of people, and the ways in which they respond to them. The result is a variety of actions and reactions under different circumstances and often under widely divergent ideological and emotional climates. Yet those actions and reactions have in one way or another brought us to the present. Institutions, patterns of behavior, systems of ideas—all have developed from something which was there before. Attitudes toward illness, theories of disease, arrangements for the care of affected individuals, modes of treatment and the practitioners who provide them—all illustrate this truism which is too often overlooked. Historical analysis makes it possible to penetrate past social structures and the changes they have experienced in the course of time so as to illuminate our understanding of the process of development which has led to the present, thus providing meaning and significance not to be found in a study restricted solely to a contemporary segment. This is a basic function of medical history, to lay bare the origins of medical institutions, their organization, ideas and operation, and to explain their significance. The translation of medical and other values is likewise historically conditioned, and historical studies can throw light on this aspect as well. An account of how it came into existence will reveal the prevailing structure of health services in sharp perspective and highlight its dynamics.

Medicine as a social activity undertaken within the context of human need and group life develops institutional forms through which ideas and practices are carried out by members of an organized society, characterized by division of labor and specialization of function. Viewed in these terms, medicine, or health care, can be studied by any means available for the investigation of social institutions. In fact, social scientists (sociologists, psychologists, anthropologists, economists) have been making such studies, and in their efforts have to a greater or lesser degree employed historical approaches and materials. In the light of this situation which is likely to expand, what can and should be the relations between history and the social sciences in the field of our common interest, health in its various aspects? No social science is a totally self-contained system, and each has areas and facets that border on other disciplines including historical studies. In this connection, it may be most fruitful to examine an area of this kind and to see what generalizations may be drawn from this discussion.

Addressing the American Historical Association in 1958, William L. Langer emphasized that the psychological effects of the Black Death were a significant historical phenomenon and he proposed that the matter he studied by means of psychoanalytic concepts and methods.[19] Since then the psychological aspects of historical events and personages have increasingly attracted attention, indeed to such an extent that this area of interest has received a specific designation, psychohistory. As this interest has grown, two problem areas have come under investigation.

One encompasses the social and psychological impact of collective stress situations, including both natural and man-made disasters, and interest has focused on the social psychopathology of major or recurrent epidemics. This problem is important not only in its own right, but also because it is a part of the larger problem of the affective history of societies. Actually, the historical investigation of such problems is not completely new. One need only recall Hecker's study of the medieval dance frenzy (1832), Crawfurd's study of 1914 on plague and pestilence in literature and art, and d'Irsay's examination in 1927 of defense reactions during the Black Death. Such studies were sporadic, however, so that a large and potentially important area still remains to be investigated.

Useful approaches to this problem area have more recently come from several different directions. Utilizing a wide range of literary and visual sources, Alberto Tenenti explored psychological attitudes toward life and death in Italy and France during the Renaissance.[20] Several years earlier, Millard Meiss had used pictorial evidence to demonstrate a change in the psychological state of a social group over a period of time following a disaster. In his study of painting in Florence and Siena after the Black Death, Meiss showed that changes in art which occurred following the epidemic resulted from the establishment of a new state of mind among the people of these cities.[21]

More provocative is the work of René Baehrel, who pointed out that from a psychological viewpoint the period during which an epidemic prevails is a period of fear, of anxiety, and may be compared with and studied like periods of revolutionary terror. Indeed, Baehrel suggested that psychological attitudes developed in earlier epidemics and famine periods were latently available during the terror of the French Revolution. Moreover, he argued further that in such psychological climates social class antagonisms, religious animosities, and other hostile attitudes towards groups and individuals may be activated and realized in violent behavior. This thesis had already been illustrated independently by Séraphine Guerchberg in her study of the controversy over the alleged plague sowers and the massacre of Jews on this ground at the time of the Black Death.[22]

The broad framework within which studies, such as those of Baehrel and Tenenti, must be seen and from which they derive in part was set forth in 1940 by the French historian, Lucien Febvre. In this programmatic statement he urged historians to turn their attention to the emotional life of men in their social environment and to reconstruct it on the basis of its manifestations as indicated by available evidence from a variety of sources, not only written records. One might study, for example, how words were used at different periods, the vocabularies available to various groups, and related aspects. Another source suggested by Febvre was iconography; a third was literature; and still another was provided by legal cases and documents. In short, any evidence that might throw light on collective and individual psychology. In this sense Febvre envisaged a history of love, of pity, of cruelty, of death. How this program was actually applied may be seen in his masterly work on the religion of Rabelais, where he showed on the basis of empirical evidence what 16th century men could have experienced and considered thinkable in relation to the supernatural.[23]

This is psychohistory on a conscious level, where the historian is aware that analysis of the manifest content of beliefs and ideas, and of the modes of expression, the intensity of emotional relationships and the selective valuation placed on different kinds of relationships reflects a certain psychological organization. Such aspects are indicative of the psychological make-up and modes of behavior of individuals and groups in relation to the larger structure of social and cultural life. Historical periods are characterized by different sensibilities, that is, modes of feeling shared in varying degree by those living at a particular time. An awareness that the public and the personal interpenetrate within the framework of society must underlie any endeavor to understand these psychological aspects. Groups and individuals cannot be divorced from the larger institutions within which they carry on their lives, since it is within this framework that their psychologies are formulated. The way in which an individual in a given historical period perceives his world, the feeling he has about it, depend on his interests, beliefs and values, on the intricate connection between his inner life, his life-pattern, and the specific social and cultural conditions which he encounters in his environment. This characteristic mode of perceiving and feeling which I call sensibility is an expression of the way in which the personality integrates these diverse elements.

Such relationships are as complex for groups as they are for individuals. In any given historical period, a society or a group within it may exhibit a characteristic pattern of emotional attitudes. A prevalent psychological orientation of this kind, which by analogy with Whitehead's concept of a climate of opinion can be called an emotional climate develops out of social and cultural conditions specific to a group or society and is related to its historical development. Numerous individual sensibilities contribute to an emotional climate, and in turn the prevalence of such a complex of feelings tends to stimulate individuals and groups to perceive their socio-cultural environment, the various aspects of society along certain lines and to act in characteristic ways.[24]

Furthermore, even when an emotional climate tends to pervade a given historical period or society, this does not preclude the presence at the same time of other, possibly opposed, complexes of feeling. Anyone who has looked into the psychological depths of the 18th century is aware that its many complexities cannot be reduced to a simple pattern or slogan. For those satisfied by a simplistic tag, the 18th century continues to remain the "Age of Reason". Under closer and more penetrating scrutiny, however, the homogeneity which the designation seems to imply dissolves. Homogeneity was no more characteristic of the 18th century than of any other historical period. Behind the seemingly serene certitude of the smile of reason lurked complexities and ambiguities. Both reason and feeling were recognized as springs of human behavior in the 18th century, and contemporaries were aware that there were complicated and intricate reciprocal relations between them. But when a rupture of the relations between the head and the heart led to a fundamental rift, the ensuing gap opened a way for the emergence of the dark, the weird and the demonic, in short, the irrational, from the depths of the 18th century psyche.[25]

One must also note that the effects of emotional climates are not limited by time or space. Emotional states created by specific historical conditions can persist for longer or shorter periods, and they may recur and evoke empathic or sympathetic responses among individuals and groups in other societies and historical situations. Certainly there seems to be an affinity between the psychological atmosphere of which Choderlos de Laclos, Restif de la Bretonne, and the Marquis de Sade are representative and the sensibilities of some among our contemporaries. Certainly it is no accident that *Les Liaisons dangereuses* is now considered by many as one of the most important novels of the 18th century, or that it has become almost a commonplace in certain circles to regard de Sade as an inspired precursor of modern thought. Whatever the reasons may be, there appear to be similarities of sensibility and emotional climate between the later 18th century and the mid-20th century.

The same point can be made about our own time as "an age of anxiety". When W. H. Auden coined the phrase, he meant it to apply to the contemporary world in terms of its social, psychological and moral insecurity. As we look at our world it is not surprising that many people feel they cannot cope with the changes to which they have been exposed at so fast a pace, nor that they feel they cannot understand what is going on about them and what it all means for their own lives. Surely it is no wonder that for many our time is characterized by widespread feelings of insecurity and a sense that we have been cast adrift without compass or charts. Viewed historically, however, our situation is neither unique nor as unprecedented as some believe. There have been other times, other periods in history, when insecurity, a sense of personal insignificance, feelings of frustration and unhappiness, and similar characteristics seem to have predominated and which have also been designated as ages of anxiety. Johan Huizinga described the "sombre melancholy" that weighed on people's souls in the 15th century France and Burgundy, and he noted that sometimes it seems "as if this period had been particularly unhappy".[26] According to Paul Tillich, "If one period deserves the name of the 'age of anxiety', it is the pre-Reformation and Reformation".[27] And Walter E. Houghton has emphasized the degree to which the mid-19th century in Great Britain was both an age of anxiety and an age of optimism.[28]

Periods so characterized are those in which the consciousness of many people, and even more so their subconsciousness, is haunted in varying degree by fear and worry, by loneliness and apathy, and by frustration, resentment, and aggression. These are periods in which many see themselves trapped in a world from which they want more than anything else to escape, either by destroying the old order and actually creating a new and better world, or by withdrawing into a compensatory inner or transcendental world.

Given the recurrence of such periods in history one may ask whether they are at all comparable: Do they exhibit behavioral or psychological similarities? Are certain forms of psychopathology, irrationality, common to such periods at different points in time? Are such periods a consequence of common or analogous factors? In my opinion questions such as these are to be answered affirmatively. Basically, what is common to such periods is that they are times when societies and their cultures, or segments within them, are changing into something else, when the accustomed structure of order, power, belief and meaning comes apart, and men confront the dark, inscrutable face of the future, not knowing what is to come. At such times the tension between outer experience and the world within, between social reality and emotional disarray, leads to the development of a type of sensibility and an emotional climate dominated by anxiety. So long as men live within an accepted structure of action, feeling, and value, as long as the majority of individuals follow customary lives and continue to think and feel as they had always thought and felt without raising fundamental questions, human energy flows without hindrance into activity. But what happens when this energy cannot be released in the usual or expected manner? These repressed, undischarged, often inchoate emotions, these energies thwarted of effective outlet in social life, create tensions which seek and find release through aberrant, often bizarre channels. Intense yearnings and frustrated social impulses are transformed into pathological aberrations. Such periods of transition and crisis, when familiar worlds are broken and anxiety is diffused in society, bring forth individuals who reach the wilder shores of sanity where some are able to maintain themselves, even though precariously, while others lose their hold and are submerged in the depths of unreason.[29]

Such developments must be viewed within a larger framework. Different societies have culturally constituted systems which are potential means through which members of the society may resolve psychological conflicts and develop defense mechanisms to satisfy unconscious neurotic needs. The ancient cult of Asclepius was such a system in which faith in the god, the practices of incubation and dream interpretation, the rituals and the therapies, together with the environment created by the priests and the other patients combined to provide an institutional framework which enabled patients such as the sophist Aelius Aristides to behave in extravagant but culturally sanctioned ways, thus protecting them from the possibly disruptive consequences of their unconscious needs and private defensive maneuvers.[30] Cynic asceticism was another such system in antiquity, as was affective mysticism in the later Middle Ages.[31] Although comprising different constituent elements, analogous culturally constituted systems were similarly employed among other groups. For Joseph Karo in the 16th century, the combination of Jewish Kabbalistic theory and practice with the concept of maggidism made available a means of dealing with his unconscious intrapsychic conflicts and of maintaining an adequate psychological balance, thus enabling him to carry on his considerable intellectual labors and to become the great scholar and codifier of normative rabbinic Judaism.[32]

Psychosocial means other than those involving religion may also be developed by psychologically troubled individuals which make it possible for them to act within socially accepted contexts. In mid-Victorian England, for example, many intellectuals exhibited strong evidences of psychological disorder. Feelings of isolation, loneliness, ennui, despair and depression recur so frequently in the letters and writings of men like Charles Kingsley, Alfred Tennyson, John Stuart Mill, Thomas Carlyle, Arthur Hugh Clough, and others as to leave the impression of endemic psychopathology. Indeed, if one is to understand the earnest busyness of the Victorians, one must comprehend its roots in an emotional climate and a sensibility in which anxiety was a major element. As George Eliot shrewdly observed, action was therapy. "No wonder the sick-room and the lazaretto have so often been a refuge from the tossings of intellectual doubt—a place of repose for the worn and wounded spirit . . . here, at least, the conscience will not be dogged by doubt, the benign impulse will not be checked by adverse theory; here you may begin to act without setting one preliminary question".[33] And work they did until they broke down and collapsed, but as Lecky remarked, the breakdowns were due to anxiety, not overwork.[34]

Donald Meyer's remarks on the plight of many middle-class women in America at the end of the 19th century seem applicable here. "After all", he says, "what was one of the results of sickness in most civilized communities? The sick got taken care of. To those who were ill, attention was paid. Was it possible that the patient was looking for such attention? Sickness might be, not ego-alien, but a project of the ego: for people who were under-employed, a form of occupation; for the lonely, a demand for intimacy. Sickness might constitute a means for bringing lives otherwise diffuse to a focus. It might paradoxically be an assertion of desire".[35]

Against the background of the preceding discussion may be set the other current psychohistorical area of interest, the use of psychological models to understand historical individuals, particularly leaders of various types in terms of the interplay between public performance and private personality.[36] This endeavor has also had earlier antecedents, medical and non-medical. On the medical side are the so-called pathographies, for example, Möbius's case history of Rousseau and Lange's account of Hölderlin. Another is Jaspers' study of Strindberg and Van Gogh in which he tried to show how the neurotic drives of his subjects contributed to their creative accomplishments.[37] These biographical studies were in essence case histories undertaken by psychiatrists or by those with psychiatric orientations. Freud's discoveries and ideas were applied very early to biographical material, indeed by Freud himself as in *Eine Kindheitserinnerung des Leonardo da Vinci* and other contributions. His example was followed by others, among them Stefan Zweig who dedicated his study of Hölderlin, Kleist and Nietzsche to Freud.[38] One of the earliest examples of the application of analytical concepts was Karl Abraham's study in 1912 of Amenhotep IV (Ahknaton).[39] Many of the early contributions were relatively crude and were frequently vitiated by the fallacy of unilateralism, that is, by an effort to establish a one to one relationship between traumatic early experiences and later behavior, as for instance in the Bullitt—Freud analysis of Woodrow Wilson.

Probably the most successful practitioner so far has been Erik Erikson with his studies of Luther and Gandhi. Erikson's work illustrates both some possibilities and limitations. One of Erikson's major achievements is that he did not fall into the trap of simply reducing Luther to his psychic traumata and weaknesses. On the other hand, his portrayal of Luther's transformation of his weaknesses into spiritual power and strength, which enabled so many of his contemporaries to identify with him and to accept his position on theological and political issues, fused quite successfully "the personal troubles of milieu" and "the public issues of social structure".[40]

But Erikson's analysis also has certain limitations, which concern both method and substance. Erikson begins his study of Luther with a story of the young monk having had a fit, a story for which there is no good evidence. Nevertheless, he uses the story, justifying his practice on the ground that if it didn't happen, it as good as happened. *Si non è vero, è ben trovato.* But unfortunately Erikson gives no criteria indicating when and where he would admit rumor and legend as evidence, and when he would not. This is not good enough. After all, historians and other social scientists have at their disposal techniques and methodologies for verifying and appraising evidence on the basis of which some understanding of human actions can be achieved. Certainly, practitioners of psychohistory cannot be exempt from applying them or developing new ones where necessary.

Another point is Erikson's emphasis on Luther's anality, apparently overlooking the fact that the whole tone of life and its expression in sixteenth-century Germany was coarse. Cursing, belching, farting, gluttony and rude behavior were common at all levels of society, the highest as well as the lowest, to judge from the testimony of such observers as Erasmus and Machiavelli.[41]

There is no doubt that psychohistorical studies in the biographical area offer rich potentialities, and there are a few outstanding contributions such as Starobinski's elegant and subtle analysis of the tensions in

Rousseau's personality and their relation to his ideas and activities.[42] However, if the potentialities of psychohistory are to be realized, certain points must be emphasized. In modern history and biography, the study of process is preeminent. This applies as well to the area of health in its various aspects. In psychohistory we want to see the character forming, its singularities taking shape in relation to inner drives and compulsions as well as to outer circumstances. The task of the psychohistorian is to represent convincingly internal processes, pressures and changes that participated in producing the phenomenon he confronts. To do this it is necessary first of all to be aware of the character of a given period. It is not enough to know about Luther; one must also know the sixteenth century and its varied aspects, particularly in Germany.

To recapitulate, one cannot investigate normal or abnormal socio-psychological phenomena without reference to the milieu in which they occur. Individuals and groups function within socio-cultural systems which define and establish the boundaries of deviance and abnormality. This requires a genuine understanding of the sociocultural system as the mutable but omnipresent arena in which behavior and other vital phenomena, normal and abnormal, present themselves. Furthermore, values are intimately related to the socio-cultural system and for which they may be functional or dysfunctional. An understanding of such systems and the kinds of personalities and social organizations they produce is necessary to comprehend the criteria employed at different periods and by various groups, lay or professional, secular or religious, for the judgment of socio-psychological phenomena. There is increasing evidence from historical, anthropological and sociological studies that human personality, perception, and modes of feeling (or sensibility) are differently organized relative to the social environment at different periods and at varying levels of complexity.

As an example, I wish to suggest that during the 18th century as compared with earlier periods there were in some respects decisive changes in forms of irrationality. In literature, art, politics and economics, the 18th century offers instances of a kind of surrealistic rationality—a rationality that is under no restraint so that when carried to its logical culmination it becomes a form of irrationality. Ideas are pushed with inexorable logic to extremes where, as if by the operation of a Hegelian dialectic, they emerge as their very opposites. One thinks of Swift's devastating satire in Gulliver's third voyage of "rational" projects pushed logically to the point of madness, or in his *Modest Proposal* where the principles of political arithmetic are developed in the same way. A counterpart to this obsessive rationality is to be found in *Les Liaisons dangereuses* where the rigor with which Valmont, a very Machiavelli of seduction, plans his conquests reminds one of academic war strategists using game theory. Similarly, appeals for a rational architecture led to visionary structures dominated by formal purity, which exemplify Wordsworth's "reason in her most exalted mood", but which from the point of view of the builder and user were impractical and irrational.[43] Analogous examples are to be found in the political arena, particularly in the evolution of the principles by which Robespierre and St. Just aspired to create a social organization and a moral order in which virtue could express itself and where harmony would reign.[44] I need not elaborate on current counterparts of these examples. They are all too evident in so many of our modern horrors.

Most of this discussion has been devoted in a broad sense to history and psychopathology. There are two reasons for this emphasis. One is that for almost two decades I have investigated various aspects of this problem area. The other is that in principle basic relations between health, history and the social sciences in this area apply to others as well, whether health institutions, systems for providing health care, or the role of health personnel in society. For this reason I shall now offer some general points that have either been implicit in my presentation, or have simply been noted in passing and should be emphasized.

First, history and the other social sciences can work together most fruitfully in collective and comparative history, or what I have called historical sociology. As an example, my studies in the historical sociology of mental illness deal with the place of the mentally ill, however defined, in societies at different periods and the factors (social, psychological, cultural) that have determined it.[45] A similar approach has characterized my investigations of specialization in medicine and public health. Specialization is today deeply ingrained in the institutional and organizational structure of health services. Why has this happened? What factors started the process which produced the situation found today? What factors have reinforced it and are likely to continue into the foreseeable future? In the early 1940s, I developed a model involving medical and non-medical factors and processes, and using data from European and American sources.[46] (This model has since been used by a German medical historian to investigate medical specialization in antiquity.)[47] Two years ago I applied it again to data on specialization in the United States over the past thirty years.[48] This study showed that trends predicted on the basis of the analysis published in 1944 have continued into the present and have even been accentuated.

In short, the use of historical analyses to study sociological problems is certainly possible, and for some problems indeed essential. Historical and sociological analysis can be pursued simultaneously. Every social phenomenon is the result of historical process, that is societal factors operating over a period of time through human interaction. Only when the social scientist examines small parts or aspects of the process is he methodologically justified in overlooking the historical aspect. As soon as large-scale phenomena are investigated, account must be taken of the historical facet. This applies as well to the results (theories, models, data et alia) of researches. Clearly, there is a need for historians to understand concepts methods, terminology, and problems of the social sciences, but conversely this point applies as well to the social scientist.

The social scientist who investigates health problems needs to know the medical or public health history relevant for his interest. Knowledge of this kind can provide perspective and insights, and may even lead social scientists to study certain problems sooner than they have done. For example, in 1935 I investigated the reception given in Europe to the research of William Beaumont, a 19th century American physician-physiologist.[49] The results showed that English, French and German scientists and physicians reacted differently to the same research data, and I noted the need for an analysis in terms of the socio-cultural background of medicine and scientific research in these countries in order to elicit those elements which brought about the observed selectivity.[50] Several years later in connection with this research I pointed more specifically to the need to investigate the relation of university organization to scientific work in Germany, France, and Great Britain in order to account for the differing approaches. Furthermore, I pointed to the importance of a pre-existing group of active researchers working on problems similar to that with which the new data or discoveries deal; in the case of Beaumont this was gastric physiology.[51] This work, as far as I can tell, remained largely if not totally unknown to social scientists. Yet the issues raised are a part of what we know now as the sociology of science, and to which a great deal of attention is being given.[52] Very likely, publication in books and periodicals concerned with medical history rendered these studies unavailable to social scientists. Moreover, the sociology of science and medicine had not yet been recognized as having great interest for social scientists. Today, however, the social scientist must be conscious of the historical literature dealing with health and its possible significance for his work.

Throughout this paper I have tried to present explicitly as well as implicitly a number of areas concerned with health in which history and the social sciences are enmeshed, as well as issues that arise from these relations. Obviously, in matters of this kind there can be no final answers. Nonetheless, an awareness of these relations and issues can help us all to greater clarity in dealing with them. If I have in some small way contributed toward this end my purpose will have been accomplished.

REFERENCES

1. Vynne-Edwards, V. C. *Animal Dispersion in Relation to Social Behavior*, New York, Hafner-Publishing Company, 1962; Stellar, E. and Sprague, J. *Progress in Physiological Psychology*, pp. 119–160. Academic Press, New York, 1968.
2. Altmann, S. (ed.): *Social Communication among Primates*, pp. 221–236. University of Chicago Press, Chicago, Ill. 1967.
3. Singh, S. D. Urban Monkeys, *Scientific American*, p. 110. July 1969.
4. Lack, D. *The Natural Regulation of Animal Numbers*, chap. 15. Oxford, 1954.
5. Schorr, Alvin L. *Slums and Social Insecurity*, pp. 31–32. Govt. Printing Office, Wash., D.C., 1963.
6. Eisenberg, Leon, The *Human* Nature of Human Nature, *Science* **176**, 123–128, 1972 (p. 127); Birch, H. G. and Gussow, J. D. *Disadvantaged Children: Health Nutrition and School Failure*, Harcourt Brace Jovanovich, New York, 1970.
7. For example see Schultz, Adolph H. Notes on Diseases and Healed Fractures of Wild Apes and their Bearing on the Antiquity of Pathological Conditions in Man, *Bull. Hist. Med.* **7**, 571 – 582, 1939; Brothwell, D. The Palaepathology of Early British Man, *Jr. Roy. Anthropol. Inst.* **91**, 318 – 344, 1961; Jarcho, S. Lead in the Bones of Prehistoric Lead-Glaze Potters, *Amer. Antiq.* **30**, 94 – 96, 1964; Ruffer, M. A. *Studies in the Palaeopathology of Egypt*, pp. 17 – 19. Univ. Of Chicago Press, Chicago, 1921.
8. Preuss, Julius. *Biblisch-talmudische Medizin. Beiträge zur Geschichte der Heilkunde und der Kultur überhaupt*, pp. 363–364. S. Karger. Berlin. 1911.
9. Xenophon. *Memorabilia* III,**9**, 6 – 7 (Loeb ed.), pp. 226 – 227.
10. Voltaire. *Correspondence* 1704–1738, texte établi et annoté par Theodore Bestermann (Bibliothèque de la Pléiade), vol. 1, p. 203. Paris, Gallimard, 1963.
11. Field, M. J. *Search for Security. An Ethno-Psychiatric Study of Rural Ghana*, p. 296. Northwestern University Press, Evanston, 1960.
12. *Goldberger on Pellagra*, Milton Terris (ed.), pp. 113 – 291. Louisiana State University Press, Baton Rouge, 1964.
13. Ibid., p. 290.
14. Farquhar, George. *The Best Plays*, edited with an introduction by William Archer (Mermaid Series), pp. 399 – 400. Ernest Benn, London, 1906.
15. Mossner, E. C. *The Life of David Hume*, pp. 66 – 91. Nelson, Edinburgh, 1954. Greig J. Y. T. (ed.): *The Letters of David Hume* (2 vols.), vol. 1, p. 14. Oxford University Press, New York, 1932.
16. [Sir William Temple]: *Miscellanea . . .* By a Person of Honour, London, 1680, p. 227. The "Essay on the Cure of the Gout by Moxa" is one of six essays which make up this volume and is to be found on pages 189 – 238; see also George Rosen: Sir William Temple and the Therapeutic Use of Moxa for Gout in England, *Bull. Hist. Med.* **44**, 31 – 39, 1970.

17. Ramazzini, Bernardino. *Diseases of Workers*, the Latin Text of 1713 revised with translation and notes by Wilmer Cave Wright, p. 449. University of Chicago Press, Chicago, 1940.
18. Thorndike, Lynn. Fifteenth Century Patients, *Bull. Hist. Med.* **28**, 252 – 258; Dean Lockwood: *Ugo Benzi: Medieval Philosopher and Physician* 1376 – 1439, pp. 67 – 68, 264 – 266, 309. Univ. of Chicago Press, Chicago, 1951, Philippe Ariès: *L'Enfant et la vie familiale sous l'ancien régime*, p. 29. Paris, Plon, 1960.
19. Langer, W. L. The Next Assignment, *American Historical Review* **63**, 283 – 304, 1958.
20. Tenenti, Alberto. *Il Senso della morte e l'amore della vita nel Rinascimento (Francia e Italia)*, Einaudi, Torino, 1957.
21. Meiss, Millard. *Painting in Florence and Siena after the Black Death*, Princeton University Press, Princeton, N.J., 1951.
22. Baehrel, René. Epidemie et terreur: Histoire et sociologie, *Annales de l'histoire de la Revolution française* **22**, 113 – 146, 1950; Séraphine Guerchberg: La controverse sur les traités de peste de l'époque, *Revue des études juives*, n.s. **8**, 3 – 40, 1948. Somewhat over a hundred years earlier, an equally terrible example of the way human beings can be sacrified to panic and fear was published by Alessandro Manzoni in his *Storia della colonna infame* (1842). This is the story of those who were accused of spreading the plague in Milan in 1630 by smearing the walls of houses with a poison. Arrested and tortured to make them confess, they were condemned to a horrible death and their houses were destroyed.
23. Febvre, Lucien. La sensibilité et l'histoire, *Annales d'histoire sociale* **2**, 5 – 20, 1940; idem: *Le Problème de l'incroyance an XVIe siècle. La religion de Rabelais*, Michel, Paris, 1962 (originally published 1942).
24. For the application of these concepts as analytic tools see George Rosen: Emotion and Sensibility in Ages of Anxiety, *American Journal of Psychiatry* **124**, 771 – 784, 1967; ibid: Enthusiasm "a dark lanthorn of the spirit", *Bull. Hist. Med.* **42**, 393 – 421, 1968.
25. Rosen, George. Forms of Irrationality in the Eighteenth Century. Read at the Meeting of the American Society for Eighteenth Century Studies, Univ. of Maryland, April, 1971. Accepted for publication in *Studies in Eighteenth Century Culture*, vol. II, Case-Western Reserve Press, 1972 (in press).
26. Huizinga, J. *The Waning of the Middle Ages*, pp. 31ff. Anchor Books, Garden City, M.J., 1954.
27. Tillich, Paul. *The Courage to Be*, Yale Univ. Press, New Haven and London, 1952. Yale Paperbound, 1965, p. 58.
28. Houghton, W. E. *The Victorian Frame of Mind*, 1830–1870, Yale University Press, New Haven and London, 1957. Yale Paperbound, 1963, p. 54.
29. For antiquity, as an example, see E. R. Dodds: *Pagan and Christian in an Age of Anxiety*, pp. 37 – 68, Cambridge Univ. Press, Cambridge, specifically 43 – 44, 55.
30. Rosen, George, *Madness in Society*, pp. 110 – 117. Univ. of Chicago Press, Chicago, 1968.
31. MacMullen, R. *Enemies of the Roman Order*, pp. 59 – 62, 93, 99, Harvard Univ. Press, Cambridge, Mass. 1966. Nock, A. D. *Conversion. The Old and the New in Religion from Alexander the Great to Augustine of Hippo*, pp. 168 – 170, Oxford University Press, London, 1933. H. Moller: Affective Mysticism in Western Civilization, *Psychoanalytic Review* **52**, 115 – 130, 1965.
32. Werblowsky, R. J. Z. *Joseph Karo, Lawyer and Mystic*, pp. 78 – 83, 149 – 150, 265 – 266. Clarendon Press, Oxford, 1962. In this connection it is of interest to note a cultural and psychological analysis of Buddhist monasticism in Burma by Spiro, Melford E. Religious Systems as Culturally Constituted Defense Mechanisms, in *Context and Mean-*

ing in Cultural Anthropology, edited by Melford E. Spiro, pp. 100 – 113. Free Press, New York, 1965.
33. Eliot, George, "Janet's Repentance", *Scenes of Clerical Life*, p. 391. Oxford University Press, London, 1916.
34. Lecky, W. E. H. *The Map of Life. Conduct and Character*, p. 309. Longmans, Green & Co., London, 1909.
35. Meyer, Donald. *The Positive Thinkers*, p. 52. Doubleday, Garden City, N.J., 1965.
36. An example is Rogow, Arnold A. *James Forrestal. A Study of Personality, Politics and Policy*, Macmillan, New York, 1963.
37. Möbius, P. J. *J. J. Rousseau's Krankheitsgeschichte*, F. C. W. Vogel, Leipzig, 1889; Lange, Wilhelm, *Hölderlin, Eine Pathographie*, Ferdinand Enke, Stuttgart, 1909; Jaspers, Karl. *Strindberg und Van Gogh. Versuch einer pathographischen Analyse unter vergleichender Heranziehung von Swedenborg und Hölderlin*, E. Bircher, Bern, 1922.
38. Zweig, Stefan. *Der Kampf mit dem Dämon. Hölderlin. Kleist. Nietzsche*, Insel Verlag, Leipzig, 1925. This volume is the second in a trilogy. The first, *Drei Meister* (1919) deals with Balzac, Dickens, and Dostoyevski; the third, *Drei Dichter Ihres Lebens* (1928) with Casonova, Stendhal, and Tolstoi.
39. Abraham, Karl. Amenhotep IV (Echnaton), *Imago* **1**, 334 – 360, 1912.
40. Wright Mills, C. *The Sociological Imagination*, pp. 8 – 9. Oxford Univ. Press, New York, 1959.
41. Friedell, Egon. *Kulturgeschichte der Neuzeit* (3 vols. in one), vol. 1, pp. 316 – 320. Phaidon Press, London and Oxford, 1947.
42. Starobinski, Jean. *Jean-Jacques Rousseau. La Transparence et l'Obstacle*, Plon, Paris, 1957.
43. Kaufmann, Emil. Etienne-Louis Boullée, *Art Bulletin* **21**, 213 – 227, 1939; idem: Three Revolutionary Architects. Boullée, Ledoux and Lequeu, *Transactions of the American Philosophical Society*, vol. 62 (part 3), pp. 436 – 473. October, 1952, idem: *Architecture in the Age of Reason*, Cambridge, Mass., 1955; Rosenau, Helen. Architecture and the French Revolution: Jean Jacques Lequeu, *Architectural Review* **106**, 111 – 116, 1949; idem: *Boullée's Treatise on Architecture*, London, 1953; Chastel, André. The Moralizing Architecture of Jean-Jacques Lequeu, in *The Grand Eccentrics*, edited by Thomas B. Hess and John Ashbery, pp. 57 – 66; Collier Books, New York, 1966. Boulée, Etienne-Louis. *Architecture. Essai sur l'art*, Textes réunis et présentés par J.-M. P. de Montclos, Hermann, Paris, 1968.
44. Malraux, Andre. "Preface" to Albert Ollivier: *Saint-Just et la force des choses*, p. 23. Gallimard, Paris, 1954.
45. Rosen, George. *Madness in Society. Chapters in the Historical Sociology of Mental Illness*, University of Chicago Press, Chicago, 1968.
46. Rosen, George. *The Specialization of Medicine*, Froben Press, New York, 1944 (Reprinted New York, Arno Press and New York Times, 1972).
47. Michler, M. *Das Spezialisierungsproblem und die antike Chirurgie*, Bern, Hans Huber Verlag, 1969.
48. Rosen, George. Whither Specialization? in *Medicine and Society. Contemporary Problems in Historical Perspective*, pp. 197 – 219. American Philosophical Society Library Publication No. 4, Philadelphia, 1971.
49. Rosen, George. *Die Aufnahme der Entdeckung William Beaumonts durch die europäische Medizin* [Abhandlungen zur Geschichte der Medizin und der Naturwissenschaften, Heft 8], Berlin, 1935. An English translation appeared as *The Reception of William Beaumont's Discovery in Europe*, Schuman, New York, 1942.
50. Rosen, *Reception* . . . ., pp. 85 – 86.

51. Rosen, George. Notes on the Reception and Influence of William Beaumont's Discovery, *Bull. Hist. Med.* **13**, 631 – 642, 1943.
52. Ben-David, E. G. J. Scientific productivity and academic organization in nineteenth century medicine, *American Sociological Review* **25**, 828 – 843, 1960.

WHAT IS SOCIAL MEDICINE?

A Genetic Analysis of the Concept

I.

Introduction

Disease is a biological process which is older than man. It is as old as life itself, for it is an attribute of life. A living organism is a labile entity in a world of flux and change, and health and disease are linked aspects of this all-pervading instability. Health and disease are expressions of changing relationships between the various components of the body, and between the body and the external environment in which it has its being. As a biological phenomenon, the causes of disease are sought in the realm of nature; but in man disease has still another dimension. Nowhere does human disease occur as "pure nature"; instead it is ever mediated and modified by social activity and the cultural environment which such activity creates.

These general conceptions are not new, and in earlier periods medical practitioners were aware of them in an empirical way. The practice of medicine has always been linked with the social and economic conditions of particular groups of people, but these relations were only rarely made the subject of theoretical discussion. Not until modern times does there appear a clear awareness that intimate bonds link social conditions and medical problems. The need for consideration of social viewpoints in dealing with problems of medicine and hygiene was recognized by various medical men during the eighteenth century. Probably best known in this connection are Bernardino Ramazzini and Johann Peter Frank. It was left for the nineteenth century, however, to develop the idea of medicine as a social science, and eventually to formulate with greater precision and clarity the concept of social medicine.

II.

Medicine—A Social Science. The Idea of 1848

In 1893, in an essay dealing with the etiological therapy of infectious diseases, Emil Behring noted as characteristic of the medical thought of the earlier nineteenth century the association in a causal relationship of social misery and disease.[1] For specific illustration of this point, he referred to Rudolf Virchow's report on the epidemic of typhus fever in 1847 in Upper Silesia. Virchow conceived of this outbreak as due to a complex of social and economic factors, and consequently expected little from any medicinal therapy. Instead, he proposed thoroughgoing social reform, which in most general terms comprised " complete and unrestricted democracy," education, freedom and prosperity. Behring passes over this with the condemnation of faint praise, remarking that while these views also had their merits, now, following the procedure of Robert Koch, the study of infectious diseases could be pursued unswervingly without being sidetracked by social considerations and reflections on social policy.[2]

What is the meaning of this profound cleavage that separates Behring and Virchow? For an answer to this question, an analysis of Virchow's conception of the nature of medicine offers a point of departure. Basic to such an analysis is the circumstance that his views originated and found explicit expression as an integral part of his activity during the revolutionary movement of 1848.[2a]

On May 1, 1848 in a letter to his father Virchow tried to explain

[1] E. Behring: *Gesammelte Abhandlungen zur ätiologischen Therapie von ansteckenden Krankheiten*, Leipzig, Georg Thieme, 1893, p. xvii (Der Beginn der socialen Aera aber macht sich in unserem Jahrhundert bemerkbar in der Zurückführung der Krankheiten auf das sociale Elend), and p. xix (Hier finden wir die Anschauungen in voller Schärfe, welche noch lange Zeit einer naturwissenschaftlichen Betrachtungsweise der Krankheitsätiologie entgegenstanden: die Zurückführung der epidemischen Krankheiten auf das *sociale Elend*).

[2] *Ibid.*, p. xix.

[2a] For an excellent analysis of the German medical reform movement of 1848 and of Virchow in relation to this movement consult the monograph of Erwin H. Ackerknecht: Beiträge zur Geschichte der Medizinalreform von 1848, *Sudhoff's Archiv für Geschichte der Medizin* 25: 61-109, 112-183.

his fundamental point of view. " I have often been deceived in people," he wrote, " but not yet in the age. As a result, I now have the advantage that I am no longer a partial man, but a whole one, and that my medical creed merges with my political and social creed." [3] That Virchow practiced what he preached is clear from his actions. The March Days in Berlin had followed hard on the heels of the victorious February Revolution in Paris. On March 18, the people of Berlin rose in revolt and threw up barricades. Among the defenders of the barricade that blocked the Friedrichstrasse from the Taubenstrasse was Rudolf Virchow.[4] Not quite four months later, on July 10, 1848 appeared the first number of the weekly, *Die medicinische Reform*, edited jointly by Virchow and R. Leubuscher. In the challenging programmatic editorial with which he launched the journal, Virchow showed that the change from the musket to the pen had in no way altered his fundamental position. He said:

> The " Medical Reform " comes into being at a time when the overthrow of our old political institutions is not yet completed, but when from all sides plans are being laid and steps taken toward a new political structure. What other task could then be more natural for it to undertake, than that of participation in clearing away the old ruins and in constructing new institutions? Severe and mighty political storms such as now roar over the thinking portion of Europe, shaking to the foundation all elements of the state, indicate radical changes in the prevailing conceptions of life. In this situation medicine cannot alone remain untouched; it too can no longer postpone a radical reform in its field.[5]

This awareness of the relations of medicine to social problems, Virchow formulated in the somewhat rhetorical but striking slogan: " Medicine is a social science, and politics nothing but medicine on a grand scale."

The idea of medicine as a social science did not originate with Virchow. Industrialization and its attendant social problems led various investigators to study the influence of such factors as poverty

[3] Rudolf Virchow: *Briefe an seine Eltern 1839 bis 1864,* herausgegeben von Marie Rabl geb. Virchow, Leipzig, Wilhelm Engelmann, 1907, pp. 144-145.

[4] *Ibid.*, p. 135.

[5] *Die medicinische Reform. Eine Wochenschrift, erschienen vom 10. Juli 1848 bis zum 29. Juni 1849,* Berlin, Druck und Verlag von G. Reimer, No. 1, p. 1.

and occupation on the state of health. This was particularly true in France where during the 'thirties and 'forties medical men such as Villermé, Benoiston de Chateauneuf, and Guépin, and social theorists like Constantin Pecqueur dealt with socio-medical questions. Arnold Ruge, a democratic German journalist, wrote in 1844 that "Every attempt to make science serviceable to the world, every association of science with politics is directly linked to France."[6] This judgment may be taken as applying also to ideas on the social relations of medicine. From Paris, the fountainhead of advanced thought, liberal ideas spread to Germany. The publication in 1842 of Lorenz Stein's book, *Der Socialismus und Kommunismus des heutigen Frankreich; Ein Beitrag zur Zeitgeschichte*, made a profound impression on the German public.[7] Virchow's contact with these intellectual currents is indicated by the quotation, in a letter of 1843 to his father, of a passage from Ruge's *Deutsche Jahrbücher*, which had been suppressed by the Prussian government.[8] Other German physicians shared Virchow's point of view, and during 1848 joined forces with him to secure long overdue medical reforms. Prominent in this group were Salomon Neumann and Leubuscher, Virchow's editorial associate. In his book, *Die öffentliche Gesundheitspflege und das Eigenthum*, published in 1847, Neumann had vigorously asserted the view that "medical science is intrinsically and essentially a *social* science, and as long as this is not recognized in practice we shall not be able to enjoy its benefits and shall have to be satisfied with an empty shell and a sham."[9] And in 1851, in a study of the medical statistics of the Prussian state, Neumann again stressed the importance of this idea.[10] The same point of view was

[6] Arnold Ruge: Plan der Deutsch-Französischen Jahrbücher, *Deutsch-Französische Jahrbücher*, herausgegeben von Arnold Ruge und Karl Marx, Paris, 1844, p. 6. [Reproduced in facsimile in the series *Neudrucke marxistischer Seltenheiten* (I) Verlag von Rudolf Liebing (L. Franz & Co.), Leipzig, 1925.]

[7] Lorenz von Stein: *Geschichte der sozialen Bewegung in Frankreich von 1789 bis auf unsere Tage* (3 vols.), München, Drei Masken Verlag, 1921, vol. I, pp. vii-viii.

[8] Virchow, *Briefe*, p. 52.

[9] S. Neumann: *Die öffentliche Gesundheitspflege und das Eigenthum. Kritisches und Positives mit Bezug auf die preussische Medizinalverfassungs-Frage*, Berlin, Adolph Riess, 1847, pp. 64-65.

[10] S. Neumann: Zur medizinischen Statistik des preussischen Staates nach den

expressed by Leubuscher in the statement that " medicine is a purely social science ";[11] but he went on to point out that the idea still lacked any practical content.[12]

Nevertheless, it is clear from contemporary discussions that the proponents of this idea were not dreaming of some medical Cloud-cuckooland, but employed it rather as a convenient formulation under which to sum up definite principles. The *first* of these is that *the health of the people is a matter of direct social concern.* Society has an obligation to protect and insure the health of its members. According to Neumann,

> It is the duty of society, i. e., of the state, as a fundamental condition for all enjoyment and activity, to protect, and when endangered to save, the lives and health of the citizens. If it is the duty of social man to combat and to help endure the dangers which develop precisely because of social life, then it is equally clear that the state is obliged to combat and where possible to destroy not only natural dangers, but as well those dangers to human life.[13]

Virchow derived the same point as a logical consequence of democratic principles.

> The democratic state [he declared] desires that all its citizens enjoy a state of well-being, for it recognizes that they all have equal rights. Since general equality of rights leads to self-government, the state also has the right to hope that everyone will know how through his own labor to achieve and to maintain a state of well-being within the limits of the laws set up by the people themselves. However, the conditions of well-being are health and education, so that it is the task of the state to provide on the broadest possible basis the means for maintaining and promoting health and education through public action. . . . Thus it is not enough for the state to guarantee every citizen the basic necessities for existence, and to assist everyone whose labor does not suffice for him to acquire these necessities; the state must do more, it must assist everyone so far that he will have the conditions necessary for a healthy existence.[14]

The *second* principle involved in the idea of medicine as a social science is that *social and economic conditions have an important effect*

Acten des statistischen Bureau's für das Jahr 1846, *Archiv für pathologische Anatomie und Physiologie und für klinische Medicin,* 3: 13-141, 1851 (see page 19).

[11] R. Leubuscher: Zur Reform der Sanitätspolizei, *Medicinische Reform,* p. 11.

[12] *Ibid.,* p. 11.

[13] Neumann: *Öffentliche Gesundheitspflege,* p. 64.

[14] Rudolf Virchow: Die öffentliche Gesundheitspflege, *Medicinische Reform,* No. 5. August 4, 1848, pp. 21-22.

on health and disease, and that these relations must be subjected to scientific investigation. For Neumann no proof was necessary to show that "the greatest number of diseases which either prevent the complete enjoyment of life or kill a considerable number of people prematurely are due not to natural causes, but rather to artificially produced social conditions."[15] He was convinced that poverty, hunger, and misery "if not identical with death, disease and chronic suffering were nevertheless, like their inseparable companions, prejudice, ignorance, and stupidity, the inexhaustible sources from which the former originate."[16]

Virchow's basic standpoint was very similar, but in expressing it his emphasis differed from that of Neumann. The investigation of the Silesian typhus epidemic of 1847 led Virchow to the conclusion that its causes were as much social, economic and political as they were biological and physical. This view he later generalized in a series of articles on *Public Health,* in which he discussed the relation of medical problems to social and political developments. "The very word 'Public Health,'" he declared, "shows those who were and still are of the opinion that medicine has nothing to do with politics the magnitude of their error."[17] Virchow conceived the scope of public health as broadly as possible, indicating that one of its major functions was to study the conditions under which various social groups lived, and to determine the effects of these conditions on their health. On the basis of this knowledge it would then be possible to take appropriate action. "For if medicine is really to accomplish its great task, it must intervene in political and social life. It must point out the hindrances that impede the normal functioning of vital processes, and effect their removal."[18]

As an extension of his views on the relations of medicine to society, Virchow developed a theory of epidemic disease as a manifestation of social and cultural maladjustment. Reasoning by analogy, he drew a parallel between the individual and the body

[15] Neumann: *Öffentliche Gesundheitspflege,* p. 64.

[16] Neumann: Zur medicinischen Statistik . . . p. 61 (see footnote 10).

[17] *Medicinische Reform,* p. 21.

[18] Rudolf Virchow: *Die Einheitsbestrebungen in der wissenschaftlichen Medicin,* Berlin, Druck und Verlag von G. Reimer, 1849, p. 48.

politic: "If disease is an expression of individual life under unfavorable conditions, then epidemics must be indicative of major disturbances of mass life."[19] These disturbances are social and economic in nature, e. g. business depressions, unemployment and the like. "Don't we see that epidemics everywhere point to deficiencies of society?" Virchow asked. "One may point to atmospheric conditions, general cosmic changes and the like, but in and of themselves these never cause epidemics. They always produce them only where, because of poor social circumstances people have lived for a long time under abnormal conditions."[20] Virchow differentiated *natural* and *artificial* epidemics, basing his distinction on the degree to which cultural factors interpose themselves between nature and man.

Living conditions [he pointed out] are either natural or artificial depending on the spatial and temporal situation of the individual. The development of culture, by multiplying the relations of individuals to each other, also complicates living conditions. . . . Consequently epidemics are *natural* or *artificial* depending on whether the change in living conditions occurs of its own accord through natural events, or artificially, because of the mode of life.

Natural epidemics have always been present whenever changes of season, of weather, etc. altered living conditions, and the great mass did not protect itself by artificial means. They recur as often as external conditions require, and remain as long as these last. Fluxes, intermittent fevers, and pneumonias have occurred epidemically at all times.

Artificial epidemics, however, are attributes of society, products of a false culture, or of a culture which is not available to all classes. These are indicative of defects produced by political and social organization, and therefore affect predominantly those classes that do not participate in the advantages of the culture. Here belong typhus, scurvy, the sweating sickness, and tuberculosis.[21]

Furthermore, these "artificial" epidemics occur not only as a result of social contradictions, but also as significant manifestations of the historical process. Such outbreaks of disease occur at nodal points in history, during periods of political and intellectual revolu-

[19] *Ibid.*, p. 46.

[20] Rudolf Virchow: Die Epidemien von 1848. (Gelesen in der Jahressitzung der Gesellschaft für wissenschaftliche Medicin am 27. Novb. 1848.), *Archiv für pathologische Anatomie und Physiologie und für klinische Medicin*, 3: 3-12, 1851 (see page 10).

[21] Virchow: *Einheitsbestrebungen*, pp. 46-47.

tion. " History has shown more than once," Virchow declared in August, 1848, " how the fates of the greatest empires were decided by the health of their peoples or of their armies, and there is no longer any doubt that the history of epidemic diseases must form an inseparable part of the cultural history of mankind. Epidemics correspond to large signs of warning which tell the true statesman that a disturbance has occurred in the development of his people which even a policy of unconcern can no longer overlook." [22] And in 1849 Virchow carried this train of thought to its logical conclusion. " Epidemic diseases exhibiting an hitherto unknown character appear and disappear," he pointed out, " after new culture periods have begun often without leaving any trace. As cases in point take leprosy and the English sweat. The history of artificial epidemics is therefore the history of disturbances which the culture of mankind has experienced. Its changes show us with powerful strokes the turning points at which culture moves off in new directions. Every true cultural revolution is followed by epidemics, because a large part of the people only gradually enter into the new cultural movement and begin to enjoy its blessings." [23] Finally, attention must be drawn to the fact that in his socio-historical theory of epidemic disease, Virchow also included the so-called psychic epidemics, a field in which interest has again been aroused by the events of our own time.[24]

If society has an obligation to protect the health of its members, and it is recognized that social and economic conditions have an important effect on health and disease, then it follows logically that *steps must be taken to promote health and to combat disease, and that the measures involved in such action must be social as well as medical.* This is the *third* principle involved in the idea of medicine as a social science, and was recognized by Virchow, Neumann and the other

[22] *Medicinische Reform,* p. 45.

[23] Virchow: *Einheitsbestrebungen,* p. 47.

[24] It is interesting to note that Temkin and Hirschfeld in 1929 called attention to Virchow's theory of epidemic disease and pointed out the astonishing proximity of his view to that expressed by Sigerist in 1928. See O. Temkin: Studien zum " Sinn"-begriff in der Medizin, *Kyklos* (1929), vol. 2, p. 103; E. Hirschfeld: Virchow, *Kyklos* (1929) vol. 2, pp. 110-111; H. E. Sigerist: Kultur und Krankheit, *Kyklos* (1928), vol. 1, pp. 60-63.

medical men who participated in the movement of 1848. The broad outlines of the program of action proposed as a result of the acceptance of this principle are probably represented best by a draft for a Public Health Law prepared by Neumann and submitted to the Berlin Society of Physicians and Surgeons on March 30, 1849.[25] According to this document: [26]

I. Public Health has as its objectives
   1. The healthy mental and physical development of the citizen;
   2. The prevention of all dangers to health;
   3. The control of disease.

II. Public Health must care for
   1. Society as a whole by considering the general physical and social conditions that may adversely affect health, such as soil, industry, food and housing.
   2. Each individual by considering those conditions which prevent him from caring for his health. These may be considered in two major categories:
      a. Conditions, such as poverty and infirmity, where the individual has the right to request assistance from the state;
      b. Conditions where the state has the right and the obligation to interfere with the personal liberty of the individual in the interest of health, e. g. in cases of transmissible disease and mental illness.

III. Public Health can fulfill these duties by
   1. Supplying well trained medical personnel in sufficient number;
   2. Adequate organization of the medical personnel;
   3. Establishing appropriate institutions for public health.

---

[25] *Medicinische Reform*, p. 227 seq.

[26] Gertrud Kroeger: *The Concept of Social Medicine as presented by Physicians and other Writers in Germany, 1779-1932*, Chicago, Julius Rosenwald Fund, 1937, pp. 14-15.

Voices were raised for governmental action, and many specific measures were proposed, all of which fall within the broad program drafted by Neumann. A very important problem was the provision of medical care for the indigent, and proposals were put forth by Virchow and others for public medical services for the poor, including free choice of physicians.[27] It was realized, however, that provision of medical care was not enough, that it must go hand in hand with social prophylaxis. In consequence, we find Virchow proclaiming the *right of the citizen to work,* as a fundamental principle to be included in the constitution of a democratic state.[28] (Here Virchow was influenced by the action of the French Provisional Government of 1848 in recognizing the right to work, the doctrine of the *Droit au travail* that Louis Blanc had been preaching since 1839.)[29]

The problem of the industrial worker also demanded attention. Although industrialization in Germany began later than in England and France, and proceeded at a slower pace during the first half of the 19th century, by 1848 the existence of a wage-earning class, an industrial proletariat, could no longer be overlooked. As in England and France, industrialization was ushered in by a slaughter of the innocents. Those that survived the cradle were given over to the tender mercies of the factory and the mine. It was plain, said Virchow, that "the proletariat in ever increasing degree became the victim of disease and epidemics, its children either died prematurely or developed into cripples."[30] To deal with this problem Leubuscher proposed a program of industrial hygiene, with emphasis on the legislative regulation of working conditions.[31] Particularly important was the question of limiting the working day. Leubuscher advocated the prohibition of child labor before the age of fourteen, reduction of the working day in dangerous occupations, protection of pregnant women, the establishment of standards for ventilation

[27] *Medicinische Reform,* pp. 127, 185, 189, 190.

[28] *Ibid.,* p. 38.

[29] J. A. R. Marriott (editor): *The French Revolution of 1848 in its Economic Aspect. Vol. I, Louis Blanc's Organisation du Travail. . . .* Oxford, The Clarendon Press, 1913, pp. xxxvi-lxix.

[30] *Medicinische Reform,* pp. 126-127.

[31] P. Leubuscher: Zur Reform der Sanitätspolizei, *Medicinische Reform,* pp. 11-12, 47-49.

of work rooms, and the prevention of industrial poisoning through the use of non-toxic materials.

Demands were also made for uniform licensure of medical practitioners entitling them to practice in every German state; appointment of physicians to official positions on the basis of competitive examinations; and the establishment of a National Ministry of Health.[32]

Very important was the recognition that for investigation of the causal relations between social conditions and medical problems it was necessary to have reliable statistics. The significance attributed by Virchow to medical statistics is indicated by his statement that "Medical statistics will be our standard of measurement: we will weigh life for life and see where the dead lie thicker, among the workers or among the privileged." [33] It was Neumann, however, who was most active in agitating for the collection of accurate statistics. In 1847, he pointed out that without medical statistics there could not be an efficient organization of medical activity.[34] Several years later, Neumann made it clear that what he wanted was not medical statistics in any narrow sense; he called for "social statistics," that is statistical information on all elements of social life that in any way have a bearing on problems of health and disease.[35] Neumann carried on statistical investigations in line with these principles, and reference will be made to these studies in the following section.

An explanation of the cleavage between Behring and Virchow emerges from the preceding analysis of the idea of medicine as a social science. For Virchow who saw medicine in its organic relations to the rest of society, and recognized health and disease as enmeshed within the web of social activity, the strict bacteriological view could not but seem narrow and limited, if not a complete intellectual aberration. Virchow recognized the discoveries of the bacteriologists, but he could never accept an unqualified causal rela-

[32] *Medicinische Reform,* pp. 13-16 (especially page 14). See also Ackerknecht, *op. cit.,* pp. 113-130.

[33] *Medicinische Reform,* p. 182.

[34] Neumann: *Öffentliche Gesundheitspflege,* p. 84.

[35] Neumann: Zur medicinischen Statistik . . . pp. 86-89 (see footnote p. 274).

tionship between bacterium and disease. For him the tubercle bacillus was not identical with tuberculosis.

The views of Virchow and his collaborators did not mature in their own day, but the seed had been sown. With the defeat of the revolution of 1848, the medical reform movement came to a quick end. Virchow had to discontinue the publication of the *Medicinische Reform,* but in his last editorial, comparing the contemporary situation with that which faced Moses after bringing Israel out of Egypt, he wrote:

> We too must wander in the wilderness and fight. Our task is an educational one; we must train men capable of fighting the battles of humanism. We have nothing more to expect from the governments so that further publication of a periodical is useless. Among the doctors, those who are capable of further education need no continuous guidance, while the indolent dullards will never be affected by reason. We can therefore only accept the task of educating the people concerning problems of public health, and problems of earning their daily living, and of assisting them through the continuous provision of new teachers to achieve the broadest basis for the winning of the final victory. The medical reform that we had in mind was a reform of science and society. We developed its principles; even without the further existence of this organ they will advance. Every moment, however, will find us occupied in working for them and ready to fight for them. Our cause remains unchanged; it is only the field of activity that changes.[36]

III.

From Virchow to Grotjahn. England, Belgium, and Germany to 1900

Beliefs of men regarding social organization and social change, and their attitudes toward the society in which they live, may be viewed as variations on the themes of desire and expectation. While the middle class in Germany was fighting for political power, the English middle class had already attained its goal. This situational difference finds its reflection in varying social philosophies. In Germany, the democratic radicals put forth a charter of liberty for the people in which they proclaimed the preeminence of human rights and human dignity, and accepted the logical consequences of this

[36] *Medicinische Reform,* p. 274.

charter in relation to health and disease. In England, on the other hand, the same doctrine of liberalism, with its implications of human rights, human dignity, liberty and equality, had already woven itself into public consciousness, but had emerged with a different emphasis as the doctrine of economic liberalism. This philosophy with its acceptance of social atomism and the predetermined harmony of man and nature manifesting itself through inexorable economic laws carried with it a stubborn insistence on the absolute necessity of submission to the supposed laws of society. Even the protests against the effects of economic liberalism on the lives of men did not substantially alter the doctrine. Discrepancy between social fact and social theory was not generally recognized as affecting the hard central core of economic liberalism, and it was not until the latter part of the nineteenth century that the gradual and peripheral erosion which had been carried on in practice began to receive conceptual recognition.

Such an intellectual environment was hardly conducive to analyses of the social aspects of health and disease, and no thoroughgoing theoretical formulations like those of the German authors were developed. And yet, certain stubborn facts insisted upon intruding themselves into public consciousness. Questions of ill-health, poor housing, dangerous and injurious occupations, excessive morbidity and mortality could not be overlooked, and investigations of these social problems were undertaken, often by medical men, to find out how they had arisen.

From this point of view it is instructive to look at a study of *The Moral and Physical Condition of the Working Classes Employed in the Cotton Manufacture in Manchester* published in 1832 by James Philips Kay, M. D. Permeating this anatomy of social misery is the bleak gospel of contemporary economic orthodoxy. At the very outset, Kay emphasizes that the immutable laws of economics cannot be transgressed. " The evils here unreservedly exposed," he says, " so far from being the necessary consequences of the manufacturing system, have a remote or accidental origin, and might, *by judicious management*, be entirely removed. Nor do they flow from any single source: and, especially in the present state of trade, the hours of labour cannot be materially diminished, without occasioning the most serious commercial embarrassment." [37] It must be kept in mind that this was the period when Richard Oastler was leading the campaign for a shorter working day.[38] In reply to this demand the employers argued that a cut in hours meant that wages would have to be cut in direct proportion. Furthermore, the interests of both workers and employers were complementary and were menaced by foreign competition. Injudicious agitation and legislation would therefore harm the workers more than it would help them. What was needed was not factory legislation, but free trade. In this spirit, Kay pointed out that

> The profits of trade will not allow a greater remuneration for labour, and competition even threatens to reduce its price. *Whatever time is substracted from the hours of labour must be accompanied with an equivalent deduction from its rewards,* and we fear that the condition of the working classes cannot be much improved, until the burdens and restrictions of the commercial system are abolished.
>
> Those political speculators who propose a serious reduction of the hours of labour, unpreceded by the relief of commercial burdens, and unaccompanied by the introduction of a *general system of education,* appear to us deluded by a theoretical chimera.[39]
>
> Believing that the natural tendency of unrestricted commerce, is to develop the energies of society, to increase the comforts and luxuries of life, and to *elevate the physical condition* of every member of the social body, we have exposed with a faithful, though a friendly hand, the condition of the lower orders connected with the manufactures of this town, because we conceive that the evils affecting them result *from foreign and accidental causes.* A system, which promotes the advance of civilization, and diffuses it over the world—which promises to maintain the peace of nations, by establishing a permanent international law, founded on the benefits of commercial association, cannot be inconsistent with the happiness of the *great mass of the people.*[40]

Nevertheless, the prevalence of disease among the poor could not be overlooked, and as Kay himself points out it was the high inci-

[37] J. P. Kay, *The Moral and Physical Condition of the Working Classes Employed in the Cotton Manufacture in Manchester,* London, James Ridgway, 1832, p. 1.

[38] Cecil Driver: *Tory Radical. The Life of Richard Oastler,* New York, Oxford University Press, 1946, pp. 118-190.

[39] Kay, *op. cit.,* pp. 59-60.

[40] *Ibid.,* p. 47.

dence of communicable disease that led to an investigation of the Manchester workers. It was found that vice, physical degradation, poverty and illness were intimately interlocked. For proof of the relation of ill health to other forms of social pathology, Kay cites the records of the medical charities of Manchester. After reviewing the statistical data, he is led to conclude for example, that more than half the inhabitants of Manchester are "either so destitute or so degraded, as to require the assistance of public charity, in bringing their offspring into the world."[41] Yet Kay can see no necessary relation between existing socio-economic organization and the various kinds of social maladjustment that he had observed. It is indeed an instructive study in the situational determination of ideas to analyze Kay's presentation, for he remains an acute observer throughout. In fact, in one respect he is much in advance of his own time. Discussing the Irish immigration and the consequent effect on conditions in Manchester, he indicates an awareness, as yet unclear and lacking precise conceptual formulation, that the dismal scenes in his portrayal are the product of a cultural cataclysm.[42] Anthropologists have recently recognized that the change that affected a large part of white society in the early days of capitalism is similar to the changes among various African peoples under the influence of contact with white civilization.[43]

Other physicians did recognize, however, that social and economic institutions, especially industrialism, had significant and necessary connections with the health problems of the factory workers. Outstanding in this respect was C. Turner Thackrah, whose pioneer treatise on occupational medicine, *The Effects of Arts, Trades, and Professions . . . on Health and Longevity . . .*, first appeared in 1831. This book became a bible among the factory reformers, and Thackrah actively supported the struggle to restrict child labor.[44]

The employment of young children in *any* labour is wrong . . . [he said] No man of humanity can reflect without distress on the state of thousands

[41] *Ibid.*, pp. 40-42.

[42] *Ibid.*, pp. 6-7.

[43] R. C. Thurnwald: *Black and White in East Africa; The Fabric of a New Civilization*, 1935.

[44] The writer has in his possession a copy of the second edition (1832) of Thackrah's book with a presentation inscription by the author to Michael Thomas Sadler, parliamentary spokesman of factory reform.

of children, many from six to seven years of age, roused from their beds at an early hour, hurried to the mills, and kept there with the interval of only 40 minutes, till a late hour at night; kept, moreover, in an atmosphere impure, not only as the air of a town, not only as defective in ventilation, but as loaded also with noxious dust. Health! cleanliness! mental improvement! How are they regarded? Recreation is out of the question. There is scarcely time for meals. The very period of sleep, so necessary for the young, is too often abridged. Nay, children are sometimes worked even in the night.[45]

In 1831, at a meeting in Leeds in support of factory legislation, Thackrah was present on the platform with Richard Oastler and Michael Sadler. He made a forceful speech condemning the lack of regulation of working conditions, and citing the cases of some of his child patients in support of his position. Was it any wonder, he demanded, that the resistance to disease of the rising generation was being undermined by prevailing conditions? [46]

During the early 'thirties, however, the climate of opinion was still unfavorable to any basic change. Economic and religious doctrine encouraged acceptance of the status quo, and discouraged any attempts to change conditions. Economic success was evidence of divine favor, while failure implied the absence of religious sanctity, and was therefore indicative of moral inadequacy.[47] Any effort to alter existing conditions was consequently an impiety and dangerous to social welfare for it meant that one was interfering with the predestined law of God.

Peter Gaskell presented in 1833 a survey of the " manufacturing population of England " in which he showed how the introduction of steam power and the consequent industrial revolution had affected the workers and their families. He saw that the conditions under

[45] C. Turner Thackrah: *The Effects of Arts, Trades and Professions, and of Civic States and Habits of Living, on Health and Longevity*, Second Edition, Greatly Enlarged, London and Leeds, 1832, p. 80.

[46] Driver, *op. cit.*, pp. 135-136.

[47] For the background out of which these ideas developed and the process by which they came into being see Max Weber: *Gesammelte Aufsätze zur Religionssoziologie* (vol. I), Tübingen, 1922, pp. 17-206; Ernst Troeltsch: *Die Soziallehren der christlichen Kirchen und Gruppen,* in his *Gesammelte Schriften* (vol. I), Tübingen, 1923, pp. 710 ff.; R. H. Tawney: *Religion and the Rise of Capitalism,* New York, 1926; Erich Fromm: *Escape from Freedom*, New York, 1941.

which the factory hands lived and worked affected their health. "Life," he concluded, "though not necessarily shortened by manufacturing occupation, is stripped of a most material portion of that which can alone render it delightful—the possession of health, and those who are engaged in it may be said to live a protracted life in death."[48] Nevertheless, he points out that "the health and physical condition of the manufacturing population have their origin, and are dependent in a great degree upon the perversion of their moral and social habits." Therefore the first step "to be made is to improve the moral condition of the labouring population—without this nothing can avail it."[49] Furthermore, in discussing child labor he says:

> The employment of children in manufactories ought not to be looked upon as an evil, till the present moral and domestic habits of the population are completely re-organised. . . . There can be no question but that very considerable practical difficulties lie in the way of any extensive change as to the hours of labour. . . . It is doubtful if any legislative interference can be effective; but on the other hand, whether it may not most materially injure the future prospects of the labourers, and accelerate a fate already too rapidly approaching them. Still some modifications might be made to satisfy the claims of nature and humanity, contradistinguishing these from fanaticism and bigoted ignorance.[50]

As the decade of the 'thirties passed, however, and the decade of the 'forties came to occupy the scene, a gradual but definite shift in thought on the social aspects of health and disease became evident. The reports to the Poor Law Commission culminating in 1842 in Chadwick's classic *Inquiry into the Sanitary Condition of the Labouring Population of Great Britain*, and in 1844 in the report of the Health of Towns Commission provided a factual base for this ideological maneuver. Indicative of the change are the comments of Arthur Helps in 1845. "However true it may be," he wrote, "that moral remedies are the most wanted, we must not forget that such remedies can only be worked out by living men"; and while "a

[48] P. Gaskell: *The manufacturing Population of England, its Moral, Social and Physical Conditions, and the changes which have arisen from the use of Steam Machinery. . . .* London, Baldwin and Cradock, 1833, p. 239.

[49] *Ibid.*, pp. 215-216.

[50] *Ibid.*, pp. 209-210.

primâ facie reluctance to all interference is most reasonable . . . , nevertheless, interference must often be resorted to " in the interests of social improvement.[51]

Recognition of the causal relations existing between social problems and medical conditions went hand in hand with programs for remedial action. Most of this activity was empirical, and hardly any effort was made to develop a theoretical foundation for such programs. On this account alone considerable credit would be due to Henry W. Rumsey for his attempt to formulate a theory of public health and medical care within the framework of social organization and social action. Yet Rumsey deserves still higher praise; not only did he undertake to formulate a social policy for medicine, but he clearly visualized and set up goals which still remain unattained. In 1856, he published a volume entitled *Essays on State Medicine,* in which among other subjects he dealt with the provision of medical care to the poor. Rumsey's position is characterized by his statement that

> upon the right ordering of a State Provision for the medical care of the poorer classes in their own dwellings, depends the stability and efficiency of the whole superstructure of Medical Police.
>
> And I say *Care* of the poor, because it is now pretty generally acknowledged that any such provision, to be permanently useful, must not be limited to mere routine attendance on cases of actual illness and accident, to a perfunctory supply of pills and potions, with a bald return of names, diseases, visits, etc., from uneasy officers to incompetent Boards.[52]

He went on to show that the promotion of health and the prevention of disease were matters of social concern and required governmental action.

> Sanative care, as well as instruction [he contended] are beyond the means of half the population. Both are imperatively necessary for the safety of the Commonwealth—for the health and happiness of the people. Both may be bestowed gratuitously, from a right source, without causing pauperism. Nay,

[51] [Arthur Helps]: *The Claims of Labour. An Essay on the Duties of the Employers to the Employed. The Second Edition. To which is added, an Essay on the Means of Improving the Health and Increasing the Comfort of the Labouring Classes*, London, William Pickering, 1845, pp. 195, 245.

[52] Henry W. Rumsey: *Essays on State Medicine*, London, John Churchill, 1856, p. 239.

5

they are the best means of preventing it, by promoting health and longevity, and by enabling the sick and the ignorant to work usefully and profitably. Both therefore should be brought home to every working man's family; and both need to be directed and administered by specially qualified authorities.[53]

Finally, Rumsey described the medical personnel whom he visualized as carrying on such a program. The functions of a " district medical officer " should be preventive in nature. In detail, his description of the duties of such an officer comprises much of the modern public health program. Rumsey insisted that the health officer would become

the sanitary adviser of the poor in their dwellings. Many removable causes of sickness within their own control would be pointed out during his beneficent visits. The miserable effects of alcoholic stimulation might be impressed on the minds of sufferers from intemperance, at times when no warnings or counsel save those of a medical visitor would be listened to.

The state of the apartments of the poor, their clothing and bedding, the choice and preparation of their food, the physical management of their children, their nursing in sickness,—would all come occasionally under his cognizance. He would often be the first to detect unwholesome occupations or trades in the neighborhoods by their effects on those under his charge. In the execution of his ordinary duties, he might often be led to suspect the adulteration or impurity or decay of some article of food, or the deleterious qualities of some pretended medicine or falsified drug taken by the poor. . . . [In short], he would be, in a peculiar sense, the Missionary of Health in his own parish or district—instructing the working classes in personal and domestic hygiene—and practically proving to the helpless and the debased, the disheartened and disaffected, that the State cares for them,—a fact, of which, until of late, they have seen but little evidence.[54]

At the time when Rumsey expressed these views the health officer was still a novelty. The first Medical Officer of Health in England was Dr. W. H. Duncan, who in 1847 was appointed to this office at Liverpool. In 1848, the Corporation of the City of London appointed John Simon to a similar post.[55] Chadwick had suggested in 1842 that a " district Medical Officer " should be appointed locally, and the Public Health Act of 1848 contained power for the appoint-

[53] *Ibid.*, p. 248.

[54] *Ibid.*, pp. 280-282.

[55] John Simon: *English Sanitary Institutions*, London, John Murray, 1897, pp. 246-248.

ment of medical officers of health in England, with the exception of London. In 1855, the Metropolis Management Act provided for the appointment of such officers in London (outside the City).[56]

The appointment of health officers for various London districts, as well as for many provincial towns, and the fact that the subject of public health had attracted considerable attention led the authorities of St. Thomas's Hospital in 1856 to establish a course of lectures on public health, the first of its kind in England.[57] Dr. Edward Headlam Greenhow was appointed to this lectureship. In preparing his first course of lectures, he realized that a good deal of the information upon which the health agitation of the preceding twenty years had been based was vague and inadequate. When he wanted to consider the preventable causes of disease, Greenhow found that statistical information on this score was defective. He determined to supply this deficiency and worked on his project for about a year. At the request of John Simon, this study appeared in 1858 as a parliamentary report of the General Board of Health.[58]

In his conclusion, Greenhow pointed out that the causes which produce the prevalent diseases of unhealthy places

> are multifarious; and that, whilst an impure atmosphere, whether the impurity arise from the defective removal of refuse and excrete matters, from the overcrowding of dwellings, or from manufacturing processes, is among the most powerful, there are many other causes of disease to which attention has hitherto been too little directed. Insufficient or unsuitable food, sedentary habits, the absence of the physical and mental stimulus afforded by variety of scene, and especially by rural prospects, the weariness caused by the monotonous character or many occupations, and, not least, the cares and anxieties of life are all of them causes which help to swell the catalogue of

---

[56] George Newman: *The Building of a Nation's Health*, London, Macmillan and Co., Ltd., 1939, p. 15.

[57] John Simon relates that the "arrangements at St. Thomas's Hospital were in adoption of proposals which I, as member of the School, had made there" (*English Sanitary Institutions*, p. 266 footnote).

[58] General Board of Health. *Papers Relating to the Sanitary State of the People of England: Being the Results of an Inquiry into the different Proportions of Death produced by certain Diseases in different Districts in England; communicated to the General Board of Health by Edward Headlam Greenhow, M.D. . . . with An Introductory Report by the Medical Officer of the Board, on the Preventability of certain Kinds of Premature Death*, London, Eyre and Spottiswoode, 1858.

illness, and to add to the register of deaths in great cities. Some of these causes of preventable sickness and premature death arise necessarily from the circumstances of our social system, and are but little, if at all, under the control of the executive government. Notwithstanding their exclusion from the catalogue of removable causes of unhealthfulness, there would yet remain ample scope for the employment of hygienic measures. . . . One of the most evident facts brought to light by the present investigation is the influence of occupation on health. This influence is either direct . . . ; or it is indirect, as where the employment of women in factories seems to aggravate the infantile mortality, and particularly that produced by the nervous diseases of childhood. It is probable that a careful examination into the nature of these employments, and the manner in which their hurtful results are produced, would show that such results are not the inevitable consequences of the several industrial occupations. . . .

It may be more difficult to deal with the other branch of this question. The withdrawal of children from their mother's care, and the consequent substitution of artificial feeding for the natural diet of infancy, which is probably one at least among the causes of a large infantile mortality in places where the female population are largely engaged in factory labor, is possibly an evil inherent in the modern factory system. Whether it can be met without an undue interference with the rights of labour is a question the consideration of which forms no part of my present duty.[59]

In his introduction to Greenhow's report, John Simon concurred in the findings of his colleague and went on to emphasize the necessity for considering,

whether the advantages of our social progress must have with them such evils as I have described; whether the higher civilization of urban life cannot be attained without a corresponding development of diseases, which depend on the non-removal of excrement, and the non-ventilation of dwellings; whether the manufacturing greatness of England be not compatible with better sanitary care for the lives of the employed, and with less enormous entail of infantine [sic] disease. . . .

Nor probably will such questions appear unimportant to the public economist. For the physical strength of a nation is no mean part of its prosperity. And with us, perhaps, that raw material may have risen in value, while eastern war and westward emigration have been draining into their respective channels so much of our English manhood.

But if the subject may justly claim to be considered by the government and the legislature of this country, it is on higher grounds than those. The sacredness of human life against unjust aggression is the principle above all others

---

[59] *Ibid.*, pp. 131-133.

by which society subsists. To have realized this principle in law and government is the first indication of a social state. . . .[60]

This document showed the necessity of constituting some machinery by which the British government might institute methodical inquiries wherever there appeared to be an excess of disease. That this argument was accepted by Parliament may be inferred from the Public Health Act of 1858, which authorized the Privy Council to institute from time to time such inquiries concerning matters of the public health as they might see fit. John Simon became Medical Officer to the Privy Council and undertook various studies on its behalf. During the period 1862-1865, Simon was particularly concerned with the investigation of "*food-supply,* of *house accommodation* and the *physical surroundings,* and of *industrial circumstances.* . . ."[61]

In the Sixth Report to the Privy Council (1863), Simon presented the results of an inquiry into the dietaries of the poor carried out by Dr. Edward Smith. Malnutrition was prevalent, Simon reported, and

from such degrees of it as Dr. Smith found existing among the lowest fed of the examined classes, there must, I feel assured, be much direct causation of ill-health, and the associated causes of disease must be greatly strengthened by it in their hurtfulness. These are painful reflections, especially when it is remembered that the poverty to which they advert is not the deserved poverty of idleness. In all cases it is the poverty of working populations. Indeed, as regards the in-door operatives, the work which obtains the scanty pittance of food is for the most part excessively prolonged. Yet evidently, it is only in a qualified sense that the work can be deemed self-supporting. All disease of such populations, and whatever destitution results from it, must be treated at public expense. . . .

How far (if at all) the described circumstances of our poorest labouring population tend to better themselves, and how far (if at all) they may be bettered by interference from without, are questions which cannot be discussed without reference to parts of political economy on which I am incompetent to speak. Indirectly, indeed, those questions are of the vastest sanitary importance, for the "public health" of a country means the health of its masses, and the masses can scarcely be healthy unless, to their very base, they be at least moderately prosperous. And although the satisfactory solu-

[60] *Ibid.*, pp. xlvi-xlvii.
[61] Simon, *op. cit.*, p. 293.

tion of those questions is a task for other sciences than the science of medicine to fulfil, yet assuredly, if that solution can be given, the ultimate result will be among the foremost gains which a department of public health can have to record.[62]

Clearly, by the decade of the 'sixties, considerable advance had been made in Britain toward a socially oriented view of health and disease. Although this position was not as sharply defined as the German idea of medicine as a social science, various medical writers and administrators had recognized that social and economic conditions were intimately related to the greater or lesser prevalence of disease, and that these relations should be made the subject of exact scientific investigation, utilizing in considerable measure statistical materials and methods. Somewhat slower to develop was an overt recognition that the health of the people was a matter of direct social concern, and that social as well as medical measures were necessary for the prevention of disease and the promotion of health. Economic liberalism was evidently still the dominant social philosophy, but in practice it was gradually being recognized as ultimately untenable for an industrial society. For example, the establishment of a system of free medical advice to all the wage-earners in England and Wales was seriously under consideration in 1870 by the Poor Law Board. "The economical and social advantages of free medicine to the poorer classes generally," said a member of the board, "as distinguished from actual paupers, and perfect accessibility to medical advice at all times under thorough organization, may be considered as so important in themselves as to render it necessary to weigh with the greatest care all the reasons which may be adduced in their favour." [63] It was in the decade of the 'eighties however, that the interplay of long term trends and particular events came to focus in a new formulation of social problems and values.[64] Out of this rephrasing of social goals and ideologies there would in time develop a theory of social medicine.

[62] John Simon: *Public Health Reports* (2 vols.), London, J. and A. Churchill, 1887, vol. II, pp. 97-98.

[63] Sidney and Beatrice Webb: *The State and the Doctor*, London, Longmans, Green and Co., 1910, p. 7.

[64] Helen Merrell Lynd: *England in the Eighteen-Eighties*, New York, Oxford University Press, 1945, pp. 3-19 and 61-112.

But while British developments were still in the future, a Belgian doctor had already presented a well-developed system of social medicine. This was the achievement of Dr. Meynne, an army doctor, whose book, *Topographie Médicale de la Belgique*, appeared in 1865. (It is interesting to note that while on the titlepage, the subtitle read: *Études de géologie, de climatologie, de statistique et d'hygiène publique*, on the wrapper this is covered by a superimposed square of paper bearing the subtitle: *Études d'hygiène publique et médecine sociale, de statistique, de climatologie et de géologie médicales.*)

Under the influence of the Industrial Revolution in England, and the urgent necessities of the Napoleonic Imperium, Belgium had early achieved a high degree of industrialization. As Clapham remarks, Belgium was the one country in Europe "which kept pace industrially with England, in the first half of the nineteenth century."[65] But as in England, industrialization was followed by grave social problems, not the least of which was wide prevalence of disease, especially in the industrial population. Studies and inquiries into the social, economic and medical status of the Belgian people had been carried out at various times during the thirty years preceding the publication of Meynne's work. As a result he had at his disposal a considerable mass of data, and this is reflected in the scope and comprehensive character of his *Topographie Médicale*.

Meynne originally undertook this treatise to provide a medical topography (or in other words, a local medical geography) of Belgium.[66] But the book can only partly be called a medical topography, for Meynne went beyond a study of the distribution of prevalent diseases in relation to causative factors. In the last analysis, he presented a treatise on the social pathology and social hygiene of Belgium. Deeply imbued with the basic importance of preventive medicine Meynne wrote:

> Curative medicine, which saves from death one person who is seriously ill here, and another elsewhere, undoubtedly accomplishes a meritorious task, but hygiene, which prevents thousands of cases of illness will always be

---

[65] Quoted in Knight, M. M., Barnes, H. E., and Flugel, F.: *Economic History of Europe in Modern Times*, Boston, Houghton Mifflin Company, 1928, p. 674.

[66] Meynne: *Topographie Médicale de la Belgique*, Bruxelles, H. Manceaux, 1865, pp. i-iii. For a discussion of medical topography and medical geography see Arne Barkhuus: Medical Geographies, *Ciba Symposia*, 6: 1997-2016, 1944-45.

superior to the former in terms of the social results achieved. The latter is medicine on a grand scale, medicine applied to the nations. . . .

Hygiene, which is based on a knowledge of morbid causes, will one day constitute the basis of all social science, because the public health will always be the primary wealth of a people, and because the national economy would soon find itself in a position of inferiority in relation to foreign countries if the physical strength of the working classes is going to be seriously affected. Hygiene will one day become the guide of the administrator, as well as of the legislator; and political economy instead of devoting itself too exclusively to investigation of national wealth will then take the sanitary status of populations as the point of departure for its doctrines.[67]

The *Topographie Médicale* is divided into four parts. The first deals with the geography, geology and climatology of Belgium; the second with the morbidity and mortality of the Belgian population, including a discussion of the causes of the most prevalent or most serious diseases; the third with the relations of the diseases to soil, climate, poverty, nutrition, housing, and alcoholism; and finally, the fourth section is concerned with a discussion of various preventive measures designed to alleviate or remove the conditions previously described. Meynne makes full use of statistical materials; for he recognized that statistics provided a formidable instrument for the study of the problems in which he was interested.

As a result of his studies, Meynne concluded that poverty was the most potent disease breeder of all, surpassing by far other alleged causes such as soil, climate, and contagion.

As a cause of the majority of serious diseases [he said] poverty surpasses all other influences, even those of soil and climate. In general, it may be said that *deaths and the diseases that lead to degeneration of the species are to be found in diverse social strata in proportion to the degree of poverty that they experience.*

We arrived at this remarkable contrast between the well-to-do classes and the laboring classes without any preconceived idea. In each chapter the results of statistics and of observation became more striking, the problem became clearer and more precise. At the end we found ourselves face to face with an important social fact: the excessive inferiority which afflicts the sanitary and physical state of the proletarian classes. Their life is very much shorter; they age prematurely; their progeny is less viable; they have twice as much chance of being attacked by tuberculosis and dyscrasic dis-

[67] Meynne, *op. cit.*, pp. iii-iv.

eases; they are much more exposed to all epidemic diseases; and they are almost alone subject to accidents and violent death. Let us note also that poverty is the primary cause in most cases of their ignorance, their lack of orderliness, and even of their debauchery and intemperance. In short, one may say that physical and moral decadence attacks fatally a large number of those who have the misfortune to be born in poverty.[68]

But, he went on, having studied the causes of disease it was now necessary to call attention to the means of preventing or controlling the majority of serious diseases. However, for one who thinks in terms of *prevention*,

the horizon expands far beyond the domain of medical prescriptions. In fact, it becomes a matter of nothing less than the suppression of prejudice, error and ignorance, the encouragement of salutary labor, the development of a sense of dignity on the one hand and the conquest of cupidity, and injustice on the other. For this immense program, it is necessary to have the collaboration of all men of good will, and above all the assistance and unified direction of the state and of the scientists.

Since we believe that the doctor is by right a member of this great scientific council, we have, as the conclusion of this study, boldly advanced our opinion regarding the most urgent capital reforms and economic remedies—at the risk of seeing some one object on the ground of our incompetence. . . . Certainly, no one can pretend to know everything, but we refuse to acknowledge the scholastic limits of each special science. All the sciences are sisters; they ought to join hands so that one day they will form a whole: the great social science.[69]

Meynne was convinced that the future belonged to public health, or, as he also termed it, preventive medicine. His conception of the field was impressively broad. It was to concern itself with the sanitation of soil and water; the hygiene of unhealthy and dangerous industries; the location, construction and operation of hospitals, prisons, schools and barracks; the supervision of food to prevent fraud and adulteration; child guidance and education; vocational guidance; premarital and family counselling—in short, it would come to play a part in education, public administration and political economy. In part, this far-sighted program has been realized in our time, but much still remains to be done.

More specifically, Meynne proposed that attention be given to

[68] *Ibid.*, pp. viii-ix.

[69] *Ibid.*, p. xii.

rendering the worker more independent, and to protecting him from exploitation. He advocated higher wages, better housing, better nutrition, and amelioration of various social evils such as alcoholism. Recognizing the outstanding importance of nutrition, he proposed that special retail outlets for workers be set up where they could purchase food at cost price. Such establishments could likewise sell clothes and household furnishings. Meynne also asked for limitation of the working day, the raising of the age for apprenticeship, and improved working conditions in factories and shops with particular regard to occupational hygiene.[70] Note should also be taken of his proposal to set up a system of rural hospitals to serve the agricultural population. This idea was not new, for the problem of providing medical care and hospital service in rural areas had received considerable attention in France and Beligum.[71] What is new is the inclusion of this question in a system of social medicine. Finally, attention must be called to chapter VI of Meynne's treatise. Here he takes up the diseases of greatest importance, analyzes each in terms of its causation, and calls attention to the social factors involved. Among the diseases considered are pulmonary phthisis, scrophula, pneumonia, bronchitis, emphysema and asthma, cardiac diseases, rheumatism, arthritis, gout, neuralgia, gastro-intestinal maladies, typhoid fever, dysentery, scurvy, anthrax, cancer, smallpox, scarlatina, mental disease, epilepsy, chorea, deaf-mutism and epidemic diseases (cholera, typhus fever, diphtheria, whooping cough). This section is unique, for not until Grotjahn's *Soziale Pathologie* do we again find this kind of analysis.[72]

During the latter half of the nineteenth century, the idea of social medicine was kept alive in Germany and in some cases developed further by a few far-seeing and socially-minded men. In some instances their ideas were derived from the thought of 1848. The leaders of 1848, Virchow and Neumann, remained active in politics and loyal to their principles. Virchow was called back to Berlin in

[70] *Ibid.*, pp. 519-547.

[71] See the articles "Hygiène Rurale" and "Médecins Cantonaux" in *Dictionnaire d'Hygiène Publique* . . . edited by Ambroise Tardieu, Paris, J.-B. Baillière, 1854 (II), pp. 216; 465.

[72] Meynne, *op. cit.*, pp. 123-235.

1856, and in 1861 he became a member of the Berlin municipal council. In 1862 he was elected to the Prussian Landtag, and from 1880 to 1893 he served as a member of the Reichstag. Throughout this period, Virchow remained firm in the conviction that matters of health and disease were social as well as medical questions. In 1860, at the meeting of the German scientists and physicians, Virchow forcefully urged the need for combating and preventing the effects of illness and infirmity.

When statistics show [he asserted], that in some localities one-third of all deaths is due to pulmonary diseases, and when phthisis in the narrower sense of the term produces 15 to 18 percent, and even more, of the deaths, it shows that disturbances exist in the development of our populations, disturbances which arise from political and social institutions, and are therefore preventable.[73]

Neumann likewise continued to study disease from a social viewpoint. Many of his investigations were statistical in nature. Between 1856 and 1866, he carried out and published three studies on morbidity and mortality in the laboring population of Berlin. When the Gesellschaft für soziale Medizin, Hygiene und Medizinalstatistik was organized at Berlin in 1905, Neumann was elected an honorary member; and at the time of his death in 1908, Alfred Grotjahn had already developed his concept of social hygiene.

During the three decades that followed 1848, the program of medical reform was transformed into a more limited program of sanitary reform, which was practically attainable. Nevertheless, the causal relationships between general social conditions and the health of individuals could not be overlooked. In 1867, Lorenz von Stein, jurist and administrator, in a treatise on public administration dealt with the administrative aspects of public health.[74] Stein pointed out that the health of individuals becomes a matter of public concern to the extent that individuals are subjected to noxious conditions over which they have no control, and to the extent that such persons become a burden on society. In these circumstances, he insisted, it is the duty of government to establish and to maintain conditions

[73] Karl Sudhoff: *Rudolf Virchow und die Deutsche Naturforscherversammlungen*, Leipzig, Akademische Verlagsgesellschaft, 1922, p. 14.

[74] For Stein see above, p. 677 and footnote 7.

that would protect the individual from any dangers arising out of social activity, and to re-establish and to promote in a positive manner the health of the affected individual.[75] Stein was considerably influenced by English health legislation, and cited the English experience in support of his thesis.

Contemporary with von Stein were a number of medical men who in varying degree recognized the importance of the influence of social conditions on health, and discussed this subject from varying points of view. One of the most interesting of these, and yet one of the least known is Eduard Reich (1836-1919), an eccentric and peripatetic medical scholar. He lived and taught in Jena, Göttingen, Bern, Strassburg, Gotha, Kiel, Würzburg, Erlangen, Koburg, and Sondershausen. In the course of his wanderings, Reich found the time to write a large number of books, the last of which appeared in 1910.[76] Most important of these is his *System der Hygieine* which appeared in 1870-71 in two volumes. In this treatise Reich offers a well-rounded presentation of what he conceived to be the field of hygiene. This work is the product of far-ranging scholarship and profound erudition. The wide reading upon which it is based may be inferred from some of the authors cited by Reich. Among these are Brillat-Savarin, P. J. G. Cabanis, Henry C. Carey, Girolamo Cardano, August Hirsch, Liebig, Paola Mantegazza, Malthus, Moleschott, Quetelet, the *Regimen Salernitanum*, Ramazzini, the economist J. B. Say, Virchow, Villermé, and J. G. Zimmermann.

The organization of Reich's *System* proceeds from his definition of hygiene. To the question " What is hygiene? " he said:

> I understand hygiene to be the totality of those principles, the application of which is intended to maintain individual and social health and morality, to destroy the causes of disease, and to ennoble man physically and morally. The concept of hygiene thus comprises far more than was formerly comprehended under dietetics and medical police. Hygiene deals with man as a whole, as an individual and as he manifests himself in the family and in

[75] Lorenz von Stein: *Die Verwaltungslehre*, III. Teil. Erstes Hauptgebiet. II. Teil, Stuttgart, J. G. Cotta, 1867, pp. 1 ff. See also Kroeger, *op. cit.*, pp. 18-19 (footnote 26 above).

[76] Alfons Fischer: *Geschichte des deutschen Gesundheitswesens*, Bd. II, Berlin, Kommissionsverlag F. A. Herbig, 1933, pp. 362-365.

society; it deals with man in all his conditions and relations. Consequently, hygiene comprises the entire physical and moral world, and collaborates with all the sciences whose subject is the study of man and his environment.[77]

Hygiene, or the theory of health and welfare, is the philosophy, science and art of healthy living for the individual, the family, society and the state. Its stream derives from three tributaries: the first arises from practical philosophy, the second from medicine, and the third from social science. Moral hygiene is an application of practical philosophy, social hygiene an application of social science, and dietetic (as well as climatic) and police hygiene are applied medicine.[78]

On this basis, Reich set up four branches of hygiene: moral hygiene, social hygiene, dietetic hygiene, and police hygiene. Within these categories, he undertook to explore human experience, both personal and social, as it bore on health. What Reich regarded as falling under each of these headings is evident from the table of contents of the *System*. It contains the following subjects:

1. *Moral Hygiene*
   - Moral acts
   - The passions
   - Intellectual life
   - Education
   - Religion and morality
2. *Social Hygiene*
   - Introduction
   - Population
   - Marriage
   - Labor and poverty
     - Labor
     - Poverty
     - Sources of poverty
     - Effects of poverty
     - Forms of poverty
     - Charity
     - Cooperative action
     - Conclusion
3. *Dietetic Hygiene*
   - Nutrition
   - Care of the Skin
     - Clothing
     - Cleanliness
     - Cosmetics
   - Gymnastics
   - Travel
   - The senses. Sleep. Reproduction
   - Habitation
   - Climate
4. *Police Hygiene*
   - The health office
   - The health law
   - Health control of food and stimulants
   - Health control of dwellings
   - Control of epidemics

From this outline it appears that while Reich's categories are not entirely congruent with those in use at present, his police hygiene

[77] Eduard Reich: *System der Hygieine* (2 vols. in one), Leipzig, Friedrich Fleischer Verlag, 1870-71, vol. I, p. xvi.

[78] *Ibid.*, p. xii.

may be regarded as equivalent to public health administration, dietetic hygiene as coinciding with personal hygiene, social hygiene as representing an early form of social medicine and social work, and moral hygiene as a combination of social psychology, sociology and health education. Of the greatest interest here is Reich's concept of social hygiene.

> Social hygiene [he asserted], is concerned with the welfare of society. On the basis of statistics it follows the phenomena of social life, surveys the population in its various states, observes marriage, studies labor, and descends into the slough of despond which is poverty, but not to bring some empty consolation, but rather to help and to save, to strengthen the weary and to awaken them to new life, and to support by means of charity those who cannot care for themselves.[79]
>
> It is the task of social hygiene to prevent diseases of society and to maintain the well-being of the civil community. In order to achieve this aim, social hygiene must examine critically the manifestations of social life, trace its currents to their source, and there undertake its regulatory and ameliorative work.
>
> There are two things which influence social life most powerfully, and give it a characteristic stamp and color. We refer to the total constitution of the individual, and to the property relationship. These two elements interact reciprocally. . . .
>
> Because social life depends, on the one hand, on the physical and moral constitution of individuals, and, on the other, on property, the measures taken by social hygiene can be effective only if they aim to improve the constitution, and at the same time make possible a natural development of the property relationship. Above all else social hygiene must wipe out poverty, for as long as this exists there can be no question either of improving the constitution, or of a normal development of economic relations. . . .[80]

To achieve his goal, Reich advocated self-help and cooperative action, measures which were widely advocated at the time, and which seem to be a reflection in some degree of Proudhonist social philosophy. In addition, he was an ardent advocate of health education for all age groups and social classes.

The ideas of Eduard Reich remained almost unknown, but similar views were expressed by his better-known contemporary, Max von Pettenkofer, and reached a wide audience.[81] On March 26 and 29,

[79] *Ibid.*, p. xxii.

[80] *Ibid.*, p. 267.

[81] Pettenkofer is too well known to require an account of his life in this paper. For those readers who wish to consult biographical details, see E. E. Hume: *Max*

1873, Pettenkofer addressed the *Verein für Volksbildung* in Munich on the value of health to a city. The purpose of these lectures was to urge the need for thoroughgoing sanitary reform in order to improve health conditions in the city. It was Pettenkofer who made hygiene and experimental laboratory science, but he was fully aware that man's health is influenced not only by his physical environment but also by the social world in which he lives. After calling the attention of his audience to the need for sanitary reform, he warned his listeners not to expect a panacea. Health was a resultant of the combined action of a number of factors, and all of these would have to be taken into account.

> At present [he said], it has become the fashion to think that the health conditions of a city are determined exclusively by good sewerage, abundant water supply and good toilets, and particularly by the introduction of water-closets. . . . [In applying these measures] we solve not even one-third of our problems, as foreign experience has shown. And so we must look around for other factors, in many other directions.
>
> Our health is also determined, to a large extent, by nutrition; not only by the quality of food but also by its quantity. What we consume may not only be good or bad, but also too much or too little. . . .[82]
>
> It is, therefore, necessary that we apply ourselves to this task which is becoming more urgent every day, since the prices of all foodstuffs are rising continuously. So long as man finds himself in circumstances that permit him to have all the food he wishes, and to select it freely, he usually finds instinctively what is good for him; but when he has to contend with poverty or when the food he receives depends on the will of another, then we need standards in order to know what kind of food is necessary and what the minimum quantity is. . . .[83]
>
> Housing conditions are also extremely important. Housing exerts a great influence on our health in two ways, in that it must, first, allow us to get the fresh air we need, and, second, protect us against heat and cold. . . .
>
> Customs and habits exert no small amount of influence on general health conditions. . . . Customs and habits include in my opinion, the amount that an individual generally spends from his earnings or income for food, drink, housing, clothing and other items, and also for luxuries. . . .

---

von Pettenkofer, New York, Paul B. Hoeber, 1927; H. E. Sigerist: *Grosse Aerzte*, München, J. F. Lehmanns Verlag, 1932, pp. 288-292.

[82] Max von Pettenkofer: "The Value of Health to a City, Two Lectures, Delivered in 1873," Translated from the German, with an Introduction by Henry E. Sigerist, *Bull. Hist. Med.* 10: 597; 602, 1941.

[83] *Ibid.*, p. 604.

Political and social conditions are also influential upon the health and mortality of a population. All over the world the rich generally enjoy better health and live longer than the poor. Every epidemic, whether intermittent fever, typhoid or cholera, takes a larger toll from the poorer classes, sometimes and in many places to such an extent, that particularly cholera was a few years ago still called a disease of the proletariat. The poor, of course, do not suffer more from disease than the rich because they have less cash in their pockets but only insofar as they are deprived of the necessities of life. . . .[84]

Pettenkofer went on to point out that the public health is a matter of community concern, and that any measures that may be taken to help those in need react to the benefit of all.

In every large community [he said], there are always many people who have not the means to procure for themselves the things that are absolutely necessary to a healthy life. Those who have more than they need must contribute to supply these wants in their own interest. . . . Whenever causes of disease cannot be removed or kept away from the individual, the citizens must stand together and accept taxation according to their ability. When a city provides good sewerage, good water supplies, good and clean streets, good institutions for food control, slaughter houses and other indispensable and vital necessities, it creates institutions from which all benefit, both rich and poor. The rich have to pay the bill and the poor cannot contribute anything; yet the rich draw considerable advantages from the fact that such institutions benefit the poor also. A city must consider itself a family, so to say. Care must be taken of everybody in the house, also of those who do not or cannot contribute toward its support.[85]

In view of this standpoint, it is not at all surprising to find Pettenkofer, in 1882, employing the term social medicine for hygiene.[86]

The significant influence that social institutions and conditions exert upon health was also pointed out by Nikolaus Alois Geigel (1829-1887). As a student, he had participated in the movement of 1848, and its ideology left a permanent impression on his thinking. In 1870, Geigel became professor of hygiene at Würzburg, and in 1874 published a monograph on public health in Pettenkofer's *Handbuch der öffentlichen Gesundheitspflege und der Gewerbekrankheiten.* The introduction to this monograph discussed the relation

[84] *Ibid.*, pp. 605, 607-608.
[85] *Ibid.*, p. 609.
[86] Hynek Pelc: La Médecine sociale et son développement en Tchécoslovaquie, *Bruxelles médical* (No. 26), April 26, 1936.

of changing social and economic conditions to health and disease. Geigel dealt with the effects of the rise of capitalism, the growth of an industrial proletariat, increasing urbanisation and the unhygienic conditions under which workers were compelled to live, the dangerous materialism of the upper classes, and the influence exerted by the church, which he regarded as pernicious and reactionary. Like many of his predecessors and contemporaries, Geigel insisted on the need for accurate statistics that would throw light on social phenomena. Thus, he felt that fluctuations of food prices, or an increase or decrease in the consumption of agricultural and industrial products could be just as important (in fact even decisive) for the prevalence of disease as climatic changes, an increase or decrease in the size of the proletariat, or of the national wealth.

These ideas were not without influence. When the *Reichsgesundheitsamt* was set up in 1876, Dr. Struck, the first director of the organization, issued a programmatic memoir in which he set forth its objectives.[87] In this program medical statistics were given an exceedingly prominent position.

> The relations of people to each other [wrote Struck], the conditions under which they are born, develop, and work, their age, environment, their territorial distribution, the soil on which they live, the water that they drink, their economic status, their nutrition and so forth, all these shall be brought into relation with the diseases that occur among them, with the span of their lives and their mortality, in order to determine the causes which lead to illness and premature death.

The significance of such information was not lost on the leaders of the industrial workers. Commenting on Struck's program, August Bebel, the Social Democratic leader, said of this passage:

> Should such statistics show, for instance, that the housing, places of work, and nutrition of large groups of the population are absolutely inadequate, it follows necessarily that steps must be taken to improve them. The discussion of social questions is thus placed in the foreground, and based on official figures and conclusions that cannot be denied, the demands and practical proposals for changing conditions will attain an irresistible power, because

---

[87] *Denkschrift über die Aufgaben und Ziele, die sich das Kaiserliche Gesundheitsamt gestellt hat,* verfasst von Struck, Berlin 1878, cited by Fischer, *op. cit.*, (II), p. 307.

6

thousands and hundreds of thousands of people from all classes of the population will support them.[88]

The relation of health and hygiene to economics was pointed out in the same year by Heinrich Rohlfs, in an article advocating that Germany adopt an economic policy based on the national protectionism of Friedrich List. In the course of his discussion, Rohlfs quoted with approval Pettenkofer's remarks of 1875 that he conceived of " hygiene as the economics of health, just as economic science regards the production and distribution of goods. Just as it is not simply the fear of loss, but even more the striving for great gain which is the driving force in economic science, so this must also become the point of view of hygiene as the science of health. It is for hygiene to investigate and to evaluate all the influences in the natural and artificial environment of the organism, so as to be able by means of this knowledge to increase its well-being." [89] Rohlfs also pointed out that the establishment of the Reichsgesundheitsamt was a great advance and would have a considerable influence on the development of hygiene.

Nevertheless, despite an awareness of the social relations of health and disease, the last three decades of the nineteenth century in Germany were characterized by a social and cultural environment which was unfavorable for the development of this awareness to a clearer concept which would admit of practical medical application. To most Germans after 1871, the movement of 1848 was something from a strange past. The national aspect of the movement was still recognized, but the social ideals had been abandoned. The German intellectuals and the middle class accepted the policy of Bismarck, and for the most part gave up their progressive program. At the same time the extraordinary rapidity with which the natural sciences developed gave them an enormous prestige in medicine. To this was added the appearance of bacteriology with what seemed to

[88] August Bebel: *Das Reichsgesundheitsamt und sein Programm vom socialistischen Standpunkt beleuchtet*, Berlin, Verlag der Allgemeinen deutschen Associations Buchdruckerei, 1878, p. 9.

[89] Heinrich Rohlfs: Ueber das Wechselverhältniss der Nationalökonomie zur Hygiene in seiner historischen Ausbildung, *Deutsches Archiv für Geschichte der Medicin und Medicinische Geographie* 1: 70-106, 1878 (see p. 85).

be the answer to the problem of disease causation. Under these conditions, it was not difficult to overlook the patient and his environment and to equate germs and disease in the relationship of cause and effect. Not the patient but the disease became the prime concern of the physician. This was the position so sharply expressed by Emil Behring in 1893.

Yet at the very peak of the bacteriological triumph, interest in the significance of social conditions in the causation of disease led various physicians to react against the exaggerated bacteriological standpoint. Hüppe summed up this point of view in 1899 with the statement: "Hygiene is a social art which has developed in response to social need; consequently it must and will always be social hygiene, or it will not exist at all."[90] Only a few years later Alfred Grotjahn put forth his concept of social hygiene, which initiated the theoretical development of social medicine during the first half of the twentieth century.

IV.

Alfred Grotjahn and After

At the very time when Behring was ardently proclaiming bacteriology as the ultimate medical truth and Koch as its prophet, a young German medical student in search of a subject for a doctoral dissertation conceived the idea of systematically investigating medical problems in the light of social science, so as "to arrive finally at a theory of social pathology and social hygiene, which with its own methods . . . would be used to investigate and to determine how life and health, particularly of the poorer classes, are dependent on social conditions and the environment."[91] The student was Alfred Grotjahn, and throughout his life he pursued this aim, as he later characterized it, with "paranoid stubbornness." As a result he developed a systematic theory of social medicine, and profoundly influenced the development of this field of medical activity.

[90] Hueppe: *Handbuch der Hygiene*, Berlin 1899, p. 11, cited by Alfons Fischer: *Grundriss der sozialen Hygiene*, Berlin, Julius Springer Verlag, 1913, p. 23.

[91] Alfred Grotjahn: *Erlebtes und Erstrebtes. Erinnerungen eines sozialistischen Arztes*, Berlin, Kommissions-Verlag F. A. Herbig G. M. b. H., 1932, p. 72.

Grotjahn's thinking was deeply affected by two currents of thought. While yet a medical student he became a member of the Social Democratic Party, and occupied himself with the literature of socialism and social problems. Later he rejected Marxian socialism, and took his stand on the basis of social reformism. A more lasting influence was exerted by the economist and historian Gustav Schmoller, whose seminar Grotjahn attended during the winter of 1901-1902. Here he learned the methodology of the social sciences, and applied this knowledge in the preparation of a paper for the seminar. This paper dealt with the changes in food consumption of workers that had occurred in Germany and other countries as a part of the process of industrialization. This study was published by Schmoller in 1902, but the views expressed by Grotjahn aroused the antagonism of Max Rubner, then professor of hygiene at the University of Berlin. Grotjahn warned against judging diets too exclusively on the basis of caloric adequacy, and Rubner who had become world famous for his studies on the caloric aspects of nutrition took umbrage at these heretical, non-experimental opinions. This was the beginning of an extended conflict which divided the world of German medicine and hygiene until after the First World War. Rubner was successful for a while in preventing Grotjahn from obtaining an academic post. In 1912, he received a minor position under Carl Flügge, and eventually in 1920 he was appointed to the first chair of social hygiene established at the University of Berlin (the full story is to be found in Grotjahn's absorbing autobiography, *Erlebtes und Erstrebtes*).

As early as 1898 Grotjahn had already published a study of alcoholism from the viewpoint of social hygiene.[92] In 1902 in collaboration with his friend F. Kriegel, Grotjahn began the publication of his annual review and bibliography of social hygiene, demography, and medical statistics.[93] The scope of the subject as envisaged by

[92] Alfred Grotjahn: *Der Alkoholismus nach Wesen, Wirkung und Verbreitung*, Leipzig, 1898.

[93] A. Grotjahn and F. Kriegel: *Jahresbericht über soziale Hygiene, Demographie und Medizinalstatistik, sowie alle Zweige des sozialen Versicherungswesen*, published by Gustav Fischer Verlag, Jena, from 1902 to 1915, and by Richard Schoetz Verlag, Berlin, from 1916 to 1923. In 1925 the bibliographical section was continued in the *Archiv für Soziale Hygiene und Demographie.*

Grotjahn at this time may be inferred from the subject headings of the bibliography: 1. Methodology and history of social hygiene; 2. Population statistics and mortality; 3. Morbidity, prophylaxis and medical care; 4. Social hygiene of labor; 5. Social hygiene of nutrition; 6. Social hygiene of housing and clothing; 7. Social hygiene of childhood, and youth; 8. Public health; 9. Theory of degeneration, constitutional pathology, and sex hygiene.

On March 1, 1904, Grotjahn presented before the German Society for Public Health a paper on the nature and purpose of social hygiene.[94] In it he sketched the scope of social hygiene, gave a preliminary definition of the subject, and indicated the lines of probable future development. At the very outset, Grotjahn indicated that he preferred not to use the term social medicine, which he regarded as being too limited in its connotation. Since the establishment of the sickness insurance system by Bismarck in 1883, it had been used to refer to insurance medicine, and Grotjahn felt that it would lead to confusion if this term were applied to the broader field that he envisaged.

Up to that time, he pointed out, hygiene both in theory and practice had occupied itself with the noxious natural factors that threaten the human organism and with the means of combating and controlling these factors. This was essentially physical-biological hygiene. In applying the results of physics, chemistry and biology, it related man to his natural environment. But, Grotjahn insisted, as a science, hygiene cannot restrict itself to this aspect. Man has yet another dimension; he is a social being, and this cannot be overlooked.

> Man has learned to make himself independent of the direct influence of nature [Grotjahn asserted.] Between man and nature there is culture, which is linked to the social structures within which alone, man can be truly man. It is bound up with the horde, tribe, family, clan, community, state, nation and race, and with their economic forms that vary so widely historically and

[94] A. Grotjahn: Was ist und wozu treiben wir Soziale Hygiene? *Hygienische Rundschau* (No. 20), 1904 (As this paper was available to me only in the form of a reprint which Dr. Bruno Gebhard, of the Cleveland Health Museum very kindly put at my disposal, I am unable to give the page references. It appeared under the Verhandlungen der Deutschen Gesellschaft für öffentliche Gesundheitspflege zu Berlin, Session of March 1, 1904).

geographically. . . . Hygiene must therefore also study intensively the effects of these social conditions in which men are born, live, work, enjoy themselves, procreate and die. It thus becomes *social* hygiene, which takes its place beside physical-biological hygiene as a necessary supplement.

Grotjahn indicated that one of the major problems of social hygiene would be that of physical and social degeneration. With this in mind he emphasized the importance of a program of eugenics.

After these preliminary considerations Grotjahn went on to define his concept of social hygiene. He regarded social hygiene as having two aspects: one, descriptive, the other, normative.

Social hygiene as a *descriptive* science is concerned with the *conditions* that affect the spread of hygienic culture among groups of individuals, and their descendants, living under the same spatial, temporal and social conditions.

Social hygiene as a *normative* science is concerned with the *measures* which are intended to spread hygienic culture among groups of individuals, and their descendants, living under the same spatial, temporal and social conditions.

To elucidate this definition, Grotjahn remarked:

If it is the task of social hygiene as a descriptive science to picture the general existing state of hygienic culture, then as a normative science it is its conscious purpose to spread the hygienic measures, which at first always benefit a preferred minority, to the entire population and thus carry on a progressive improvement of existing conditions.

If social hygiene as a descriptive science has already shifted away from the natural sciences and has recourse to such ancillary sciences as statistics, economics, and so forth, as a normative science it is completely independent of the methods of natural science, and utilizes those of the social sciences. Cultural-historical, psychological, economic and political elements all enter into the calculus of social hygiene. Naturally, the goal as ever is to prevent as far as possible any damage to the health of the greatest number, or even of the entire community.

Finally, Grotjahn went on to discuss some of the ancillary sciences upon which social hygiene would have to rely. These were medical statistics, demography, anthropology (in particular anthropometry), economics and sociology.

This paper on the nature and purpose of social hygiene was also published in a somewhat revised form as a preface to the third volume of the *Jahresbericht.*[95]

The sketch first presented in 1904 was later expanded by Grotjahn in the best known of his many publications, the classic *Soziale Pathologie,* which first appeared in 1911 and went through several editions. The book consists of two major parts, the first dealing with eighteen groups of diseases where the social relations of each group are discussed, the second with the general aspects of social medicine. In the first section, Grotjahn does on a larger scale what Meynne had attempted more than forty years earlier. A list of the subjects treated by Grotjahn is instructive. These are: acute communicable diseases, chronic communicable diseases, venereal diseases, skin diseases, cardiovascular diseases, diseases of the respiratory organs, gastrointestinal and metabolic diseases, occupational intoxications, rheumatism, dental diseases, gynecological and obstetrical conditions, diseases of infancy and childhood, nervous and mental diseases, surgical conditions, cancer, ophthalmic diseases, and diseases of the ear and the throat. In the general section, Grotjahn considered the following topics: the social evaluation of individual groups of diseases, the social value of medical activity in relation to social medicine, the social causation of disease, degeneration as the central problem of studies in social pathology, qualitative planning of human reproduction in relation to eugenics, quantitative planning of human reproduction in relation to decline of population, and the social value of hygienic activity in relation to social hygiene.

Preceding the two major sections of *Soziale Pathologie* is an introduction which contains a number of fundamental principles that help to round out our presentation of Grotjahn's ideas. After a brief review of the history and the definition of social hygiene (or social medicine), he sets forth six points that are important for systematic study of human disease from a social viewpoint.[96]

[95] A. Grotjahn and F. Kriegel: *Jahresbericht über die Fortschritte und Leistungen auf dem Gebiete der Sozialen Hygiene und Demographie. Dritter Band: Bericht über das Jahr 1903,* Gustav Fischer, 1904, pp. i-xv.

[96] Alfred Grotjahn: *Soziale Pathologie. Versuch einer Lehre von den sozialen Beziehungen der menschlichen Krankheiten als Grundlage der sozialen Medizin und der sozialen Hygiene.* Zweite neubearbeitete Auflage, Berlin, August Hirschwald Verlag, 1915, pp. 9-18.

1. The significance of a disease from a social point of view is determined in the first place by the *frequency* with which it occurs. Medical statistics are therefore the basis for any investigation of social pathology.

2. A disease becomes socially significant not only through the frequency of its occurrence. It is necessary to know also the *form* in which the particular disease occurs most frequently. As a rule the characteristic textbook form is not the one in which the disease occurs most frequently, nor is it generally the form which is most affected by social conditions or in turn affects them. Consequently, it is necessary to determine the socio-pathological typical form.

3. The most important relations between the diseases and social conditions are naturally in the realm of causation. The etiology of disease is biological and social. So far only the biological etiology has been studied extensively. The same must be done for the social etiology of disease. The social basis of disease may be considered under the following heads: Social conditions (a) may create or favor a predisposition for a disease; (b) may themselves cause disease directly (c) may transmit the causes of disease; and (d) may influence the course of a disease.

4. Not only are the origin and course of diseases determined by social factors, but these diseases may in turn exert an influence on social conditions. This influence is exerted particularly through the outcome of the disease. This may manifest itself in death, recovery, chronic infirmity, predisposition for other illness, and finally, in degeneration.

5. In the case of a disease which is important from a social viewpoint, it must be established whether medical treatment can exert an appreciable influence on its prevalence, and whether such therapeutic success as may be achieved is important from a social point of view.

6. How can we prevent diseases or influence their course by social measures? This requires attention to the social and economic environment of the patient.

Grotjahn realized that many diseases of social importance were chronic in character. He recognized, however, that a large number of these were preventable, and that health education could be an extremely important factor in this connection. He also accepted the fact that the voluntary health agency had a significant rôle to play in solving questions of social hygiene. Similarly, he was of the opinion that the physician should use his position to promote developments in medicine and social hygiene so that social hygienic measures could be applied to all the people. For the physician to understand these responsibilities, Grotjahn saw that the teaching of social hygiene would have to become a part of the medical curriculum. He himself taught at the University of Berlin, and academic instruction was also given at other German and Austrian medical schools.

Grotjahn was not an isolated phenomenon. He was only the outstanding figure of a group of men who during the first two decades of the twentieth century developed the concept of social medicine so that it could be used in medical education and medical practice. An important initial impulse toward the development of the field had derived from Bismarck's social insurance program. Many of the physicians realized, however, that to restrict the concept of social medicine to the medical aspects of social insurance was to take too restricted a view of the matter. Consequently, we find many of the men who wrote on social medicine attempting to define the field so as to broaden it and yet keep it within practical bounds.

The literature on social medicine that appeared during the period from 1900 to 1920 is extensive, and we can do no more in this survey than to select several authors who in some respect contributed to the development of the concept of social medicine.

At the opening of a course on social medicine in 1909 in Vienna, Ludwig Teleky discussed the tasks and the aims of social medicine.[97] "The task of social medicine," he said, "is to investigate the relations between the health status of a population group and its living conditions which are determined by its social position, as well as the relations between the noxious factors that act in a particular form or with special intensity in a social group and the health condi-

[97] Ludwig Teleky: Die Aufgaben und Ziele der sozialen Medizin, *Wiener klinische Wochenschrift*, 1909.

tions of this social group or class." With this definition, Teleky added an important element for an understanding of the nature of social medicine. By making use of the concept of social class, and calling attention to its significant rôle in the study of health differentials, he introduced an important methodological tool. In this sense he emphasized that the origin of social medicine and practical activity in this field derived from the existence of separate classes that are differentiated from each other not only through their social functions, but also by the different standards of life that characterize the members of these classes.

If this be the task of social medicine, for what purpose are these investigations to be carried out? To this Teleky's reply is that the goal of social medicine, on the basis of the knowledge obtained in special studies, is to contribute to the elimination of all elements that exert a deleterious influence on health and to the elevation of the general state of health. In order to accomplish this, it becomes necessary to go one step further and analyze the vague concept " social condition " (*soziale Lage*) into its component elements. When the sources of the malady have been uncovered, ways and means must be found to control these.[98]

Finally, Teleky summed up the matter in the following statement.

> Social medicine [he said] is the borderland between the medical and the social sciences. It determines the effect of given social and occupational conditions on health, and indicates how, by means of sanitary or social measures, such noxious influences can be prevented, or their effects eliminated or ameliorated. It is also the task of social medicine to indicate how the achievements of individual hygiene and clinical medicine can be made available to those who are unable individually and on the basis of their own means to take advantage of these achievements. Social medicine must provide physicians with the scientific tools that they need in order to be active in the fields of social insurance and social welfare. Finally, it must study the changes in the position of the medical profession, as well as the developmental trends that become apparent.

A survey of social medicine as it had developed in Germany prior to the First World War is contained in the collaborative volume,

[98] Teleky also points out that the effects of social conditions on health can be determined by 1) direct observation, and 2) with the help of statistics.

Krankheit und Soziale Lage edited by M. Mosse and G. Tugendreich which was published in 1913.[99] This book consists of three parts. The first is a general section dealing with history and statistics. The second section is devoted to the social etiology of disease, and the third to the social therapy of disease. In each section the chapters are contributed by individual authors who deal with some specific factor, such as housing, nutrition, occupation, or with a particular group of diseases—infectious diseases, venereal diseases, tuberculosis, nervous and mental diseases, neoplasms, dental diseases, alcoholism. Under social therapy the contributors discuss the influence of social legislation on the prevention, diagnosis and course of disease, the respective tasks of governmental and private agencies, and the control by the state of the social causes of disease.

On the whole, Mosse and Tugendreich follow the ideas of Grotjahn. But where the latter believed that social hygienic measures should culminate in eugenic action, the former regarded the equalization of life expectancy for all socio-economic classes as the goal of social medicine. They likewise designate statistical methods and materials as of the highest importance for the investigation and practice of social medicine, and devote a separate chapter to this topic.

The advance made in the theory and practice of social medicine in Germany up to the outbreak of the First World War is summed up in the statement of Adolf Gottstein: "Social etiology can now be regarded as accepted."[100] This opinion is strengthened by the fact that a number of significant books on social medicine appeared at this time. Some of these have been discussed above. Others were: Walter Ewald: *Soziale Medizin* (1911); A. Grotjahn and J. Kaup: *Handwörterbuch der Sozialen Hygiene* (1912); Adolf Gottstein: *Einführung in das Studium der Sozialen Medizin* (1913); L. Teleky: *Vorlesungen über Soziale Medizin* (1914).

Characteristic of all these authors, and of the fact that they were dealing with a relatively new field is the circumstance that the subject of research methods receives little attention. All agree on the

[99] M. Mosse und G. Tugendreich (editors): *Krankheit und Soziale Lage*, München, J. F. Lehmanns Verlag, 1913 (880 pp.).
[100] *Ibid.*, p. 722.

preeminent significance of statistical materials and methods. Fischer devotes a section to methods. Most of his discussion is concerned with statistics, but he goes on to mention that for specific problems the investigator may use methods taken from various social and other sciences. Among these are anthropometry, epidemiology, genealogy, sociology, economics, occupational technology, legal study, and in general health education and community organization.[101]

The period following the First World War did not add much to the theory of social medicine. Manuals and handbooks for medical administrators, students of social medicine, and practising physicians were published, but for the most part these did not concern themselves extensively with theory. The publication in 1932 of the *Grundriss der Sozialen Medizin* by Franz Ickert and Johannes Weicksel is noteworthy, for the first section of this work deals at length with the concept of social medicine.[102] This section was written by Ickert, and in defining the field of social medicine he divides it into four parts: social physiology and pathology, social diagnosis, social therapy, and social prophylaxis.

The meaning of these divisions is clarified by the subjects discussed under each. Under social physiology and pathology come the various aspects of income, nutrition, housing, and occupation. By social diagnosis Ickert comprehends a " case-work " type of approach in relation to health. Of interest is his reference to Mary Richmond's concept of social diagnosis which had been introduced into Germany by Alice Salomon. From this flow social therapy and social prophylaxis. The former comprises measures intended to make possible the achievement of medical therapeutic aims. These may be financial or social, and may be classified under the general headings of social welfare, social insurance, and attention to special groups such as the physically handicapped. Social prophylaxis includes legislative action in relation to housing and labor (labor legislation, safety measures, accident prevention), health education, physical education, and eugenics. Ickert was impressed by the

[101] Fischer, *op. cit.*, pp. 7-13 (see footnote 90).

[102] Franz Ickert and Johannes Weicksel: *Grundriss der Sozialen Medizin*, Leipzig, Johann Ambrosius Barth, 1932, p. 1 ff.

emphasis on health education in the United States, and urged the importance of action in this field.

In discussing the social relations between individual diseases and the environment, Ickert follows the six-point outline that Grotjahn had set up. As a fundamental basis for any work in social medicine he insists on a knowledge of statistics, and emphasizes the importance of statistical data for dealing with populations in terms of age, sex, morbidity, mortality and migration.

The concepts of social medicine developed in Germany, in particular the ideas of Grotjahn, had a wide influence on the theoretical development of this field in other countries, notably in Central and Eastern Europe. Noteworthy is the development of social medicine in Czechoslovakia.

The concept of social medicine as understood in Czechoslovakia may be illustrated by the definition given by Pelc in 1936.

> Medicine in its broadest sense [he said] is the science which studies the factors on which the health of man is based, as well as the means of maintaining, improving and promoting health. We consider social medicine as a discipline which permits us to recognize the physical and mental maladies of human groups, and to determine the means—almost always of a general nature—which enable us to treat and to control these diseases, and to improve the health status of human groups. In social medicine two fundamental aspects may be distinguished, one descriptive, the other normative.[103]

The scope of social medicine as envisaged by Pelc may be seen from the description of the course that he gave at the University of Prague.[104] This course was given over a period of two semesters at the Institute of Social Medicine in Prague. Two hours a week were devoted to theoretical lectures and three hours to practical demonstrations. The first semester covered social pathology and social hygiene, and dealt with the following topics: methods of statistical demography and their application in evaluating the physi-

[103] Pelc, *op. cit.* See above footnote 86.

[104] Hynek Pelc: Les méthodes d'enseignement de la médecine sociale à l'Université Charles à Prague, Reprint from *Bruxelles Médical* (no. 11), January 10, 1937. See also Hynek Pelc: Le problème de la création de l'Institut de médecine sociale près la Faculté de l'Université de Prague, Reprint from *Revue d'Hygiène et de Médecine sociale*, October 1936.

cal and sanitary condition of a population; health education; nutrition; housing; maternal and child health, and school hygiene; handicapped children; mental hygiene; control of tuberculosis and venereal disease; alcoholism and chronic illness; occupational hygiene. The second semester dealt with the organization of public health and curative medicine in Czechoslovakia under the following divisions: the hygienic and social organization of the country; hospital organization and administration; organization of the medical profession (including medical ethics); and social insurance.

Social medicine has also been extensively developed in the Scandinavian countries, the Soviet Union, Italy, France, Switzerland, Holland, Belgium and Yugoslavia. Thinking on social medicine in the Soviet Union was considerably influenced by the ideas of Grotjahn.[105] In general, developments in specific countries may be regarded as exhibiting specific characteristics due to conditions in the particular country.[106] Italians, for instance, have tended to emphasize the physiology and pathology of occupation; in France and Belgium attention has been focussed on the social hygiene of childhood, control of tuberculosis and venereal disease, and medical problems of labor. In Yugoslavia, under Andrija Stampar, the emphasis was on the problems of a rural population.

Social medicine in Belgium has an outstanding representative in René Sand, and it is of interest to present his concept of social medicine before turning to recent developments in Great Britain and the United States. In his book, *L'Économie humaine par la médecine sociale,* which appeared in 1934, Sand defines social medicine as "the preventive and curative art considered, both in its scientific foundations as well as in its individual and collective applications, from the point of view of the reciprocal relations which link the health of man to his environment."[107] He divides social medicine into the following subdivisions:[108]

1. *Social anthropology* is concerned with the study of physical and mental inequalities in different social classes.

[105] Grotjahn: *Erlebtes und Erstrebtes,* p. 270.

[106] René Sand: *L'Économie humaine par la médecine sociale,* Paris, Les Editions Rieder, 1934, pp. 11-13.

[107] *Ibid.,* p. 14.

[108] *Ibid.,* pp. 15-17.

2. *Social pathology* studies in the same classes variations in the incidence, course and outcome of disease, or in other words social inequalities of disease and death.

3. *Social etiology* seeks the causes of these differences in heredity and environment.

4. *Social hygiene*, which includes both social therapy and social prophylaxis, deals with the application of palliative, curative and preventive measures to diseases of social origin. In this, social insurance and occupational medicine play important parts.

Sand's concept of social medicine is broad, and it is important to note also the central rôle that the concept of social class plays in his view.

Interest in social medicine has developed slowly in Great Britain and the United States, and only recently has an awareness arisen of the need for formulation of a concept of social medicine. The social relations of health and disease had been recognized by physicians and laymen, but owing to a number of causes no concerted effort had been made to organize such knowledge on a coherent basis and thus make it available for practical application. In part this was due to the dominant rôle that laboratory sciences and techniques had come to play in medicine, in part to the concurrent rise and expansion of medical specialism, and in part to the limited view of public health that has been current in both countries. Furthermore, the bias created by these factors was reinforced by powerful social ideologies still rooted in the nineteenth century version of natural law.

During the past two decades, however, influences within medicine itself and in society as a whole have acted to overcome these obstacles. The development of psychiatry, of medical social work, and of various branches of medicine such as endocrinology and nutrition, tended to break down the compartmental thinking of the physician, and to bring back into mental focus the sick person, the patient. Moreover, within society as a whole the ideology of complacent individualism was wearing thin and consciousness of social problems, including those involving health, became exceedingly acute. The concept of the welfare state achieved articulate prominence during the threatening 'thirties and culminated during the next decade in the famous Beveridge Report.

In Britain, various studies on social aspects of health and disease appeared during the 'thirties. Among these may be mentioned G. C. M. M'Gonigle and J. Kirby: *Poverty and Public Health* (1936); J. B. Orr: *Food, Health and Income* (1936); and R. M. Titmuss: *Poverty and Population* (1938). The subtitle of the last book—*A Factual Study of Contemporary Social Waste*—with its reference to the wastage of human lives, characterizes the point of view of most of these writers.

Another significant undertaking was the work of the Peckham Health Centre in London, which was started in 1926 by G. Scott Williamson and Innes H. Pearse.[109] At this institution the attempt was made to develop health as a positive social value on the basis of a fundamental social unit, the family. These workers defined health as the product of "a progressive mutual synthesis participated in by both organism and environment." Thus health is not a something that is passively acted upon by social conditions, but is the product of a functional dynamic process which is an integral part of a healthy social life.

By 1943, these ideas had advanced so far in Great Britain that an Institute of Social Medicine was set up at Oxford with John A. Ryle as the first Professor of Social Medicine. (The working life of this Institute began in the spring of 1944.) Some two years later F. A. E. Crew was appointed to a chair of social medicine at Edinburgh. It is therefore of considerable interest to see what concepts of social medicine have been put forth by Ryle and Crew.

In 1943, Ryle defined social medicine as embodying

> the idea of medicine applied to the service of man as *socius*, . . . with a view to a better understanding and more durable assistance of all his main and contributory troubles which are inimical to active health and not merely to removing or alleviating a present pathology. It also embodies the idea of

---

[109] For the story of the Peckham Health Centre and its work see I. H. Pearse and G. S. Williamson: *The Case for Action*, London, Faber and Faber, 1931; *Biologists in Search of Material. An Interim Report on the Work of the Pioneer Health Centre Peckham*, London, Faber and Faber, 1938; I. H. Pearse and Lucy H. Crocker: *The Peckham Experiment. A Study in the Living Structure of Society*, London, George Allen and Unwin, Ltd., 1943.

medicine applied in the service of *societas*, or the community of men, with a view to lowering the incidence of all preventable disease and raising the general level of human fitness.[110]

The *Annual Report* of the Institute of Social Medicine, published in 1945, contains a statement of the purposes of the Institute which may be regarded as representing Ryle's view of the scope of social medicine. This purpose is

(a) To investigate the influence of social, genetic, environmental and domestic factors on the incidence of human disease and disability. (b) To seek and promote measures other than those usually employed in the practice of remedial medicine, for the protection of the individual and of the community against such forces as interfere with the full development and maintenance of man's mental and physical capacity.

[In summary, then], Social medicine is a comprehensive term. It may, in fact, be held to include the whole of the public and industrial health services, the social services and the remedial services of a community. But just as clinical medicine may be considered not only in terms of "medical practice," but also as an "academic discipline," so too may social medicine be considered. Its observations and researches are in connection with groups or populations rather than with individuals. It requires different methods and collaborations. . . . Social pathology is the related science of social medicine. . . . The problems of social pathology must be sought in the field.

As methods to be used for expanding the knowledge of social medicine, Ryle lists: 1. statistical studies of morbidity and mortality; 2. the socio-medical survey; and 3. the social experiment (this refers to studies such as that of M'Gonigle and Kirby (1936) mentioned above.

Recently (March 7, 1947), at the centennial celebration of the New York Academy of Medicine, Ryle spoke on "Social Pathology and the New Era in Medicine." [111] In this address he characterized social medicine, in contradistinction to public health, as "deriving its inspiration more from the field of clinical experience and seeking always to assist the discovery of a common purpose for the remedial and preventive services, places the emphasis on man, and endeavors to study him in and in relation to his environment."

[110] John A. Ryle: Social Medicine: Its Meaning and its Scope, *British Medical Journal*, Nov. 20, 1943, vol. II, p. 633.

[111] "City Seen as Heart of Medical World," *New York Times*, March 7, 1947.

In social medicine the environment is extended to include

> the whole of the economic, nutritional, occupational, educational, and psychological opportunity of experience of the individual or of the community. . . .
>
> Social medicine is concerned with all diseases of prevalence, including peptic ulcer and chronic rheumatic diseases, cardiovascular disease, cancer, the psychoneuroses and accidental injuries—all of which have their epidemiologies and their correlations with social and occupational conditions and must ultimately be considered to be in greater or less degree preventable.
>
> [Finally, social medicine] properly takes within its ambit the whole of the work of a modern social service department. This includes social diagnosis and social therapeutics—the investigation of conditions, the organization of after-care and the readjustment of the lives of individuals and families disturbed or broken by illness. The almoner or medical social worker also has an important part to play in teaching and in the follow-up activities of a clinical research unit.

The remarks on social medicine published by Crew in 1944 add nothing to the views set forth by Ryle.[112] In January, 1947, there appeared the first issue of the *British Journal of Social Medicine*, edited by F. A. E. Crew and Lancelot Hogben. The editors define social medicine as

> that branch of science which is concerned with: (a) biological needs, interactions, disabilities, and potentialities of human beings living in social aggregates; (b) numerical, structural, and functional changes of human populations in their biological and medical aspects. To a large extent its methods must necessarily be statistical, involving the use of numerical data obtained either from official sources or from special field investigations, and interpreted in the light of established findings of the laboratory and of the clinic. Social medicine takes within its province the study of all environmental agencies, living and non-living, relevant to health and efficiency, also fertility and population genetics, norms and ranges of variation with respect to individual differences and, finally, investigations directed to the assessment of a regimen of positive health.[113]

While these British developments are no doubt of great interest and hold considerable promise for the future, the conceptual ap-

[112] F. A. E. Crew: Social Medicine. An Academic Discipline and an Instrument of Social Policy, *Lancet*, November 11, 1944, p. 6.

[113] *British Journal of Social Medicine*, Vol. 1, no. 1., January 1947. The definition quoted is to be found in the " Notice to Contributors " on the back of the cover.

paratus of the authors quoted above does not yet seem to be as well developed as that of the German writers previously discussed. Although the word " social " is used repeatedly, there is no effort to define precisely what is meant by " social." Thus in one statement social medicine is " to investigate the influence of social, genetic, environmental and domestic factors on the incidence of human disease and disability," while another statement defines environment to include " the whole of the economic, nutritional, occupational, educational and psychological opportunity of experience of the individual or of the community." Clearly if the environment is defined as broadly as it is here it will also include social and domestic factors. And if it does not include them then social and domestic factors must be clearly defined. By comparison, however, with the definition advanced by the editors of the *British Journal of Social Medicine*, the concepts of Ryle are models of clarity. The former is a catch-all, apparently intended to accommodate all sorts of studies that have something to do with mass aspects of health and disease.

Furthermore, despite the frequent use of the word social, the statement by Crew that " social medicine is rooted both in medicine *and in sociology* " [italics mine, G. R.], and that " it includes the application to problems of health and disease of sociological concepts and methods," the bias of such studies as have been published seems still to be clinical and statistical. It still remains to be seen to what extent the British workers will actually utilize sociological concepts and methods for the exploration of specific problems; and whether they will endeavor to see how the available knowledge of the social sciences can be put to use to improve health. For the present it is significant, however, that in 1945 the Institute of Social Medicine at Oxford had a medical social worker on its staff, but no social scientist (sociologist, anthropologist or economist).

The trend toward the development of a concept of social medicine in the United States, as in Great Britain, is a recent phenomenon. Physicians had long been aware in a general way of the social relations of medicine. Daniel Drake in his *Discourses* pointed out that: " Medicine is a physical science, but a social profession. What skeletons are to the comparative anatomist, and plants to the botanist, people in health and disease are to the physician. Both his elementary studies and his after duties are prosecuted in their midst and can be pursued nowhere else." At the same time some laymen were aware that public necessity could well require state action to provide social services. Abraham Lincoln, for instance, in 1854 quoted with approval Jefferson's statement that a legitimate object of government is "to do for the people what needs to be done, but which they cannot by individual effort, do at all, or do so well, for themselves."

The roots of social medicine in the United States are to be found in organized social work which emerged out of organized charity during the 'nineties of the last century.[114] It was here that medicine and social science found a common ground for action—in the prevention of tuberculosis, securing decent working conditions in factories, better housing, and the like. It was also as a part of this trend that Richard Cabot in 1905 introduced medical social service. (The term "medical sociology" was first used in 1902 by Leartus Connor in America, and by Elizabeth Blackwell in England.)

Out of this background Francis Lee Dunham in 1925 tried to develop a concept of social medicine.[115]

> Whether as a separate field or as an adjunct to other fields [Dunham wrote], Social Medicine has a clearly defined function—social here referring to the problem's public character, and medicine to the knowledge and practice of welfare. Defined, its purpose is to further the application of scientific methods, of organization to man's social habits in order to determine their usual biological characteristics, to discover the sources, causes and effects of instability and to establish a sympathetic equilibrium between the organism's innate and acquired tendencies.[116]

Basic to the origin of this concept, according to Dunham, was the need in welfare work "for a field of preventive medicine to which social science, psychology, psychiatry and various other de-

[114] See Edward T. Devine: *When Social Work was Young*, New York, Macmillan Company, 1939; Alice Hamilton: *Exploring the Dangerous Trades*, Boston, Little, Brown and Company, 1943, pp. 53-117.

[115] Dunham, a psychiatrist, was Lecturer on Social Medicine at the Johns Hopkins University. He gave a course to students of social economics in the clinical study of the personality.

[116] Francis Lee Dunham: *An Approach to Social Medicine*, Baltimore, Williams and Wilkins Company, 1925, p. 30.

partments shall contribute but upon none of which shall the entire burden of responsibility fall. Such a field functions more naturally as an attitude, a point of view, rather than as a specific department. It may be called *Social Medicine* and its technic *An Approach to the Field of Social Medicine.*" Furthermore, " destitution and sickness are old companions and since the former is so often the result of the latter the continued administrative separation of the two problems of poverty and sickness . . . is inconsistent with official responsibility." [117]

In defining the scope and function of social medicine, Dunham put the emphasis on social and personal adjustment. Social medicine, he said, helps to harmonize human behavior and to organize conduct.

> [It] attempts to bring about a harmonious organization between personal tendencies and their surroundings. Definite departments of Social Medicine include various agencies dealing with the family as a neighborhood unit, with the interests of infancy, childhood, and youth; with educational and industrial hygiene in its relation to conduct, with the administration of justice through courts of law; with punitive and corrective institutions and with other social phenomena. General and Preventive Medicine are more strictly analytical fields from whose data Social Medicine seeks to synthesize or construct an adequate social adjustment.[118]

The approach of Dunham is markedly influenced by the biological and social thought of the period. The eugenic approach is clearly evident, and the shadow of William Graham Sumner still falls on this pioneer American attempt to formulate a concept of social medicine.

Similar ideas were expressed by a few other physicians at this time. Lewellys F. Barker commented in 1926 in this sense on broadening conceptions of the task of the practising physician.[119] Yet these attempts remained stillborn. It may well be that the almost exclusive concentration of the economic aspects of medical care, which began with the work of the Committee on the Costs of Medical Care militated against the development of a theory of social medicine.

[117] *Ibid.*, pp. 14-15. [118] *Ibid.*, p. 20.

[119] Lewellys F. Barker: Comments on Health and Life, and on Broadening Conceptions of the Tasks of Practising Physicians, *Annals of Clinical Medicine* IV: 525-534, 1926.

One might expect that the advent of the depression with its profound effect on the health of the unemployed and their families might have turned the minds of some in this direction. Nevertheless, with one outstanding exception this was not the case. The exception was Edgar Sydenstricker, who, in 1933, brought out his study on *Health and Environment.* In this monograph, he carried out a masterly analysis of the idea of environment into its component aspects, and then showed the relation of each of these to health problems. Sydenstricker thus laid the basis for a theory of social medicine, but unfortunately he never went on to develop such a theory.

Sporadic references to social medicine during the 'thirties are to be found. In 1937, Gertrud Kroeger presented a survey of the development of the concept of social medicine in Germany.[120] Michael M. Davis in 1938 called the attention of sociologists to social medicine as a field for research.[121] In 1940 Joseph Hirsh and Elizabeth G. Pritchard reporting on a survey of the teaching of social medicine in liberal arts colleges and universities gave the following definition of social medicine.[122]

> Since current public health and medical problems have their roots in the evolutionary changes which have occurred in many and diverse fields of thought and action, the term " social medicine " has been adopted to designate a total concept of the social, economic, and psychological problems which affect the health of man . . . " social medicine " refers to the economic, social, and psychological problems of public health and medical care, including collective attempts to solve them through public health legislation, tax-supported medical care, voluntary and compulsory health insurance; medical institutions and organizations; and the history of public health and medicine in relation to society.

The importance of a concept of social medicine has been repeatedly emphasized by Henry E. Sigerist. In his proposed plan for a new medical school, published in 1941, the place of social medicine in the curriculum was recognized. In 1945, Sigerist again called atten-

[120] See footnote 26.

[121] Michael M. Davis: Social Medicine as a Field for Social Research, *American Journal of Sociology*, XLIV: 274-279, 1938.

[122] Joseph Hirsh and Elizabeth G. Pritchard: Teaching of Social Medicine in Liberal Arts Colleges and Universities, *Public Health Reports* 55: 2041-2060, 1940.

tion to the important rôle that the social sciences have to play in the medical school, and pointed out that "Social medicine is not so much a technique as rather an attitude and approach to the problems of medicine," which no doubt "will some day permeate the entire curriculum." [123]

The need for a conceptual formulation, a theory, of social medicine is gaining recognition in the United States at present. In support of this contention one may cite the publication of such studies as Henry B. Richardson's *Patients Have Families* (1945), the three-day Institute on Social Medicine (March 19-21) held as part of the centennial celebration of the New York Academy of Medicine, and the recent article of Winslow Carlton on the problem of social medicine.[124] According to Carlton,

> The restoration of medicine as a social institution to a state of equilibrium within itself is a job crying for the participation of the most highly qualified physicians. Thus far, leaders in the profession of medicine have taken an active part in only a few communities; leaders in the business of medicine have taken rather too great a part. Why is this not a subject for the medical schools? It is as much a matter of concern to medicine as foreign policy is to government. Statesmanship is needed, and where else should one look than to the medical schools?
>
> What is required is the creation of a new discipline within medicine—it might properly be called "social medicine," which would concern itself with the relation of the medical arts and sciences to society. It is not a subject to be handled as an extracurricular activity at occasional institutes and conferences; it demands the same kind of concentrated attention and experts as any major field of investigation and practice. Training in medical administration will not answer, useful though administrators would be, for something worth administering is necessary. Nothing less than an organized staff of men and women working in the community, observing medical conditions with painstaking care, consulting the experience of representative people, examining the results of local medical plans and interpreting their findings as scientists will produce sound answers to the fundamental questions at issue.

From these specimen definitions, it is evident that American

[123] Henry E. Sigerist: *The University at the Crossroads*, New York, Henry Schuman, 1946, p. 130; see also pp. 106-126.

[124] Winslow Carlton: The Problem of Social Medicine, *New England Journal of Medicine* 236: 496, 1947.

thought on social medicine is in a fluid condition. Much of the thinking is still too vague and fuzzy to be of practical value. Goethe said, *Die Geschichte der Wissenschaft is die Wissenschaft selbst*, and if he was right the genetic analysis of the concept of social medicine that we have attempted can contribute to a better understanding of the complex problems of this field by providing a point of departure for further exploration.

V.

What is Social Medicine?

Historically, the appearance of a concept of social medicine has occurred in response to problems of disease created by industrialism. To a very considerable extent the history of social medicine is also the history of social policy (welfare). Concerned at first primarily with the new class of industrial workers and their problems, social medicine can today be conceived in a broader sense to include various social groups.

Based on the twin pillars of medicine and social science, the concept of social medicine could become more precise only with the advance of medicine and the development of social science. One cannot emphasize sufficiently that social medicine rests equally upon the social *and* the medical sciences. Anthropology, social psychology, sociology and economics are as important for this field as the various branches of medicine.

Fundamental to a concept of social medicine is its concern with what is true of the health of man by virtue of the fact that he leads a group life. In the light of this concern social medicine has two broad aspects: 1) descriptive and 2) normative. As a descriptive science it investigates the social and medical conditions of specific groups, and establishes such causal connections as exist between these conditions; as a normative science it sets up standards for the various groups that are being studied, and indicates measures that might be taken to relieve conditions and to achieve the standards that have been advanced.

The scope of social medicine may also be delimited in terms of three significant sociological aspects: 1) health in relation to the community, 2) health as a social value, and 3) health and social policy.

In terms of the community, social medicine is concerned with the relation of health and disease to community institutions, to population movements within large communities (that is, the invasion and succession of different population groups in specific areas), to the racial and ethnic patterns of communities, to standards of living, and to the social and economic status of different groups.

In considering health as a social value, the point of interest would be to know how this value has been defined by various social groups, the nature of the desires and expectations of different groups in respect to health, and the extent to which these ends are achieved or frustrated. Naturally, this involves an understanding of the hierarchy of values in our society, and of the place which health as a value occupies in different social classes. It will be immediately apparent that knowledge of this type has fundamental implications for such fields as medical care, nutrition, and health education.

Research which will contribute to the formation of social policy is the third major aspect of social medicine. To begin with, attention might be turned to the problem of how far legislation keeps pace with increasing knowledge of the relations between health and other aspects of social life. It is known that standards and measures once accepted tend to acquire vested interests and may become obstacles to further progress. The investigations of such lags would be of considerable interest for it would undoubtedly throw light on the power relationships between pressure groups, and the influence which they exert in legislative bodies in matters of health and welfare. Furthermore, the development of concepts of public responsibility in relation to matters of health for various socio-economic groups also falls under this head.

The concept of the social group, or more specifically of the social class, is basic to social medicine. It is therefore concerned not with the individual *per se*, but with the individual as a member of a group, of a certain economic group, or more broadly as a member of a social group, who because of this membership is exposed to various external influences deleterious to his health, influences and factors that occur exclusively, predominantly, with special intensity, or in peculiar form in his social group and are closely linked to the economic status of this group. Consequently, it is the purpose of social medicine to study all the factors that make up the social condition of a particular group, and that affect the health status of any members of this group; and on the basis of this knowledge to propose such measures of a medical, sanitary or social nature as are necessary to improve health and to make available to the people in the greatest possible degree the achievements of science in the prevention and treatment of disease.

The further development of social medicine requires also that those concerned with this subject devote attention to the achievement of greater conceptual precision. There is a definite need for more precise definition of terms, and for some agreement on the way in which certain terms will be used. There should be some understanding of what is meant by the adjective "social." It must be made clear that social does not mean environmental. Environment is a much broader term, of which the social is only one aspect.[125] The concepts of social science—for instance, social structure, institution, social organization and disorganization—must be examined to determine how useful they can be in dealing with problems of health and disease. In general, Adolf Meyer's pattern of inquiry based on critical common sense will probably be most useful: "What is the fact? The conditions under which it occurs and shows? What are the factors entering and at work? How do they work? With what results? With what modifiability?"[126]

On methods of research and application not very much need be said. Statistical methods and materials will of course play an important part, but social medicine as a synthetic science will make use of any methods that may be necessary or appropriate to the problem in hand.

Finally, important aspects will be the determination of ways and

[125] R. M. MacIver: *Society. A Textbook of Sociology*, Farrar and Rinehart, 1937, p. 102.

[126] Adolf Meyer: Spontaneity, in *A Contribution of Mental Hygiene to Education*, Program of the Mental Hygiene Division of the Illinois Conference on Public Welfare, Chicago, 1933.

means of teaching the subject to medical students and of making the knowledge acquired available to medical practitioners. In this connection it will be important to determine the rôle of the practitioner in social medicine.

We live today in a world of complex social, economic and political organization. To deal most efficiently with problems of health and disease in this world, the development of social medicine will be a necessary condition. It is as a modest contribution toward that end that this survey is presented.

CAMERALISM AND THE CONCEPT OF MEDICAL POLICE

I

In 1779, there appeared the first volume of the monumental *System einer vollständigen medicinischen Polizey* of Johann Peter Frank (1745-1821). During his lifetime six more volumes were issued, with two volumes appearing posthumously. This work is today considered a landmark in the history of thought on the social relations of health and disease. Nevertheless, to assess correctly the significance of Frank's work it is important to see it in terms of the social, political, and ideological context within which it appeared. Central to Frank's thought is the concept of medical police. The origin and growth of this idea require exploration. This essay seeks to study the development of the concept of medical police in the thinking of various individuals, and to show how the idea and the proper methods for achieving it grew in clarity and power until they reached their highest form in the work of Johann Peter Frank.

II

Admiration for the virtues of a growing population, and an intense desire to increase the number of people within a country mark the political and economic views of the later seventeenth century and of most of the eighteenth century.[1] This enthusiasm for increased numbers found expression in many quarters. In 1668, Johann Joachim Becher, a German physician, chemist, promoter of projects, and a writer on political and economic subjects, published a discourse on the rise and fall of cities and states.[2] This work lays great stress on the necessity of populousness. Becher's brother-in-law, the Austrian lawyer and privy councillor Philipp Wilhelm von Hörnigk, took the view that creation of population was the prime function of the state. All measures possible should be taken to

[1] Eli F. Heckscher: *Mercantilism* (2 vols.), London, George Allen and Unwin, Ltd., 1934, vol. II, pp. 158-161.

[2] Johann Joachim Becher: *Politischer Discurs von den eigentlichen Ursachen des Auf—und Abnehmens der Städte, Länder und Republiken, in specie, wie ein Land Volkreich und Nahrhaft zu machen und in eine rechte Societatem civilem zu bringen,* Frankfurt, 1668. For Becher see Wilhelm Roscher: *Geschichte der National-Oekonomik in Deutschland,* second edition, München und Berlin, R. Oldenbourg, 1924, pp. 270-289.

achieve as large a population as can be maintained.[3] Similar views were strongly advocated in England and Scotland. An elaborate economic program prepared for Queen Anne around 1707 by Nehemiah Grew, physician and botanist, concludes with a chapter entitled "Of the Means of Multiplying Your Majesties People for the Speedier Progress of the Aforesaid Improvements." [4] David Hume, the philosopher, urged that the state actively foster the growth of population by encouraging all institutions that favored this process and eliminating those that did not.[5] French thinking on this problem expressed itself even more in deeds than in words. In terms of actual measures taken to stimulate an increase in population, France outstripped all other countries.[6] As part of his economic program, Jean Baptiste Colbert, the minister of Louis XIV, sponsored laws to grant tax exemptions for early marriage. Indeed, in an act of 1669 applying to Canada, he went so far as to impose fines on fathers who did not marry off their daughters before the age of sixteen and their sons before twenty. A year earlier, Colbert had written to the Intendant in Canada that "An Intendant must not believe that he has done his duty unless he has made sure of a yearly increase of at least 200 families." In the same spirit a French official in 1711 proposed that a subsidy of 30 *livres* be given for every marriage, urging his proposal on the ground that "since this assistance will be given only to young people, it is not entirely useless to the state, for it will supply subjects at a cheap price."

This almost fanatical emphasis on a dense population was justified on political, economic, and military grounds. The commonly held view is neatly summed up by John Bellers, a Quaker cloth merchant of London. "Regularly laboring people are the Kingdom's greatest treasure and strength, for without laborers there can be no lords; and if the poor laborers did not raise much more food and manufacture than what did subsist themselves, every gentleman must be a laborer and every idle man must starve." [7] A larger population meant greater production as well as greater consumption, two ideas aptly phrased by Daniel Defoe. "The

[3] Philipp Wilhelm von Hörnigk: *Oesterreich über Alles, Wann es nur will* . . . , 1684. See Roscher, *op. cit.*, pp. 289-293.

[4] E. A. Johnson: *Predecessors of Adam Smith*, New York, Prentice-Hall, Inc., 1937, 1937, p. 136.

[5] *Ibid.*, p. 178.

[6] Heckscher, *op. cit.*, pp. 160-161.

[7] John Bellers: *An Essay towards the Improvement of Physick, in twelve proposals, by which the lives of many thousands of the rich, as well as the poor may be saved yearly*. . . . London, J. Sowle, 1714, p. 37.

more mouths, the more wealth," he said. With regard to consumption he argued that " Multitudes of people if they can be put into a condition to maintain themselves, must increase trade; they must have food, that employs land; they must have clothes, that employs a long variety of trade." [8] Another weighty point in favor of a large population was that more people meant a greater revenue for the monarch. Furthermore, that ingenious physician, scientist, and economist, William Petty, urged that greater administrative economy would be yet another fiscal advantage of increased numbers.[9]

These examples taken from a host of others obviously are not the opinions and actions of men concerned with imaginary conditions and abstract problems. For any adequate appreciation of their relevance to practical affairs, they must be seen as part of something broader and more comprehensive, as part of a scheme of policy and organization whose supreme aim was to place social and economic life in the service of the power politics of the state. This was the system that came to be known generally as *mercantilism,* or as *cameralism* in its more politically-oriented, specifically German form.[10]

From a political standpoint, mercantilism has often and properly been described as the policy of power. The idea of mercantilism is not exhausted, however, in such a description of its content. Mercantilism was much more than this; it was also a conception of society. As such it comprised certain ideas of the social relations of individuals and groups, and of the way in which they should be treated in matters of social policy.

The attitude of mercantilist thought to organized society is characteristically revealed in its relation to the state. The welfare of society was regarded as identical with the welfare of the state. Since power was considered the first interest of the state, most elements of mercantilist policy were advanced and justified as strengthening the power of the realm. Politically, *raison d'état* was the fulcrum of social policy.[11]

[8] Johnson, *op. cit.*, pp. 249-250.

[9] *The Economic Writings of Sir William Petty,* edited by C. H. Hull (2 vols.), Cambridge, at the University Press, 1899, vol. 1, pp. 255-256.

[10] For discussion of mercantilism every student is deeply indebted to the monumental study by Heckscher cited above. Variant views are to be found in *Lecture Notes on Types of Economic Theory,* as delivered by Professor Wesley C. Mitchell (2 vols.), New York, Augustus M. Kelley, 1949, vol. I, pp. 15-23, 48-61; and in Maurice Dobb: *Studies in the Development of Capitalism,* London, George Routledge & Sons, 1946, pp. 177-220. See also Louise Sommer: *Die Österreichischen Kameralisten in dogmengeschichtlicher Darstellung,* Wien, Carl Konegen, 1920-25, especially part one, pp. 43-56.

[11] For discussion of the history of raison d'état see Friedrich Meinecke: *Die Idee der Staatsräson,* München und Berlin, Verlag R. Oldenbourg, 1924.

What national power required, as the rulers and their advisers saw it, was first of all a large population; second, that population should be provided for in a material sense; and thirdly, that it should be under the control of government so that it could be turned to whatever use public policy required. While mercantilist doctrine in its application received varying emphasis at different times and in various places, it was recognized everywhere in some degree that effective use of population within a country required attention to problems of health.

III

The framework for the development of German thought and action on the social relations of health was provided by *cameralism*, the German variety of mercantilism. The term cameralism has two connotations. On the one hand, it designates the ideas that appeared to explain, justify, and guide the centralizing tendencies and practices in administration and economic policy of the absolute monarchy in the German states during the later seventeenth and eighteenth centuries. On the other hand, it refers to the various attempts of the same period to work out in terms of emerging contemporary political and social science a systematic account of the functioning of the various administrative services as a basis for the training of public officials.

Historically, cameralism was part of the process of legal and administrative consolidation in the growth of the modern state. Proceeding from the household of the sovereign as a point of crystallization, the modern state in its evolution advanced from a loose federation of provinces united by the person of a monarch to actual territorial amalgamation by means of institutional unification and administrative centralization. The task of cameralism as a discipline was to supply the positive content for the occasions of state action, and to systematize the growing number of state functions. This development is characterized by the establishment, in 1727, by Friedrich Wilhelm I of the first two professorships for the teaching of cameralism, one at Frankfurt a. d. Oder, the other at Halle.[12] Indeed, the entire process is not unlike that which in our own time led to the appearance of schools of business and business administration following upon the rapid expansion of industry in the later nineteenth century, which centered attention on the organizational and directive features of business.

[12] Albion W. Small: *The Cameralists. The Pioneers of German Social Polity*, Chicago, University of Chicago Press, 1909, pp. 207-210, 222.

Within the framework of cameralism, the idea of *police* is a key concept in relation to problems of health and disease. Derived from the Greek *politeia,* the constitution or administration of a state, the term police (*Policey*) was already employed in a related sense during the sixteenth century by several German writers who deserve to rank as forerunners of the seventeenth and eighteenth century cameralists. One of these was Melchior von Osse (1506-1556) who, in 1556, at the command of the Elector of Saxony prepared a monograph containing his reflections and observations on the proper conduct, organization, and function of a "Christian magistracy."[13] This document, know as Osse's *Testament,* begins with the following paragraph:

> It is among all wise people beyond dispute, [says Osse], that every magistracy (*Obrigkeit*) may prove and make evident its virtue and aptitude in two ways. First, in time of war, through manly deeds, good sagacious projects, and protection of their lands and subjects, second, in time of peace, through ordering and maintaining of good godly righteous government, judiciary and Policey.[14]

In Osse's time administration was unspecialized and not systematized. Governmental activities were relatively inchoate and confused. In keeping with this situation, Osse's presentation of the police concept is general and diffuse. A good *Policey* of a state or city requires a ruler, wise counsel, unpartisan judiciary, and a pious obedient people.

> Everything should be directed toward keeping these four parts in good condition, if one is to maintain a good *Policey,* for a lord and ruler is in three respects under obligations to the people divinely intrusted to him; namely, that he should maintain the same in good prosperous circumstances, which occurs when the people (*das Volck*) lives virtuously, and some among them are promoted to learning, and to good arts, and many wise and learned people are in their number, from whom the rest may receive good instruction, and they are not left to wander in the darkness of ignorance, and everything through which such promotion of things useful to the community is hindered is either prevented or averted by the ruler.[15]

This statement is significant in that it contains in embryo the assumptions of cameralism.

Another early form of the police concept appeared some sixty years later in a posthumous work by Georg Obrecht (1547-1612), professor of law at Strassburg.[16] Written at the request of his friend Emperor

[13] *Ibid.*, pp. 21-25.

[14] Cited by Small, *op. cit.*, pp. 25-26.

[15] *Ibid.*, pp. 37-38.

[16] See Roscher, *op. cit.*, pp. 151-158; Small, *op. cit.*, pp. 40-59; Axel Nielsen: *Die Entstehung der deutschen Kameralwissenschaft im 17. Jahrhundert,* Jena, 1911.

Rudolf II and published in 1617 under the title *Fünff underschiedliche Secreta Politica,*[17] it set forth Obrecht's economic views. Of the five monographs contained in this work, the fourth outlines a scheme of police (*Ein sondere Policey-Ordnung, und Constitution . . .*). The underlying concept is presented in a preface:

> The following Police Order and Constitution, with its seven Sanctions (*Sanctionibus*) is ordained by us especially that we may every year, and as far as practicable at all times, have reliable information how matters stand with all our subjects, young and old, rich and poor, in all parts of our jurisdiction and territory, and also how matters stand with our whole *Policey,* and all of its branches, and how, in this later wholly perverted time, they may be protected against ruin, and may be sustained in constant integrity; and how we may bring it about, after ascertaining all the facts, that our subjects may rightly, well and usefully bring up their children, and themselves lead a Christian, worthy life, and thus so conduct themselves that they may be to their children, to us their divinely appointed rulers, to their neighbor, and to the common weal, a blessing and an honor, to their own temporal and eternal advantage.[18]

Toward this end Obrecht proposed an elaborate plan for registration and regulation of the people from birth to death. Actually, in this proposal he outlined a complete system of population statistics. Furthermore, in connection with this scheme, Obrecht also suggested a plan of savings and endowment insurance for children.

From these beginnings, the police concept was expanded and carried further by a number of German writers and public officials.

An early but pregnant formulation of the cameralistic approach to the health problems of social life was presented by Veit Ludwig von Seckendorff (1626-1692), whose writings were well received by his contemporaries and exercised considerable influence even after his death. Throughout most of his life, Seckendorff served in various administrative posts at the ducal courts of Gotha and Sachsen-Zeitz.[19] His most persistent influence was exerted through his book, *Der Teutsche Fürsten Staat,* a compendium of civil law and administrative practice, which first appeared in 1655 and passed through eight editions, the last published in 1754.

According to Seckendorff, the appropriate aim of government is to establish such ordinances as will assure the welfare of the land and the

[17] Five different political secrets.

[18] Quoted by Small, *op. cit.,* p. 57.

[19] See Small, *op. cit.,* pp. 60-106; Roscher, *op. cit.,* pp. 238-252; Alfons Fischer: *Geschichte des deutschen Gesundheitswesens* (2 vols.), Berlin, F. A. Herbig, 1933, vol. I, pp. 327-328.

people. Since prosperity and welfare manifest themselves in growth of population, means must be taken to guard the health of the people so that their number may increase. A governmental program must concern itself with the maintenance and supervision of midwives, care of orphans, appointment of physicians and surgeons, protection against plague and other contagious diseases, excessive use of spirituous beverages and tobacco, inspection of food and water, measures for cleaning and draining towns, maintenance of hospitals, and provision of poor relief.

Seckendorff has been called the Adam Smith of cameralism,[20] an illuminating if not entirely apt comparison. His work already contains in embryo a program for the management of material and human resources, which at the hands of his successors was developed into a significant branch of public administration. Known as the science of police (*Polizeywissenschaft*), this branch of administrative theory and practice provided the basis upon which the concept of medical police could be developed.

The same may be said of Becher, another writer of this period to whom we have already referred. For Becher the object of a proper police is attained through good administration and social regulation. It is the office of the rulers "by good laws to maintain, protect, govern and control their subjects in the true religion; love and knowledge of God; in good morals, discipline, honor and integrity; in good and various sciences; with respect to their support and legitimate earnings, their health and life, also legitimate increase. In these five points consists the origin of all laws and the foundation of authority and obedience." How are these five departments of government to be carried on? The answer is that five *collegia* or bureaus should be created to have charge of these areas of administration. One of these should be a *collegium vitale* with the responsibility of protecting the health of the subjects.[20a]

Even more specific proposals along the lines suggested by Obrecht, Seckendorff, and Becher were made during the latter half of the seventeenth century by Gottfried Wilhelm von Leibniz (1646-1716), the great German philosopher, scientist, and politician. In all his many sided practical activities, Leibniz on numerous occasions referred to health problems and to modes of government action in such matters. A memorandum of September 1678, prepared for Duke Johann Friedrich of Hannover and headed "Thoughts on State Administration," proposed the creation of a "political topography or a description of the present

[20] Small, *op. cit.*, p. 69.

[20a] Small, *op. cit.*, pp. 124-125.

condition of the country." [21] This should include the number of cities, towns, villages and where necessary individual houses, as well as the total population of the country and its acreage. There should also be an enumeration of the number of soldiers, merchants, artisans, and journeymen, as well as information on the relation of the crafts to each other. Then there should be a listing not only of the numbers of deaths but also of the causes as in England.[22] One of the first to lay stress on statistical investigation, Leibniz's analyses of statistical materials formed the basis for later developments along such lines. Although acknowledging his indebtedness to Petty, he apparently formed his plan for a political topography independently.[23]

As to the manner in which this could be done, Leibniz had various proposals. He realized that such matters fell within the sphere of police. Thus, in 1680, in a series of notes prepared for the Emperor, he suggested the creation of a chief administrative office for police affairs. This office should include a health council.[24] Also during the eighties, Leibniz published several essays in which he indicated the need for adequate population and mortality statistics. In one of these essays he dealt with the establishment of a registration office, pointing out that in England and France mortality records were available and that information useful for politics and medicine had been derived from these sources. In a " Proposal for a Medical Authority," Leibniz again insisted on the significance of birth and death registration, the latter to include age, cause of death, and related circumstances. Having given much thought to the questions on which statistical data might supply the answers, he presented 56 questions under the heading, " Questions in political arithmetic concerning the life of man and related matters." [25] He was in-

[21] Gottfried Wilhelm Leibniz: *Sämtliche Schriften und Briefe*, Erste Reihe, *Allgemeiner politischer und historischer Briefwechsel*, herausgegeben von der Preussischen Akademie der Wissenschaften, Zweiter Band. 1676-1679, Darmstadt, Otto Reichl, 1927, pp. 74-77.

[22] John Graunt's *Natural and Political Observations upon the Bills of Mortality* first appeared in 1662 and the fifth edition in 1676, it is said under William Petty's supervision. Leibniz probably refers to this work.

[23] Essai de quelques raisonnemens nouveaux sur la vie humaine et sur le nombre des hommes, *Die Werke von Leibniz*, herausgegeben von Onno Klopp, 1. Reihe, Bd. 5, Hannover, 1866, pp. 326-337.

[24] Leibniz, *Sämtliche Schriften*, Dritter Band, 1680-1683, Leipzig, K. F. Koehler Verlag, 1938, p. 405.

[25] In the original the three essays mentioned are entitled: *Von Bestellung eines Registratur-Amtes; Vorschlag zu einer Medizinal Behörde; Quaestiones calculi politici circa hominum vitam, et cognatae.* See *Die Werke von Leibniz*, herausgegeben von Onno Klopp, 1. Reihe, Bd. 5, Hannover, 1866, p. 315 ff.

terested in the total number of people in a country, their distribution according to age and sex, the number of women of child-bearing age, the number of men capable of bearing arms, the seasonal and local prevalence of disease, the causes of death differentiated according to acute or chronic diseases, and the relation of births to deaths.

It is not possible to point to any specific result produced by Leibniz's ideas and writings. Nevertheless, it is worth noting that, in 1688, the Great Elector undertook to determine the number of marriages, births, and deaths in Prussian cities and villages. Similarly, in 1685, a *Collegium sanitatis* was established in Prussia, perhaps in connection with Leibniz's proposal for a medical authority to supervise the public health.[26]

By the beginning of the eighteenth century, the police concept had gradually developed to a point where programs could begin to crystallize in institutional forms. This situation was well portrayed, in 1717, by Christian Thomasius (1655-1728), German jurist and political philosopher. These remarks occur, in Thomasius's edition of Osse's *Testament*, which he issued with a commentary. Taking Osse's chapter on police as his cue, Thomasius continues:

> This very year there appeared at *Franckfurth am Mayn* a book entitled *Entwurff einer wohleingerichteten Policey*.[27] . . . The author, who does not give his name, assumes that the flourishing condition of the financial system of a state must rest upon four chief pillars, namely *Policey*, fiscus, commerce, and taxation. The Policey has to do with the internal and external condition (*Verfassung*) of the state. The internal condition consists in part of a vigorous society, namely, (1) in a vigorous growth of the inhabitants, partly in a joyous life, both of the soul, namely, (2) in a religious worship, (3) in virtuous conduct, and (4) praiseworthy education; and of the body, in its sustenance, and satisfaction, through (5) abundance of necessary, useful, and superfluous means-of-life, (6) robust health, and (7) peaceful security. The external condition consists (8) in the good order of people, things and places, and (9) in a convenient ornamentation of city and country. On the contrary, every state is disintegrated and disordered through (1) decline of population, (2) disregard of religion, (3) vicious life, (4) neglect of education, (5) lack of sustenance and increase of the pauper class, (6) epidemics and plagues, (7) turbulence, revolts, and private quarrels, (8) irregular confusion of social strata, affairs, and places, (9) uncultivated lands and badly ordered towns. For promotion of the different kinds of good works, and removal of the evil, the author proposes in general the establishment of a *Policey* bureau, the members of which should be charged with (1) giving their earnest attention to the above points, (2) averting harmful occurrences, (3) controlling disorder, or (4) bringing complaints before the proper tribunals, (5) maintaining reliable

[26] Alfons Fischer: *Geschichte des deutschen Gesundheitswesens* (2 vols.), Berlin, F. A. Herbig Verlag, 1933, vol. 1, pp. 295-296, 328.

[27] Sketch of a well-ordered police.

watchmen and detectives, (6) conducting unexpected visitations and inquisitions, (7) keeping a watchful eye on peaceful persons, things, and places in the state, (8) to that end drawing useful ordinance relating to persons and things, (9) responsibility for observance of same.[28]

The philosopher Christian Wolff (1679-1754) pointed out the close relation between the general welfare, which he identified with the welfare of the state, and the health of the people. In his *Vernünftige Gedanken von dem gesellschaftlichen Leben der Menschen*, published in 1721, Wolff showed that power consists above all in a rich and populous state. Lengthening the average life is important if it is desired to increase the number of people. It is clear, therefore, that good sanitary regulations are as necessary as prosperity. Contagious diseases must be prevented, and all known methods for improving the health of the community should likewise be employed.[29]

Still another indication of the development and systematization of cameralism and the police concept was the establishment by the King of Prussia, in 1727, of two chairs for the teaching of cameralism. The occupants of these positions were to teach the principles of economic management and of police, as well as other subjects so that the students would be well prepared to deal with administrative matters and to be candidates for the Prussian civil service.

Justus Christoph Dithmar (1677-1737) was designated to the chair of cameralism at Frankfurt a. d. Oder. Four years after he assumed his duties, he issued an outline of his academic lectures entitled *Einleitung in die öconomischen, Policey—und Cameralwissenschaften.*[30] Dithmar takes it for granted that the welfare and power of a state rest on a well-ordered economic, police and cameral system, and devotes Part IV of his work to the science of the police. How Dithmar conceived this subject is evident from his statement that the science of police "teaches how the internal and external nature of a state is to be maintained, with a view to general happiness, in good condition and order, and accordingly that the supreme magistracy of the country must have a care that their subjects shall not only be kept in good numbers, God-fearing, Christian, honorable,

[28] Quoted by Small, *op. cit.*, pp. 34-35.

[29] Christian Wolff: *Vernünftige Gedancken von dem gesellschaftlichen Leben der Menschen*, Halle, 1721, 275 and *passim*. See also C. E. Stangeland: *Pre-Malthusian Doctrines of Population: A Study in the History of Economic Theory* (Studies in History, Economics and Public Law, Vol. XXI, No. 3), New York, Columbia University Press, 1904, pp. 209-211.

[30] Introduction to the economic, police and cameral sciences.

and healthy life and conduct, and that their support and surplus of temporal goods shall be promoted by flourishing rural and town occupations; but also that a land shall be improved with well-laid-out cities, country districts and towns, and all kept in good conditions." [31]

In the chapter entitled "On the Maintenance of the Health of the Subjects," Dithmar discusses in some detail matters concerning the health of the community. Basing his comments on Seckendorff and Wolff, he urged the need for a large population and advocated measures to increase marriages. Healthy subjects could be expected only if the parents were healthy. Provision should be made for the training of skilled midwives. Preventive measures must be taken against contagious diseases, and care should be given to keep the streets clean, food pure, and the air clean. Trained physicians should be available to treat the sick, and hospitals and apothecary shops should be in proper condition. Finally, the conduct of health matters should be placed under a *Collegium medicum et chirurgicum*, in other words, an administrative authority to supervise the public health.

As the century advanced, the earlier idea of police was transformed more and more into a theory and practice of administration. This process was intimately related to the needs of the absolute state, and its most distinguished representatives were associated with the monarchs of Prussia and Austria. Outstanding in this connection are the names of three men—Darjes, Justi, and Sonnenfels.

Joachim Georg Darjes (1714-1791) was professor of law, first at Jena and later at Frankfurt a. O. According to Roscher, he was the most important of the cameralistic professors patronized by Frederick the Great.[32] Indeed, it was at his invitation that Darjes migrated in 1763 to Frankfurt. As a teacher he was distinguished by a capacity for systematization, attributable in part at least to his training under Christian Wolff. This faculty characterizes his *Erste Gründe der Cameral—Wissenschaften*,[33] published in 1756 at Jena. In it he created out of an encyclopedic mass of materials an orderly text suitable for the instruction of university students.

Encompassing the basic presuppositions of Darjes is the political theory developed by Samuel Pufendorf and further elaborated by Thomasius and Wolff. According to this doctrine, the theoretical basis of enlightened

[31] Quoted by Small, *op. cit.*, pp. 226-227.
[32] Roscher, *op. cit.*, pp. 419-420; Small, *op. cit.*, pp. 267-284.
[33] First principles of the cameral sciences.

absolutism, the state arose out of a social contract entered upon for self-preservation, a situation which impelled men to renounce their freedom. The purpose of the state is to secure for its people the greatest welfare and security, but it is left to the ruler of the state to determine what the greatest welfare is. The state is therefore entitled to intervene in the affairs of the people when this appears in the general interest. Consequently, the officials of the state must be trained to handle the manifold problems arising out of state action and regulation. Hence for Darjes cameralism embraced *Polizeiwissenschaft* as a science of management. He was aware that the welfare of men is related to three factors—to riches, to health, and to the enjoyment of rights. For this reason, the science of police is concerned with the population of the state, establishment of schools and universities, stimulation of subjects to work, arrangements of the state to preserve the health of the people, care of the poor, promotion of security, and preservation of the beauty of the country.

The leading representative of eighteenth century cameralism was Johannes Heinrich Gottlob von Justi (1717-1771). His development of the concept of police and of its attendant administrative technology sums up the views of his predecessors and represents the most characteristic expression of cameralism during the later eighteenth century. Justi taught at the *Collegium Theresianum* in Vienna from 1750 to 1753, where he gave a course on "economic and cameralistic sciences." From 1755 to 1757 he was active in Göttingen where he combined the office of *Polizeidirektor* with that of lecturer on cameralistic subjects. Later, in 1765, Justi entered the service of Frederick the Great as an administrator of mines. In 1768, he was arrested because of alleged irregularities in the financial administration of his office, and died, in 1771, while confined in the prison of Küstrin.

An advocate of enlightened despotism justifying the policies of Maria Theresa of Austria and Frederick II of Prussia, Justi based his administrative ideas on the political theory developed by the school of Pufendorf and Wolff. Accepting the doctrine that the state arose out of a social contract as a result of which men gave up their freedom, he made use of the postulate of the general happiness to provide an ethical basis for the regulation imposed by the absolute monarch. The relation between the ruler and his subjects was regarded like that of a father to his children. The people were not much more than the object of governmental care. In matters of health as in all other spheres of activity, the ruler knew what was best for his subjects, and by means of laws and administrative measures ordered what they should or should not do. The absolute patriarchal state is the ever-present working assumption in Justi's handling of social problems.

Justi's concept of administration and its application to matters of health are presented in two works—*Staatwirthschaft, oder systematische Abhandlung aller oekonomischen und Cameral—Wissenschaften, die zur Regierung eines Landes erfordert werden*, 1755, and *Grundsätze der Policey-Wissenschaft*, 1756.[34] In Justi's view, the internal administration of the state is the center of gravity of its power relationships. Since the paramount aim of the state is to preserve and to extend its means, the monarch has the responsibility for taking such action as will maintain and expand the available resources and make the subjects happy. It is with this objective that the science of police is concerned, namely, the maintenance and increase of the wealth of the state through appropriate institutional organization, for instance, through improved cultivation of the land, aiding the laboring class, and maintenance of order in the community.

Problems of health and disease are considered in connection with the aim of augmenting the population. Justi's treatment of the matter in his *Grundsätze der Policey-Wissenschaft* occurs in the chapter entitled "On the internal cultivation of countries or the increase of population." Among the measures proposed to promote this aim, he urges that people with hereditary diseases or who are unable to procreate should not be permitted to marry; that vice should be treated severely since it diminishes fecundity and discourages marriage; and that dissipation and disease should be prevented when at all possible. Specifically, through improved sanitary administration the government should try to lengthen the life of the people.[35]

The same problem is discussed by Justi in his *Staatwirthschaft*, where the military focus of interest is specifically brought to bear on the matter. Before engaging in war, he argues, a wise monarch will give serious attention to his population, that is, to his human resources. Through his administrative apparatus the monarch will do all he can to diminish sickness among his subjects and prevent the outbreak of contagious diseases. In relation to this aim, medicine must be improved and encouraged by the government. The same is true of surgery, midwifery, and pharmacy.

[34] State Management; a systematic treatise on all the economic and cameral sciences necessary for the government of a country, 1755; Fundamentals of Police Science, 1756.

[35] J. H. G. von Justi: *Grundsätze der Policey-Wissenschaft*, Göttingen, 1756, pp. 64-76.

To avoid quackery and abuse, the exercise of these arts must be regulated by the authorities. Provision must also be made for pure food and water. Environmental hygiene must be assured, and to accomplish this in towns and cities, building regulations must be instituted.[36]

In passing from Justi to Sonnenfels, there is a definite feeling of having passed from one intellectual climate to another. While Sonnenfels stood squarely on cameralist ground, adhering to the idea of enlightened absolutism, he also reflected the contemporary humanitarian demand for social justice as well as the enlightenment of the French *philosophes*. Illustrative of his position at the conflux of these trends is the circumstance that in his chief work, *Grundsätze der Polizey, Handlung, und Finanz*, the center of the titlepage in each of its three volumes is occupied by a vignette; that in the first volume portrays Montesquieu,[37] the second Forbonnais,[38] and the third Sully.[39] Similarly, the motto of the first volume in the fifth edition is from Cicero, the second takes its motto from Rousseau, the third from Horace.

Joseph von Sonnenfels (1732-1817) studied law at the University of Vienna and, in 1763, was appointed professor of cameral science.[40] As advisor to Maria Theresa, Joseph II, and Leopold II, he played an influential rôle in shaping Austrian political, social, and economic policy. His views were widely accepted, in large measure through his popular textbook, *Grundsätze der Polizey, Handlung, und Finanz* (first edition, 2 vols., 1765).

Like his predecessors and contemporaries, Sonnenfels considered a large population to be of central significance for the economy of a country. To accomplish this purpose the state should use all the means in its power to encourage fecundity and to preserve life. In this connection for instance, Sonnenfels recommended the establishment of maternity hospitals and foundling asylums. In the light of this approach, he defined the science of police as the science of founding and maintaining the internal security of the state. For our purpose Chapter V, " On the Security of the Person,"

[36] J. H. G. von Justi: *Staatwirthschaft* . . . (2nd edition), Leipzig, 1758, vol. I, pp. 173-176.

[37] Charles de Secondat, Baron de la Brède et de Montesquieu (1689-1755), French political theorist, best known for his *De l'ésprit des lois*, 2 vols., 1748.

[38] François Véron Duverger de Forbonnais (1722-1800), French economist and a leading representative of mercantilism in the eighteenth century.

[39] Maximilien de Béthune, Duc de Sully (1560-1641), French statesman under Henri IV. His principal work was concerned with financial administration, and contributed to the consolidation of the power of the French monarchy.

[40] Small, *op. cit.*, pp. 481-524.

is of the greatest interest in this connection. This chapter discusses in detail a large number of activities and topics that affect public welfare and the health of the subjects. Among these are crimes of violence, poor relief, care of the sick, prevention of epidemics, regulation of medical and surgical practice, securing of pure food, cleanliness of cities, methods of procuring abortions, and duelling.

Clearly, by the third quarter of the eighteenth century there had come into being in the German states a system of administrative thought and behavior which referred all activities to the welfare of the absolute state as the norm. This was the science of police. Taking very practical conditions of security as a point of departure, the theoreticians and practitioners of *Polizeiwissenschaft* evolved a body of ideas and practices designed to be used by statesmen in the pursuit of clearly specified political objectives. This concept of public administration also encompassed problems of health and welfare, accepting these as the responsibility of the state.

This political and administrative line of development was paralleled by an equally significant growth of interest among medical men in the relations of health problems to society and in particular to the state. Beginnings of this trend are already present in the early seventeenth century. Among the physicians who concerned themselves with the relations of government to health, the Tyrolean Hippolyt Guarinonius (1571-1654) deserves attention.[41] Descended from a Milanese family that had settled in Trent, he studied medicine at Padua, and later became physician to a home for women at Hall in the Tyrol. There he wrote his work on hygiene of which the first part was published, in 1610, at Ingolstadt under the title *Greuel der Verwüstung menschlichen Geschlechts*.[42] A continuation of this work, prepared over forty years later, is extant only in manuscript. Guarinonius was a devout Catholic and his book is imbued with religious ideas, a circumstance which finds most explicit expression in the close connection between hygiene and morals. Various problems of personal and public hygiene are discussed, abuses are indicated, and improvements are proposed.

In the first part of his " little book," as he called it, of 1350 folio pages, Guarinonius treated such general questions as the average duration of life, the relation between body and mind, and so on. He then proceeds to discuss housing and dwelling hygiene, food control, the use and abuse

[41] Fischer, *op. cit.*, vol. 1, pp. 282-292.

[42] The Abomination of the Devastation of the Human Race.

of alcoholic beverages, the hygiene of procreation, the protection of the health and welfare of children, school hygiene, problems of hospital supervision, and finally the problem of medical care with particular attention to quackery and malpractice.

His approach to some of these problems may be indicated briefly. In questions of housing hygiene, Guarinonius advocated various views already intimated by Hippocrates. Thus, he emphasized that settlements located on high land were more salubrious than those in the plains because people lived longer there. He recommends that in the low-lying plains, the houses should be built high, and that the streets and squares should be wide to provide for good ventilation. The problem of ventilation occupies Guarinonus also in discussing school and hospital hygiene. The air in the living rooms was bad because the rooms were small and overheated in winter. Furthermore, the atmosphere in the houses was poisoned by the unsuitable installation and poor functioning of toilets. In a like manner, school rooms are unhealthy because, due to laziness or in order to save firewood, windows are never opened and no care is taken to provide ventilation. Also, the janitors are too lazy to clean the rooms thoroughly.

These statements characterize only a small part of the contents of this book which, with censure and admonition, explanations and demands, deals with the entire field of public health as it was understood at the time. Guarinonius insists on the need for governmental action to improve health conditions and cites with approval the Augsburg police ordinance of 1530, entitled *Reformation guter Policey zu Augsperg Anno 1530*. His position is succinctly put in his demand for a "Christian police."

Another early contribution to the development of thought on governmental responsibility for the health of the community is the *Politia medica* of Ludwig von Hörnigk (1600-1667), municipal physician at Frankfurt a. Main.[43] Published in 1638, this work is noteworthy on several grounds. First, the exceedingly lengthy title presents almost a table of contents. The title reads as follows:

> Medical Polity, or a Description of the Physicians, both the ordinary ones as well as the appointed Court, Municipal, Military, Hospital and Plague Physicians, Apothecaries, Druggists, Surgeons, Oculists, Hernia and Stone Operators, Confectionery Bakers, Shopkeepers and Bathmen,

---

[43] Ludwig von Hörnigk: *Politia Medica oder Beschreibung dessen was die Medici . . . zuthun und was auch wie sie in Obacht zu nehmen . . .* Franckfurt am Mayn, Bey Clemens Schleichen, 1638; Fischer, *op. cit.*, vol 1, pp. 325-327.

Also of the women appointed to supervise midwives, midwives, lesser female attendants and nurses,

As well as all kinds of unauthorized fraudulent and impudent healers such as old women, cutpurses, crystal gazers, hedge parsons, hermits, jugglers, urine prophets, Jews, calf doctors, tramps, charlatans, informers, fanatics, pseudo-Paracelists, quacks, rat catchers, charmers, exorcists, sorcerers, gypsies, etc.

And then finally the patients or the sick themselves

What these have to do and how they are to be supervised

For the particular use and advantage of all Lords, Courts, Republics and Communities

Collected from the Holy Scriptures, Canon and Secular Law, Police Ordinances and many reliable works by Dr. Ludwig von Hörnigk. . . .

From this summary, which gives the flavor of the book, it is evident that Hörnigk touches on numerous aspects of health and disease that have social implications. Especially noteworthy in this connection are the first two words of his title, *Politia medica*, which may be translated as medical police. Furthermore, his exposition is based on a number of medical ordinances and regulations, particularly those of the cities Frankfurt and Worms, and of the state of Hessen-Kassel. In fact, he chose to present his book in the form of a medical ordinance, to which he added his discussion in the guise of a commentary. Hörnigk's book is not original in its views, but it does emphasize that health is a community problem and that it is up to the constituted authorities to act when necessary to preserve it.

Governmental supervision of public health was also advocated at the end of the seventeenth century by Conrad Berthold Behrens (1660-1736), a physician of Hildesheim. His book, *Medicus legalis oder Gesetzmässige Bestell—und Ausübung der Artzney-Kunst*,[44] published at Helmstedt in 1696, does not deal with legal medicine as one might suspect from the title, but rather with matters of community health. Based on the premise that governmental authorities are obligated by the law of nature to care for the health of their subjects, Behrens argues that such provision must rest on two major forms of action, prevention of disease, and its treatment when it occurs.[45] Prevention must concern itself with the constitution of the air and with nutrition. Behrens also deals with the subject of infection and other matters of public health interest.

Attention to the obligations of the state in matters of health and disease expanded still further in the eighteenth century. This is clearly indicated by the circumstance that a number of medical students wrote dis-

[45] Fischer, *op. cit.*, vol. I, p. 327.

[44] The Legal Physician, or the legal organization and practice of the art of medicine.

sertations on the subject. One of the earliest by Elias Friedrich Heister is entitled *De principum cura circa sanitatem subditorum* (On the care of the ruler for the health of the subjects). Published in 1738 at Helmstedt, this essay treats of various measures that a prince ought to take to maintain the health of his people. Among the subjects considered are nutrition, abuse of alcoholic beverages, and contagious diseases. Heister's essay does not refer to any of the earlier writers on the subject, nor does it exhibit any original features, but it does show that matters of public health were already being discussed at universities.

Dissertations on related subjects were also presented at other German universities. In 1753, J. G. Sonnenkalb graduated at Leipzig with a dissertation on hindrances to public health.[46] The topics with which he dealt comprised impure air, poor hospital conditions, inexperienced midwifery, brothels, and frauds and abuses in the sale of food. The ruler's concern in preserving the health of his subjects is the subject of a dissertation with which A. C. Hammer graduated at Marburg in 1768.[47] Finally, attention may be called to two dissertations published at Leipzig in 1771, both dealing with the removal of obstacles to public health.[48] These writings do not contain anything original, but they show that teachers at the universities were imparting to their students an interest in problems of public health. This is very clear in the case of the Leipzig dissertations which were all written under the influence of Anton Wilhelm Plaz (1708-1784) who was professor from 1733 till his death and, for the last ten years of his life, was Dean of the Faculty of Medicine. Among his writings is also a *Dissertatio de removendis sanitatis publicae impedimentis*, Leipzig, 1771.

Interest in health as a question of public policy entered upon a new stage of development during the second half of the century through the creation of the concept of *medical police*. Influenced by the doctrines of the political philosophers and the theoreticians of police science, physicians adopted the police concept and began to apply it to medical and health problems. As far as is known, the term medical police was first employed in 1764 by Wolfgang Thomas Rau (1721-1772) in his book *Gedanken von dem Nutzen und der Nothwendigkeit einer medicinischen Policeyordnung in einem Staat*.[49] Rau was for a time municipal physician in his

[46] J. G. Sonnenkalb: *De sanitatis publicae obstaculis*, Leipzig, 1753.

[47] A. C. Hemmer: *De principum ratione subditorum conservandi sanitatem*, Marburg, 1768.

[48] J. G. Arnold: *De removendis sanitatis publicae impedimentis*, Leipzig, 1771; Christian Liebing: *De amoliendis sanitatis publicae impedimentis*, Leipzig, 1771.

[49] Thoughts on the utility and necessity of a medical police ordinance for a state.

native city of Ulm and occupied similar posts in other communities.[50] Basing his argument on the political theory of Wolff, he went on to point out that every monarch needs healthy subjects who will be able to fulfill their obligations in peace and war. For this reason, the state must care for the health of the people. The medical profession is obligated not only to treat the sick, but also to supervise the health of the population. But the value of these activities on the part of the medical profession is in large measure cancelled out by the obnoxious and nefarious acts of charlatans and quacks. As Rau put it, the misuse of medicine by untrained persons is as harmful as the discovery of gunpowder. In order to have competent medical personnel, it is necessary to enact a medical police ordinance which will regulate medical education, supervise apothecary shops and hospitals, prevent epidemics, combat quackery, and make possible the enlightenment of the public. Rau was quite aware of the difficulties that such a program would encounter, especially in the matter of public health education. Concerning this problem, he remarked that the mass of the people could not be reached through books since " no one reads anything." He did propose, however, to use the almanacs which were very popular to spread useful precepts on diet and the maintenance of health, on the care of pregnant women, nursing mothers, and women in childbed, on the care of children, and protecton aganst endemic or epidemic disease. All these considerations clearly indicated the need for a medical police code. Rau's small book (44 octavo pages) passed through several editions and received considerable attention.

The idea of medical police, that is, the creation of a medical policy by government and its implementation through administrative regulation, rapidly achieved popularity. The influence of Rau's book is evident in the work issued in 1771 by Christian Rickmann, professor at Jena.[51] Entitled *Von dem Einfluss der Arzneiwissenschaft auf das Wohl des Staats und dem besten Mittel zur Rettung des Lebens.*[52] Rickmann's book made a strong and demonstrable impression upon his contemporaries. Based on the writings of Sonnenfels and Rau, he also advocated the creation of a code of medical police, and urged the need for a physician to compile a complete treatise on medical police. Such a work would have to show how to care for the health of the people through improvement or removal of many conditions harmful to the community, furthermore

[50] Fischer, *op. cit.*, vol. 2, pp. 14, 39, 122-123.

[51] *Ibid.*, pp. 14, 39, 123.

[52] The influence of medicine on the welfare of the state and the best means for saving lives.

how the sick and the infirm may obtain the assistance they need, and how to combat and control epidemics. Rickmann also dealt vigorously with the problem of quackery, and suggested a number of reforms. Of considerable interest is his plan for a sickness insurance scheme.

Another noteworthy point is his division of diseases into two major groups based on causation. The one he calls *natural*; it includes particularly the contagious and epidemic diseases. The second group Rickmann terms *man-made*. These diseases occur more frequently than those in the first group and are "simply the physical consequences of moral laxity." Among the *man-made* diseases, he distinguishes between those due to the patient's own derelictions and those caused by the transgressions of others. These distinctions are significant because they present in a crude and undeveloped manner an early formulation of the concept of disease as a product of social and cultural maladjustment, a view which was developed more fully and concretely in the nineteenth century.

Other physicians also turned their attention to various problems of medical police during this period. In 1773, J. F. Zückert (1737-1778), a Berlin physician, published a book on the best means to prevent the depopulation of a country when epidemics prevail.[53] He attributed the origin of epidemics to meteorological conditions as well as to the effects of such elements as famine, fear, and other misfortunes that result from poor harvests, earthquakes, wars, and sieges.[54] Nevertheless, Zückert felt that an epidemic could be nipped in the bud, given a sufficient number of hospitals and the necessary medical police ordinances. Indeed, through good medical police organization it may even be possible to prevent the spread of an epidemic to a neighboring state. Zückert also called attention to the need for popular enlightenment in health matters, but he was aware that the common people were often apathetic to their own best interests. They must therefore be regarded as children in whose interest and for whose welfare the necessary measures must be taken. When affected by contagious diseases, they must be isolated and supplied with food and medical attention.

Two years later, Ernst Gottfried Baldinger (1738-1804), professor of medicine at Göttingen (1773-83), one of the best known physicians of his time, began to issue his journal, the *Magazin vor Ärzte*.[55] In the preface he announced that the periodical would devote itself preeminently

[53] Joh. Friedrich Zückert: *Von den wahren Mitteln, die Entvölkerung eines Landes in epidemischen Zeiten zu verhüten*, Berlin, 1773.

[54] Fischer, *op. cit.*, vol. 2, pp. 123, 136.

[55] *Ibid.*, pp. 39-40.

to questions of medical police. Later, in 1782, Baldinger issued one of his official addresses under the title *Über Medicinal-Verfassung*. In it he emphasized that medicine was in considerable measure a political science (*Staatswissenschaft*), and that the best medical legislation would remain ineffective unless physicians were well-trained and the people enlightened.

The increasing concentration of interest in problems of medical police at this time is further evidenced by the appearance in rapid succession of several other significant works, each contributing to the subject in its own way.[56] In 1777 there appeared the *Fundamenta politiae medicae* [57] by J. W. Baumer (1719-1788). Although this book dealt at length with public health matters, it also included legal medicine and veterinary medicine, indicating that these fields were still incompletely differentiated. It is worth noting that Baumer employed the works of Wolff and Justi in his book. More important was the publication at Düsseldorf, in 1778, of the *Patriotische Vorschläge zur Verbesserung der Medicinalanstalten* . . .[58] by J. P. Brinkman (1746-1785). After practicing at Cleves and Düsseldorf for many years, Brinkmann went to Russia, in 1784, as personal physician to two grand dukes, but died soon after.[59] Throughout his career, he was concerned with problems of public health and welfare. In his book, Brinkman offers suggestions to improve the health of the rural population, with particular attention to the quality of surgery and midwifery. Like Rickmann, to whom, however, he does not refer, Brinkmann distinguishes diseases that are natural and therefore unavoidable, and those that are man made. In order to increase the security of the state, government should endeavor to prevent misery, disease, and death. Mortality can be decreased through appropriate medical police measures in various areas of public health. All causes that prevent the population from obtaining the means of existence must be removed through public action. Likewise, the moral behavior of the people must be regulated by law so that dissipation will not sap their vital energies. Medical care must be provided and epidemics controlled. Throughout his book, Brinkmann frequently made use of the term medical police.

IV

Having surveyed the origin and development of the concept of medical police up to the last quarter of the eighteenth century, let us assess the

[56] *Ibid.*, pp. 40-41, 124.

[57] Foundations of medical police.

[58] Patriotic proposals for the improvement of medical institutions.

[59] Karl Sudhoff: *Joh. Peter Brinkmann, ein niederrheinischer Arzt im 18. Jahrhundert*, Düsseldorf, 1902.

significance of this process. For this purpose, medical police is the concept referable to those theories, policies, and practices arising from the political and social basis of the absolute, mercantilist German state during the seventeenth and eighteenth centuries for action in the sphere of health and welfare, so as to secure for the monarch and the state increased power and wealth. To some, such a view may perhaps be oversimplified, but it is certainly more realistic and historical than a position which regards the idea of medical police *in vacuo*, and as a result tends to overemphasize the proximity of its outstanding exponents, such as Johann Peter Frank, to modern views on public health and the social problems of health and welfare. The development and exploration of the concept of medical police was a pioneer endeavor in the systematic analysis of the health problems of community life. This trend culminated in the outstanding work of Johann Peter Frank and Franz Anton Mai, which are thus seen as products of an ongoing social process operating in a particular political, economic, and social system. Upon this basis, it becomes possible to assess more clearly the significance of the work of Frank and other German writers of the later eighteenth and early nineteenth centuries, and to understand better why the impact of these ideas on practice was limited.

THE FATE OF THE CONCEPT OF MEDICAL POLICE 1780–1890

I.

The publication of Johann Peter Frank's *System einer vollständigen medicinischen Polizey* exerted an unusually strong influence on the further fate of the concept of medical police. As the successive volumes of this encyclopedic work appeared from 1779 on, their impact became evident in several directions. Naturally, this effect was felt most strongly within the German language area, and in such areas as Italy that were in close political and cultural contact with the German states. There can be but small doubt, however, that Frank also helped to spread the term and the idea of "medical police" beyond the borders of the Germanies. During the later eighteenth century and well into the nineteenth century, the idea of medical police appears not only in Germany, Austria and Italy, but also in France, Great Britain and the United States. In fact, it was used as late as 1890 in Italy[1].

Frank established the concept of medical police more firmly. His contemporaries were impressed by the fact that he had worked out in singularly systematic and finished form solutions for problems which were matters of concern quite as much in other countries as they were in the German states. Nevertheless, neither his concept of medical police nor the solutions developed on this basis were equally applicable in all countries. The idea of medical police as employed by Frank was rooted

Centaurus 1957: vol. 5: no. 2: pp. 97–113

in a particular political, economic and social system. At the end of the eighteenth century, this system differed substantially from conditions obtaining in Great Britain, France and the United States. Based upon cameralistic[2] premises, medical police as developed by Frank and other German writers was authoritarian and paternalistic character; when applied to specific problems it was concerned with the laws that must be passed and the details of what ought to be done. It was inevitable, therefore, that the concept would be materially altered by impact with fundamentally different political and social institutions. At the end of the eighteenth century, for instance, the British were already taking for granted a degree of individual freedom and initiative which was almost wholly lacking in German life. Consequently, insofar as the concept of medical police was adopted outside of Germany and brought to bear upon specific problems, it tended to be limited to those areas of community living where governmental action was most easily accepted, chiefly in the control of communicable disease and in sanitation of the environment.

In the Germanies, and also in Italy, economic progress and the social change which it entailed did not keep pace with the example set by England and France. German political, economic and social life remained in many respects narrow, conservative and particularist in spirit. While Great Britain and Western Europe moved away from the pattern woven out of absolutism and mercantilism, this evolution was retarded in Central Europe. Reinforced by the inertia of inherited relations, the ideal of orderly efficiency remained the goal of public administration, and the concept of medical police continued to be applied within this framework. Measured in terms of the progressive social aspirations connected with the French Revolution, and of the problems created by the emergent industrial civilization, the idea of medical police faced the past. As part of an ideological and administrative structure whose chief function was to buttress an antiquated edifice, it lost the creative aspects which characterized it during the eighteenth century. German writers and administrators of the first half of the nineteenth century continued to deal with questions of medical police along the lines indicated by Frank and his contemporaries. By the middle of the nineteenth century, however, the concept of medical police had in large measure become a sterile formula. Such practical significance as it still retained resided largely in administrative and regulatory activities concerned with communicable disease control, organization and supervision of medical personnel, environmental sanitation and the provision of medical care to the indigent. However, the broad social approach, the awareness of the social relations of health and disease which had characterized the thinking and writing of Johann Peter Frank and his more significant contemporaries, all this had been drained from the idea of medical police. The result was that when Germany encountered the health problems connected with the new industrial order, it became evident that a new approach to these problems was necessary.

II.

In Germany, the appearance of Frank's volumes stimulated other physicians to write on medical police. Many of these leaned heavily on the *Medicinische Polizey*. Its influence is clearly evident in several medical journals published after 1779. From 1783 to 1787, J. C. F. Scherf issued the *Archiv der medizinischen Polizey und der gemeinnützigen Arzneikunde*. This journal was continued under a somewhat different title from 1789 to 1797, and then made a brief and final appearance as *Allgemeines Archiv der Gesundheitspolizey*. That Scherf was inspired by Frank emerges clearly from his review of the first volume of the *System*. Not only did he devote more than twenty pages to this subject, but also characterized Frank's work as a masterpiece "which did Germany such great honor and which would yield such important advantages if the rulers of the German states would employ it in accordance with their duty to be the father of their country"[3]. A similar influence is detectable in the *Magazin für gerichtliche Arzneywissenschaft und medicinische Polizey*, a journal founded by C. T. Uden and J. T. Pyl and published in 1782 and 1783, then continued from 1785 to 1788 under Pyl's editorship. In Zürich, J. H. Rahn began in 1799 to issue a *Magazin für gemeinnützige Arzneykunde und medicinische Polizey*. This journal was likewise influenced by Frank's *System*[4].

A number of books published during this period also reflect the impact of Frank's writings. In 1786, Z. G. Huszty published a *Diskurs über die medizinische Polizei*, in which he paid high tribute to Frank. While he made considerable use of the *System* for his own work, Huszty also utilized a number of contemporary articles and added a section on the hygiene of mines and workships. Other writers simply copied or abstracted Frank's treatise. In 1795, for example, Franz Schraud published at Budapest a book entitled *Aphorismi de politia medica*[5]. Dedicated to Johann Peter Frank, this volume consists essentially of selected passages from his *Medicinische Polizey* translated into Latin. A similar compendium in German had been published by J. J. C. Fahner in 1792 at Berlin[6]. In

1800, Johann Benjamin Erhard, physician and philosopher, published a volume entitled *Theorie der Gesetze, die sich auf das körperliche Wohlseyn der Bürger beziehen, und der Benutzung der Heilkunde zum Dienst der Gesetzgebung*[7]. Erhard was then lecturing in Berlin and this book was intended as a guide to lectures on medical legislation[8]. In very large measure it is based on Frank. A similar work was published by Friedrich August Röber at Dresden in 1805, under the title *Von der Sorge des Staats für die Gesundheit seiner Bürger*[9]. Röber defined medical police as the care of the state for the health of its citizens, pointing out that this sphere of activity could be considered under two heads—preventive and curative. In general, this book is a popularized version of Frank's treatise. Interestingly enough, in the same year, Andreas Röschlaub, professor of medicine at Landshut, published an article discussing the tasks of hygiene. He made it clear that hygiene had not only a preventive, negative aspect, but that it must also occupy itself with what he termed "positive hygiene". By this Röschlaub meant that positive steps must be taken to promote and advance health to an optimum state. He emphasized that this idea was not new, having already been expressed by Johann Peter Frank and several of his contemporaries[10].

During the last two decades of the eighteenth century, courses on medical police began to be given at some of the German universities, and a number of books on the subject were prepared in connection with academic lectures. One of the most significant of these was by E. B. G. Hebenstreit, professor at Leipzig, which appeared in 1791 under the title *Lehrsätze der medicinischen Polizeywissenschaft*[11]. In it medical police was defined as "the science which teaches how to apply dietetic and medical principles to the promotion, maintenance and restoration of the public health". Hebenstreit's book is comprehensive in scope, as indicated by some of the topics covered—procreation, maternal and child welfare, nutrition and food sanitation, housing, hygiene of clothing, recreation, occupation, accident prevention, control and prevention of epidemics, organization of the medical profession, provision of medical care, nursing of the sick, and enlightenment of the public in health matters. A similar volume entitled *Systematisches Handbuch der öffentlichen Gesundheitspflege*[12], was published in 1818 at Vienna. The author was Joseph Bernt, professor of state medicine at the Vienna Medical School, and he intended his book to be a guide to lectures on health police for physicians, lawyers and police officials. Although Bernt defined his terms somewhat differently than other writers, such as Frank or Hebenstreit, the basic point of view and the topics covered are the same. It is to the interest of the state to see that its citizens are healthy, and this is accomplished through a well organized health police or public health organization[13]. Among the topics considered are population, vital statistics, maternal and child health, housing, clothing, nutrition, accidents, occupation, recreation, and the harm caused to health by superstitions[14].

At the universities, the teaching of medical police appears to have been initiated by Frank himself. In 1784, he lectured on the subject at the University of Göttingen[15]. At Heidelberg, lectures on legal medicine and medical police were started in 1786 by Oberkamp, who had been Frank's teacher and had encouraged him in his intention to write a treatise on medical police[16]. From the winter semester of 1786–1787 on through the succeeding decade, F. A. Mai, at various times, gave courses that dealt with aspects of medical police. In the winter semester of 1797–1798 he gave a course of this kind under the title "Medical Police Legislation". Also at Heidelberg, two physicians named Schmuck and von Leveling are reported to have taught medical police in 1793–1794 and 1794–1795 respectively. At Leipzig, the subject was taught during the eighties by Hebenstreit, who has been mentioned above. During the same period lectures on medical police were given at Ingolstadt by H. M. von Leveling, who has already been mentioned for his later teaching at Heidelberg. Despite these efforts, however, the teaching of medical police remained limited to only a few German universities.

How did the concept of medical police affect legislation and administration in the German states, an area with which by its very origin and avowed purpose it was intimately concerned? This influence may be sought in two directions, in proposals for legislation and in terms of laws actually passed and regulations instituted. Proper evaluation of this influence requires us to remember also that physicians and public officials concerned with these matters were interested chiefly in one or more of three major health problems: to maintain population growth, to provide a sufficient number of competent physicians and other medical personnel, and to enact such laws as might be necessary for the maintenance and promotion of public health. It is in these areas that the impact of the concept of medical police may be observed.

Even before the appearance of Frank's treatise, efforts had been made in various German states to enact health legislation and to put these laws into effect. Noteworthy, for example, are the activities of Christoph Ludwig Hoffmann (1721–1806) in reorganising the medical profession in two of the smaller states, in the Bishopric of Münster and in Hessen-Kassel. Hoffmann felt that medical quackery was an important health hazard, but he realized that under contemporary conditions such irregular practitioners could not be completely abolished. For this reason he proposed to train these inadequately educated healers so that there would be a satisfactory supply of physicians. All medical practitioners would be examined and divided into six classes depending on their knowledge and ability. The same would be done with the surgeons. The people would then be able to ascertain the particular class to which a physician or a surgeon belonged. These principles were incorporated in the Münster medical ordinance of May 14, 1777. In July 1777, Hoffmann held a lecture on medical organization at which the Landgrave of Hessen was present. In the course of his remarks, he pointed out that population is the important element through which a state can be made to flourish. To promote and increase population competent physicians are necessary and quackery must be combatted. As a result, on July 11, 1778, Hessen-Kassel was given a new medical ordinance modeled after that of Münster. Hoffmann's ideas were put into effect and received a good deal of attention throughout Germany, but these endeavors were limited to a relatively narrow area.

Other German states and cities enacted medical ordinances during the later eighteenth century and in the earlier nineteenth century. For the most part these were concerned with the qualifications and duties of medical personnel, control of epidemics, supervision of food supply, control of prostitution, and supervision of hospitals. No government of a German state, however, enacted a comprehensive health code to coincide with the broad scope of medical police as conceived by Frank and other German writers. Nevertheless, several proposals for legislation of this kind were made and these deserve to be noted.

In 1799, J. H. Rahn, whose journal for medical police has already been noted, presented in this publication a "Proposal and Draft of Medical Police Laws for the one and indivisible Helvetic Republic"[17]. The core of this proposal is the creation of a government agency to supervise the entire sphere of medical police. This board, to be composed of seven professors of medicine, would watch over all medical institutions and extend its vigilance and care to all areas of the health field, including such matters as nutrition, housing, clothing, procreation, protection of mothers and infants, prevention of epidemics, measures against diseases of animals, health education, and supervision of orphanages and work houses. Furthermore, each district would have a health officer, trained in the science of medical police, who would see that the sanitary laws were carried out and would gather data on vital statistics.

Even more significant than Rahn's proposal was the draft of a health code submitted to the government of the Palatinate in 1800 by Franz Anton Mai[18]. Born in Heidelberg in 1742, Mai studied in his native city, receiving his medical degree in 1765. The following year he received a teaching appointment at the school for midwives in Mannheim. His desire to create health laws was evidenced as early as 1777 when he proposed to his sovereign, the Elector Palatine, that young women who had given birth and were venereally infected should be protected against mistreatment, but they should be prevented from taking employment as wetnurses, so as not to spread infection. Mai was also active in enlightening the public on health matters. In 1781 the Elector approved Mai's proposal for a nursing school open to all who wished to be instructed in the care of the sick. At the same time Mai also organized a sickness insurance fund for the poor, and a fund to pay for nursing care for the sick poor. In 1785, he became professor of obstetrics at Heidelberg. Throughout his career, Mai was active in proposing measures to improve the health of his countrymen. In numerous publications he dealt with a variety of medical and public health problems, among them the prevention of infanticide, the elevation of standards of medical practice, the use and abuse of bathing, and the interrelation of hygiene and religion. Mai died in 1814, highly esteemed by his fellow citizens and professional colleagues.

Mai's most significant achievement, however, at least on the theoretical side, was his *Entwurf einer Gesetzgebung über die wichtigsten Gegenstände der medizinischen Polizei also ein Beitrag zu einem neuen Landrecht in the Pfalz*[19]. Mai was thoroughly conversant with Frank's *Medicinische Polizey*, for which he had a very high regard, and he complements it through his effort to encourage application of the sociomedical knowledge available at the time. The scope of Mai's code is a broad as that of Frank's treatise. Composed in 1800 it was approved by the Elector, the medical faculty of the University of Heidelberg, and the medical officials of Mannheim. Nevertheless, Mai's proposal was not realized. In considerable measure this was due to political conditions, the alarums and excursions of war, and the ineffectual character of government in the Germanies in the early nineteenth century. Yet the meaning of Mai's legislative draft is clear. Its value resides in the effort to put into practice what Frank preached—the creation of an integral code of law governing all aspects of health and intended not only to maintain but positively to promote health.

The comprehensive character of this proposed health code is indicated by the topics considered in it. These include hygiene of housing and of the atmosphere, hygiene of food and drink, medical aspects of recreation, hygiene of clothing, the health of various occupational groups, health and welfare of mothers and children, accident prevention, first aid, prevention and control of communicable disease, both human and animal, organization of medical personnel and provision of medical care, and health education.

Mai placed great emphasis on education, not only of the people, but also of physicians and other medical attendants. He felt that doctors, midwives and others who dealt with questions of health and disease were the logical health educators. His code therefore provided for such instruction. In fact, the first law of the code, dealing with the duties of a health officer, proposed that this official instruct either the children in the schools or their teachers in the maintenance and promotion of health. Furthermore, the health officer would enlighten the adolescent youth on the dangers of sexual excesses. Indeed, as one reads this section it appears that Mai intended the health officer to be a kind of community health educator who would provide instruction in health matters for young couples about to marry, for wandering students and journeymen, and such other groups or individuals as might require it.

Although Mai's proposed health code was well received by the authorities and his colleagues, it was never enacted. Foreign invasion, political weakness and disorganization pushed such matters into the background. When peace and more settled conditions returned after Napoleon's downfall, Mai was dead and the stage was being set for a new approach to the social problems of health and disease.

The achievements of Johann Peter Frank and Franz Anton Mai represent the high points in the development, exploration and attempted application of the concept of medical police. The ideas promulgated by these men continued to exist in a limited and attenuated form. Thus during the 'thirties and 'forties of the nineteenth century a number of compilations of medical police legislation appeared in the German states. In 1834, for instance, A. L. Dornblüth issued such a volume for the Grand Duchy of Mecklenburg-Schwerin[20]. A similar publication appeared in 1837 for the Kingdom of Saxony[21]. It was intended for the use of district physicians and surgeons, veterinarians and judicial and police officials. In 1841, a collection of medical police legislation for the Kingdom of Württemberg, up to and including the year 1840, appeared at Stuttgart[22].

This publication apparently answered a real need, for a second, enlarged edition, including additional material through 1846, was issued in 1847.

Various textbooks on medical police were also published during this period[23]. In 1838, A. H. Nicolai dealt with medical and veterinary police. In 1848, J. H. Schürmayer published a handbook of medical police in which he considered public health, public medical care and the work of governmental agencies. A volume on medical police for physicians, apothecaries and police officials was issued by Carl Vogel in 1853. Similar texts were prepared by Hauska in 1859, and Haeckermann in 1863. Indeed, as late as 1877 a volume dealing with the application of chemistry to the practice of medical police and forensic medicine appeared at Stuttgart[24]. None of these publications contributed anything new.

III.

At this point, it is necessary to consider the spread of the idea of medical police beyond the German borders to other countries. As one might expect, evidence of such influence is to be found in countries such as Russia, Hungary, Denmark and Italy where cultural contact with the Germanies was close. Welzien's *Grundriss der medicinischen Polizey*, published in 1800 at St. Petersburg; R. Frankenau's *Die öffentliche Gesundheitspolizey unter einer aufgeklärten Regierung* issued at Copenhagen in 1804; and the *Elementa politiae medicae* by F. Bene, published in 1807 at Budapest are all indicative of the German influence[25]. In Italy, a tradition of government action in health matters had long preceded the development of the concept of medical police. This was the case particularly in the control of communicable and epidemic diseases, as indicated by such publications as Alaimo's *Consigli medico-politici del senato Palermitano* (1652), Maurizio's *Trattato giuridico e politico sulla peste* (1684)[26]. This trend continued into the eighteenth century to merge with other influences such as the humanitarianism of the later Enlightenment. Representative of this period is Lodovico Antonio Muratori, friend of Ramazzini and Morgagni, who was active as jurist, philosopher and philanthropist. His *Trattato governo-politico medico e ecclesiastico delle peste*, published in 1720, reflects the older tendency, but a later book, *Della Publica Felicità*, which appeared in 1749 deals with the broader social problems of health much as the German writers before Frank had done[27]. Muratori pointed out that the best way to improve the condition of the people is to protect their health through hygienic measures and to restore it through medical care. Consequently, it is necessary on the one hand to control the spread of communicable diseases, to provide pure food and water, to maintain the hygiene of cities, and on the other to provide a sufficient number of physicians, surgeons, midwives and hospitals to insure the availability of medical care to all citizens. The poor should receive free medical care, and the treatment of venereal disease should be free to all[28].

Similar views were expressed by other non-medical Italian writers[29]. In general, the mercantilist point of view is the prevalent one. All agreed that populousness meant strength and prosperity. In 1765, Antonio Genovesi, professor of economics at Naples, published his *Lezioni di Economia Civile*, in which he discussed population at length. He indicated that social conditions as well as epidemic diseases may cause de-population. The question of population in relation to industry and agriculture was discussed in 1769 by Cesare Beccaria, professor at Milan, who is best known for his efforts to reform criminal law. In his *Elementi di Economia Pubblica* he pointed out that lack of subsistence and absence of well-being are among the physical causes that decrease population. Nevertheless, the force of such factors can be diminished by careful attention on the part of medical men and the public authorities concerned with sanitary control. The Milanese count Pietro Verri was a friend of Beccaria and his treatment of these questions in his *Meditazioni sulla Economia Politica* which appeared in 1771 is similar. He emphasized the disastrous effects of contagious diseases caused by want and misery. In the same year Giambattista Gherardo d'Arco, a protégé of Frederick II of Prussia, published a book entitled *Dell'Armonia Politico-Economica tra la Città e il suo Territorio*, in which he discussed what should be the proper balance between the population of a city and the surrounding territory from which it supplies its needs. In this connection d'Arco asserted that too great a concentration of population in cities is harmful because it leads to insanitary conditions which cause a higher death-rate in cities than in the country.

In view of this climate of opinion it is not surprising to find the concept of medical police readily adopted in Italy. Through his position at Pavia and the Italian translation of his *System*, Frank exerted a strong influence on Italian physicians. A number of books by Italian authors on medical police are indicative. Among these may be mentioned Barzelotti: *Polizia di sanita* (1806), Omodei: *Polizia economico-medica* (1806), and by the same author, *Sistema di polizia medico-militare* (1807). In 1824, Lorenzo Martini published his *Elementi di Polizia Medica* based largely on Frank's work. Ten years later Martini reissued this book as *Polizia Medica*, and dedicated it, interestingly enough to the American Philosophical Society of Philadelphia. In 1835, Martini published a third revised version entitled *Manuali d'Igiene e Polizia Medica*[30]. Throughout the influence of Frank is evident. In Italy, as in Germany, the term medical police continued to be used throughout the nineteenth century. As late as 1890, Giuseppe Ziino published a manual of medical police for the use of health officials and administrators. By this time, medical police was defined as concerned with the practical application of knowledge obtained experimentally or otherwise by the science of hygiene[31].

The concept of medical police was apparently not transplanted to Great Britain until the end of the eighteenth century. So far as is known, Andrew Duncan, professor of the institutes of medicine at the University of Edinburgh, was the first in Great Britain to adopt the idea and to attempt its employment in medical education. In 1798, Duncan addressed a memorial to the Patrons of the University on the importance of medical jurisprudence in medical education. From this memorial it appears that he had been lecturing on the subject since 1795 and that medical police was dealt with as a part of this course. Duncan defined medical police as consisting of "the medical precepts which may be of use to the legislature or to the magistracy, relating not only to the welfare of individuals but the property and security of nations, being perhaps the most important branch of general police, since its influence is not confined to those whom accidental circumstances bring within its sphere, but extends over the whole population of the State"[32]. While the concept of police, in the sense of public administration, was familiar in Scotland—witness Adam Smith's *Lectures on Justice, Police, Revenue and Arms* of 1763[33]—the immediate source of Duncan's lectures on medical police was the *Medicinische Polizey* of Johann Peter Frank, an indebtedness which he acknowledged repeatedly. In his memorial of 1798, Duncan outlined what he considered a suitable course of instruction in medical police for medical students. From the topics listed: hygiene of procreation, personal and environmental sanitation, control of communicable diseases, accident prevention, occupational hygiene, and administration of hospitals and other public institutions concerned with health problems, it is obviously derived from the first four volumes of Frank's work. There is no suggestion in this proposed curriculum, however, that Duncan shared Frank's social philosophy. This is not a matter for surprise since Britain had not developed the administrative absolutism prevalent on the Continent, and while mercantilism had long dominated British political and social thought, by the end of the eighteenth century this system was disintegrating, a process hastened by the unique social transformation known as the Industrial Revolution, whose cumulative effect was to establish the new industrial order.

However, the immediate effect of Duncan's representations seems to have been the establishment in 1807 of a professorship of medical jurisprudence and medical police in the Faculty of Law at Edinburgh. Medical police remained subordinate to medical jurisprudence, and the occupants of this chair continued to give a course of instruction very much like that initiated by Duncan. A comparison of the topics considered in 1863 with those listed by Duncan fails to reveal any considerable change. At about the same time a similar course in medical police was being offered by the professor of medical jurisprudence at Glasgow. It was not until the last quarter of the nineteenth century that the term "medical police" began to give way in academic circles to designations such as "public health" or "hygiene".

It was also in Scotland that the first notable treatise in English on medical police was published. This was the *Medical Police: or, the Causes of Disease, with the Means of Prevention: and Rules for Diet, Regimen, etc. adapted particularly to the Cities of London and Edinburgh, and generally to all large towns* by John Roberton of Edinburgh. First published in 1809, a second edition appeared in 1812. In his grasp of the social relations of health and disease, Roberton is closer to Frank than to Duncan. In general he deals with the same subjects.

Awareness of the social problems of health and disease is evident throughout the earlier nineteenth century and is often found expressed in terms of medical police. Thus Gordon Smith in his *Principles of Forensic Medicine*, published in 1821, defined medical police as "the application of medical knowledge to the benefit of man in his social state"[34]. Robert Cowan, professor of medical jurisprudence and police in the University of Glasgow, pointed out that the prevalence of epidemic disease depended on a variety of causes "but the most influential of all is poverty and destitution". In 1837 he advocated the establishment in Glasgow of a system of medical police[35].

Nevertheless, the idea of medical police was being limited more and more to control of epidemic disease and supervision of environmental sanitation. Thus in 1842 a writer in the *British and Foreign Medical Review* complained that in England "People are apt to think ... that medical police implies nothing more than the seizure of stinking fish or unsound meat; or at most a fear-spreading contrivance termed a Board of Health, and brought into action when cholera rages"[36]. Similarly, in 1844, James Black published a series of lectures on public hygiene and medical police from which it appears that the sphere of activity or medical police encompasses regulatory action relating to the hygiene of food, drink, occupation, disposal of the dead, water supply and environmental sanitation[37]. This restricted point of view is evident also in the discussions which preceded the enactment of the Public Health Act of 1848[38].

The employment of the term "medical Police" in the United States during the nineteenth century was generally like that in Great Britain. Thus, David Hosack in 1820 presented his *Observations on the Means of Improving the Medical Police of the City of New York*, in which he recommended improvement of the municipal water supply, better housing for the poor, introduction of a sewerage system, widening of the streets, limitation of burials within the city, and substitution of stone for wood in the construction of wharves and docks. A broader view of medical police was taken in 1862 by Louis Elsberg in a paper entitled "The Domain of Medical Police"[39]. Based in part on Schürmayer's handbook of medical police and Mohl's treatise on the science of police, Elsberg defines his subject "to be that science which teaches the application of every branch of medical knowledge ... to the purposes of police". He divides the domain of medical police into three parts: preservation of public health; removal of disease; and administration of medical affairs. In Elsberg's opinion the first of these areas of activity forms, par excellence, the domain of medical, or, as it is (in this connection) also called Sanitary Police. Elsberg's further discussion of the subject is concerned chiefly with measures to be taken against health deterioration and for the control of existing disease. In some respects, such as emphasis on measures to insure healthy offspring, Elsberg seems to echo faintly the earlier German writers on medical police. In view of his use of Schürmayer's handbook, the source of this influence seems clear.

Mercantilism played a major role in shaping the seventeenth and eighteenth centuries, and French views on the social relations of health are marked by its influence. While the French did not during this period arrive at a systematic formulation like the concept of medical police, they were nevertheless aware of the implications of the police concept in relation to health matters. (In fact the term *police* is itself of French origin). As early as 1711, for instance, the Abbé Claude Fleury, tutor to the grandsons of Louis XIV, referred to the subject of health police, indicating its significance for the welfare of the state and the duty of the monarch to concern himself with its problems[40].

However, the term "medical police" was not generally accepted in the French literature. While a few men, like F. E. Fodéré and C. C. Marc, were in some degree influenced by Frank, the majority of French medical men interested in the social aspects of health and disease pursued an independent course. Mention, should be made, however, of two publications which indicate that during the early nineteenth century limited efforts were made to apply the idea of medical police to specific problems. In 1819, a military doctor named Bidot published a proposal for a code of sanitary and medical police. In scope, it was limited to the prevention and control of epidemic disease[41]. A decade later, Étienne Sainte-Marie surveyed the problems faced by the Health Council of Lyon. In his *Lectures relatives à la police médicale*, he discussed alcoholism, prostitution, abortion, floods, factories, construction of buildings, and poisoning.

A survey of the French literature makes it clear, however, that when French hygienists studied the relations of social and political conditions to health they did so within a framework very different from that in which the concept of medical police had originated and developed. While enlightened absolutism prevailed in most of Europe, the old order was violently overthrown in France and painfully replaced by a world of capitalist enterprise and parliamentary constitutionalism.

IV.

After this survey of the fate of the concept of medical police, it is perhaps not amiss to attempt to assess its significance. In practice, the concept of medical police meant a program of social action for health grounded on a primary calculation to augment the power of the state rather than to increase the welfare of the people. Within these limits, there was undoubtedly a real concern for social welfare, and some concrete results were achieved. In 1817, for example, Johann Peter Frank commented in relation to the practical effect of his *Medicinische Polizey*: "Even though my name does not occur in them, I have stimulated the enactment of various salutory health laws in Europe". Seen in retrospect, however, the imposing concept of medical police was already hollow when Frank made this statement. Theory notwithstanding, the social purposes and ends of medical police were already outmoded and reactionary. During the early decades of the nineteenth century this concept was an ideological superstructure set upon the crumbling foundations of absolutism and cameralism. In short, to undertake to apply this concept to the dilemmas of the new industrial society was to offer a solution in terms of a remedy even then ready to be discarded.

This does not mean, however, the denial of any important achievements and permanent effects to the idea of medical police. These are to be sought not only in specific laws, but also in certain trends and tendencies. For one, the development and exploration of the concept of medical police was a pioneer endeavor in the systematic analysis of the health problems of community life. This trend culminated in the outstanding works of Johann Peter Frank and Franz Anton Mai. Secondly, a definite body of knowledge was collected and these efforts stimulated further study of such problems. To France and England, however, fell the task of developing under the new conditions of the early and middle nineteenth century the fundamental problem defined by Johann Peter Frank and the other workers who created the concept of medical police.

REFERENCES

1. Giuseppe Ziino: *Manuale di Polizia medica ad uso degli Ufficiali Sanitari del Regno e degli Amministratori*, Milano, Leonardo Vallardi, Editore, 1890, p. 2 ff.
2. George Rosen: Cameralism and the Concept of Medical Police, *Bulletin of the History of Medicine* 27: 21–42, 1953.
3. Anzeigen neuer in die medizinische Polizei und in die Volksarzneikunde einschlagenden Schriften, *Archiv der medizinischen Polizey under der gemeinnützigen Arzneikunde* 1: 363, 1703.
4. Alfons Fischer: *Geschichte des deutschen Gesundheitswesens* (2 vols.), Berlin, F. A. Herbig Verlag, 1933, vol. II, p. 133.
5. Aphorisms on medical police.
6. *System einer vollständigen medicinischen Polizey. In einem freyen Auszuge* (des P. Frank Systems), von Dr. J. Joh. Fahner, Berlin, 1792.
7. A theory of the laws relating to the physical well-being of citizens, and the utilization of medicine in the service of legislation.
8. *Denkwürdigkeiten des Philosophen und Arztes Johann Benjamin Erhard.* Herausgegeben von K. A. Varnhagen von Ense, Stuttgart und Tübingen, J. G. Gotta'sche Buchhandlung, 1830, pp. 42, 47; Fischer, *op. cit.*, (see no. 4), (II), p. 131.
9. The care of the state for the health of its citizens.
10. Andreas Röschlaub: Untersuchungen über die eigentlichen Aufgaben der Hygiene, *Hygiea* 1: 245 ff., 1805, cited by Fischer, *op. cit.*, (see no. 4), (II), p. 437.
11. Principles of the science of medical police.
12. Systematic handbook of public health.

13. Joseph Bernt: *Systematisches Handbuch der öffentlichen Gesundheitspflege ...*, Wien, Franz Wimmer und Carl Kupffer, 1818, pp. 1–2, 35.
14. Ibid., pp. XIII–XVI.
15. *Biographie des D. Johann Peter Frank.* Von ihm selbst geschrieben, Wien, 1802, p. 91.
16. *Ibid.*, p. 58; Fischer, *op. cit.*, (see no. 4), (II), p. 134.
17. »Vorschlag und Entwurf medizinischer Polizeygesetze für die eine und untheilbare helvetische Republic«, cited by Fischer, *op. cit.*, (see no. 4), (II), pp. 139–140.
18. For Mai see Max Oeser: *Geschichte der Stadt Mannheim*, J. Bensheimer, 1908, pp. 359–370; Fischer, *op. cit.*, (see no. 4), (II), pp. 47–49, 149–152.
19. Draft of a law on the most important objects of medical police – a contribution toward a new law code for the Palatinate.
20). A. L. Dornblüth: *Darstellung der Medicinal-Polizei-Gesetzgebung und gesammter Medicinal- und Sanitäts-Anstalten für den Civil- und Militärstand im Grossherzogthume Mecklenburg-Schwerin*, Schwerin, 1834.
21. *Handbuch der im Konigreich Sachsen geltenden Medicinal-Polizeigesetze, sämmtliche Gesetze enthaltend, welche der unterm 30. Juli 1836 erschienenen allgemeinen Instruction der Bezirksärzte, Gerichtsärzte und Amtschirurgen zum Grunde liegen ...*, Leipzig, 1837.
22. *Handbuch der in dem Konigreiche Württemberg geltenden Gesetze und Verordnungen in Betreff der Medizinal-Polizei nach dem Stande am Schlusse des Jahrs 1840 ...*, Stuttgart, 1841.
23. A. H. Nicolai: *Die Medicinal- und Veterinär-Polizei*, Berlin 1838; J. H. Schürmayer: *Handbuch der medizinischen Polizei*, Erlangen, 1848, second edition, 1856; Carl Vogel: *Die medizinische Polizeiwissenschaft, theoretisch und praktisch dargestellt*, Jena, 1853; Ferdinand Rauska: *Compendium der Gesundheitspolizei*, Vienna, 1859; W. Haeckermann: *Lehrbuch der Medizinalpolizei*, Berlin, 1863.
24. Leo Liebermann: *Anleitung zu Chemischen Untersuchungen auf dem Gebiete der Medicinalpolizei, Hygiene und Forensischen Praxis*, Stuttgart, 1877.
25. Joseph Bernt: *Systematisches Handbuch der öffentlichen Gesundheitspflege*, 1818, pp. 30–31.
26. J. Uffelmann: Die öffentliche Gesundheitspflege in Italien, *Deutsche Vierteljahresschrift für Gesundheitspflege*, 1879, p. 191.
27. Rosen, *op. cit.*, (see no. 2), pp. 37–41.
28. Rene Sand: *Vers la médecine sociale*, Paris, J. B. Baillière et Fils, 1948, pp. 205–206; Uffelmann, *op. cit.*, (see no. 26), p. 194.
29. C. E. Stangeland: *Pre-Malthusian Doctrines of Population: A Study in the History of Economic Theory* (Studies in History, Economics and Public Law, Vol. XXI, No. 3), New York, Columbia University press, 1904, pp. 290–298.
30. Lorenzo Martini: *Elementi di Polizia Medica*, Torino, 1824; *Polizia Medica*, Capolago, 1834, *Manuali d'Igiene e di Polizia Medica*, Firenze, 1835.
31. Giuseppe Ziino: *Manuale di Polizia Medica*, Milano, Leonardo Vallardi, Editore, 1890, pp. 2–3.
32. Cited by F. A. E. Crew in »Social Medicine as an Academic Discipline«, *Modern Trends in Public Health*, edited by Arthur Massey, New York, Paul B. Hoeber, Inc., 1949, p. 48.
33. *Lectures on Justice, Police, Revenue and Arms*, delivered in the University of Glasgow by Adam Smith reported by a student in 1763 and edited with an introduction and notes by Edwin Cannan, Oxford, Clarendon Press, 1896. See Part II: Of Police.

34. Cited by Crew, *op. cit.*, (see no. 32), p. 51.
35. Thomas Ferguson: *The Dawn of Scottish Social Welfare*, London and New York, Thomas Nelson and Sons, 1948, pp. 57, 97.
36. *British and Foreign Medical Review* 14: 446–461, 1842. See p. 446.
37. James Black: Lectures on public hygiene and medical police, *Provincial Medical and Surgical Journal*, 1844, pp. 275–280; 327–332; 259–364; 391–396; 551–557.
38. W. Strange: On the Formation of a System of National Medical Police and Public Hygiene . . ., *London Medical Gazette*, n. s. II, 452–457, 1846; *The Health and Sickness of Town Populations, considered with reference to proposed Sanatory Legislation, and to the Establishment of a Comprehensive System of Medical Police and District Dispensaries* . . . London, John W. Parker, 1846.
39. Louis Elsberg: The Domain of Medical Police, *American Medical Monthly*, 1862, pp. 321–337.
40. Sand, *op. cit.*, (see no. 28), p. 205.
41. M. Bidot: *Projet d'un Code de Police Sanitaire*, Paris, 1819. See pp. 65–69, 87 ff.

MEDICAL CARE AND SOCIAL POLICY IN SEVENTEENTH CENTURY ENGLAND

When Tudor England moved out of the Middle Ages, one result of the disappearance of the old order was an increase in poverty.[1] This problem was a matter of grave concern, for poverty was regarded as a potential danger to the security of the State. Various acts designed to deal with the poor were passed during the sixteenth century, and these measures were finally consolidated in the Elizabethan law of 1601 (43 Elizabeth, Chapter 2), which remained the basis of English poor law administration for over two centuries.

Administrative responsibility for the relief and government of the poor was assigned to the parish. As the unit of ecclesiastical administration, it was found to be a convenient division for local government. Thus when it became necessary to make systematic provision for the poor, the parochial machinery was adapted to the purpose; and the relation between the poor and the parish became peculiarly close and intimate.

While the law of 1601 makes no specific mention of health matters, it was intended to relieve the "lame, impotent, old, blind, and such other among them being poor and not able to work." As time went on, however, this simple statement was expanded in practice to include the provision of medical and nursing care.

It appears probable that the policy laid down in 1601 was followed until the outbreak of the Civil War. Wartime conditions and official neglect led to a disorganization of poor law administration. This situation was further aggravated by the necessity of providing for wounded soldiers and their dependents.[2] These urgent and exceptional matters demanded attention, and emergency measures were taken to deal with them. In the main, however, poor law policy under the Commonwealth followed along lines previously laid down. Nevertheless, a changed attitude toward the problem of poverty was developed during the period.

There is small doubt that during these years poverty came increasingly to be regarded as a disgraceful social disease. In this respect, the Interregnum anticipated the earlier eighteenth century. This position may in considerable measure be attributed to the influence of Puritanism, that is, the core of common values accepted by the Protestant sects of seventeenth century England. Within this value system certain doctrines are fundamental, among them predestination and justification through good works. Intimately associated with these theological values was an insistence on diligence and industry as necessary and worthwhile, with definite stress on utilitarian considerations. Richard Baxter in his *Christian Directory* justified this principle in these terms: "The public welfare, or the good of the many," he says, "is to be valued above your own. Every man therefore is bound to do all the good he can to others, especially for the church and the commonwealth. And this is not done by idleness, but by labour! As the bees labour to replenish their hive, so man being a sociable creature must labour for the good of the society which he belongs to, in which his own is contained as a part."[3] Furthermore, since methodical, constant labor makes possible success in one's calling, and such success is a sign of salvation, constancy in labor becomes a worthwhile end in itself. From this viewpoint poverty was an abomination, due to lack of moral stamina and systematic application.

But while poverty was regarded as an individual vice and condemned on ethical grounds, it was also discovered to be a potential source of profit to the state and therefore a public convenience. Projects for dealing with the poor and for utilizing their labor were proposed during the Commonwealth, and the number of these proposals increased greatly in the decades following the Restoration. Apparent in these proposals is a mingling of motives, among which mercantilistic considerations and the prospect of profits are prominent. With an insight which is quite remarkable, efforts were made to compute the national cost of idleness, and elaborate calculations were developed as to the increase in national wealth which would result if England's poor were made productive.

Among the proponents of such schemes some were aware of the health needs of the poor. In 1641 there appeared *A Description of the Famous Kingdome of Macaria* by Samuel Hartlib. In this Utopia, Hartlib was interested mainly in proposals for social and economic reform. A special feature of Macaria, however, is a "College of Experience, where they deliver out, yearly, such medicines as they find out by experience; and all such as shall be able to demonstrate any experiment, for the health or wealth of other men, are honourably rewarded at the publick charge."[4] Hartlib also felt that some parish priests would be more useful if they acquired some knowledge of healing, and he pointed out that in Macaria "they think it as absurd for a Divine to be without skill of Physick, as it is to put new wine into old bottles." These comments should not be considered simply as quaint conceits, but must rather be regarded as serious proposals to improve the provision of medical care, especially to the poor. In Caroline England and under the Commonwealth the number of trained physicians was small. During this period medical practitioners more and more formed a group marked by steadily increasing status and remuneration so that their services generally were not available to the poor.[5] At the same time, there is evidence from parish registers and other sources that the clergy did provide home remedies and advice on medical care.[6]

Clearly Hartlib's proposals were in line with these contemporary realities and needs. Evidence for such a view is provided from several different directions. The existence of a medical care problem is confirmed by John Cooke, a conservative and a former member of Charles I's government. In his pamphlet *Unum necessarium*, published in 1648, Cooke pleads for relief of the poor including free medical service.[7] A further indication of the apposite and constructive character of Hartlib's scheme is provided from the opposite end of the political spectrum, from the extreme left wing of the Puritan movement. In 1652 there appeared a book entitled *The Law of Freedom in a Platform or True Magistracy Restored*. The author was Gerrard Winstanley, spokesman for the group called Diggers or True Levellers, an offshoot of the popular democratic party known as the Levellers.[8] This book set out a plan for an agrarian socialist commonwealth. In Winstanley's plan a prominent place was assigned to the clergy. To a large extent the function of the minister was to be an educator. Among his duties would be the instruction of his parishioners in the arts and sciences, including medicine and surgery. It may be that Winstanley was acquainted with Hartlib's suggestion about the clergy and adopted it.

Meanwhile, Hartlib had developed another scheme to deal with the needs of the poor. He proposed, in 1647, the establishment of an Office of Addresses "for the Relief of Human Necessities."[9] This projected Office would function as a labor exchange, information bureau, and a place for the transaction of commercial business. Here would be maintained various registers, of which the most important would deal with the needs of the poor. These would include a list of physicians willing to give their services gratis. Efforts to set up such offices were made in 1650 by Henry Robinson in London, and about the same time in London and Westminster by Hartlib himself. It is not clear, however, whether lists of physicians were maintained at any of these offices.

In 1648, there was published in London a small book of thirty pages entitled *The Advice of W. P. to Mr. S. Hartlib for the Advancement of Some Particular Parts of Learning*. The author was William Petty, then "twenty-four years of age, a perfect Frenchman, and a good linguist in other vulgar languages, besides Latin and Greek; a most rare and exact anatomist and excelling in all mathematical and mechanical learning. . . ."[10] Directly inspired by Hartlib, this booklet presented several proposals for the reform of education. Petty's proposals are in line with a trend found among the Puritans of both the right and left, namely, a desire to apply knowledge to the immediate and practical needs of society. Education is a matter of vital concern to all revolutionary parties, and the leaders and spokesmen of the English revolution were fully aware of this fact. Indeed, the advent of the Long Parliament was the signal for an outburst of discussion and action on the reform of education.[11] The positive proposals for reform reflect the chief aspirations of the rising English middle class: utilitarianism, individualism, and the experimental philosophy. These ideals find concrete expression in Petty's scheme. Of special interest is his proposal for a hospital where physicians and surgeons would give and receive instruction. The hospital would be fully equipped with an anatomical theater, a chemical laboratory, an apothecary shop, a garden and a library. Among the chief personnel would be a physician, "skilled at large in the phenomena of Nature," who "shall either dissect, or overlook the Dissection of Bodies dying of Diseases; and, lastly shall take care that all luciferous Experiments whatsoever may be carefully brought to him, and recorded for the Benefit of Posterity." In addition, there would be an assistant physician who would maintain suitable records on all patients, a surgeon, and an apothecary who would be in charge of the garden. The young medical student would learn the practical side of his profession by accompanying the members of the medical staff from patient to patient.

More clearly than anyone else, perhaps, Petty represents that combination of utilitarianism, commercial drive and experimental philosophy which characterized the approach to social problems in the period following the Restoration and during the eighteenth century.[12] Petty's proposals for educational reform and advancement of knowledge stem in a straight line from Bacon's *New Atlantis* by way of Hartlib's *Macaria,* and point to the enthusiastic promulgation of elaborate projects for commercial undertakings, technological innovations and social reforms during the later seventeenth and earlier eighteenth centuries. This penchant for projects when applied to the burning issue of the poor was to be one of the significant factors determining the framework of theory and practice within which social problems of health would be viewed in the eighteenth and early nineteenth centuries.

Petty is representative, however, not only as a projector, but equally as a pioneer in the quantitative study of social phenomena. The application of the numerical method to the analysis of social problems was a development of first-rate importance, and destined to prove extraordinarily fruitful for the study of the social relations of health and disease. Petty was convinced that social and economic problems could be dealt with most effectively in terms of functional analysis and measurement, what he termed political arithmetic. His employment of this method was not merely a happy chance; he was keenly aware of the end he wished to achieve and of the means by which he proposed to do so.

In the preface to the *Political Anatomy of Ireland*, Petty says: "Sir Francis Bacon, in his *Advancement of Learning*, hath made a judicious parallel in many particulars, between the body natural, and body politic, and between the arts of preserving both in health and strength: and it is as reasonable, that as anatomy is the best foundation of one, so also of the other; and that to practice upon the politick, without knowing the symmetry, fabrick, and proportion of it, is as casual as the practice of old-women and empyricks. Now, because anatomy is not only necessary in physicians, but laudable in every philosophical person whatsoever; I therefore have attempted the first essay of political anatomy."[13]

The means for such study is political arithmetic. Petty's posthumously published work, *Political Arithmetick*, describes it in these terms: "The method I take," he says, "is not yet very usual; for instead of using only comparative and superlative words, and intellectual arguments, I have taken the course (as a specimen of the political arithmetic I have long aimed at) to express myself in terms of number; weight, or measure; to use only arguments of sense, and to consider only such causes, as have visible foundations in nature; leaving those that depend upon the mutable minds, opinions, appetites, and passions of particular men, to the consideration of others."[14]

While Petty coined the term political arithmetic and indicated the significance of a quantitative study of social fact, the most valuable pioneer work in this area was done by his friend John Graunt (1620–1674), a London haberdasher. Graunt's classsic contribution appeared in 1662 and was called *Natural and Political Observations . . . upon the Bills of Mortality*. While Graunt's work was not without antecedents, he was a statistical pioneer blazing a new trail.

Far back in the Middle Ages, numerical data had been collected for specific purposes. The Domesday Book, for instance, provided a complete review of the resources of the kingdom conquered by the Normans, but no statistical use was made of this information.[15] Later, political writers, such as Machiavelli, made use of figures, and mathematical calculations began more and more to be employed in public affairs, particularly by rulers in making surveys of the resources and revenues of their domains. Typical is the survey carried out by a German prince, Wilhelm IV, Landgrave of Hessen-Cassel, who ruled from 1567 to 1592. At the same time, advances in mathematical knowledge and expansion of scientific interests intermingled with these political and economic influences to bring about a still greater employment of numerical information. Two other streams of influence reinforced this trend. One was an increasing awareness of regularity and order in the world of human affairs. The perception of law and order in the physical realm undoubtedly provided a basis for this view. Recognition of an orderly universe made it seem logical to infer that the same might be true for society. The other stream of influence came from the effects of everyday thought and practice. Throughout this period, more and more people were learning how to do simple calculations and make measurements. This spread of the knowledge of elementary mathematics helped to prepare the way for the numerical study of social facts.

Thus it was not a matter of chance that a man like Graunt began to search for mathematical regularities in such human events as births and deaths, the incidence of disease, and related matters. Nor was his search in vain, for Graunt brought to light a number of very important facts. In the first place, he demonstrated the regularity of certain social and vital phenomena. Thus he noted "That among the several casualties some bear a constant proportion into the whole number of burials; such are chronical diseases, and the diseases whereunto the city is most subject; as for example, consumptions, dropsies, jaundice, gout, stone, palsie, scurvy, rising of the lights or mother, rickets, aged, agues, fevers, bloody flux, and scowring: nay, some accidents, as grief, drowning, men's making away themselves, and being kill'd by several accidents, &c. do the like; whereas epidemical and malignant diseases, as the plague, purples, spotted fever, smallpox and measles do not keep that equality; so as in some years, or months there died ten times as many as in others."[16] Secondly, Graunt was the first to note the excess of male over female births as well as the eventual approximate numerical equality of the sexes. Thirdly, he called attention to the excess of the urban over the rural death rate.

In making these discoveries, Graunt clearly demonstrated the usefulness of the statistical approach which Petty advocated. But while he indicated some of the social relations of vital phenomena, as well as the social significance of his studies, Graunt did not pursue further this aspect of the matter. It was precisely in this area, however, that Petty made his most significant contribution.

The inspiration of Petty's interest in political arithmetic is not far to seek. He was concerned with all sorts of practical affairs: fiscal matters, trade, population, education, the plague. Full of the idea that numerical data could throw light on such problems, he employed figures and calculations wherever he could. At all times, however, the focus of interest is not on calculation for its own sake, but always in relation to the specific political, economic or social problem involved. This characteristic orientation is clearly revealed whenever he deals with matters of health, in his discussions of population, and in his various statistical proposals.[17] Throughout his numerous published and unpublished writings occur schemes to increase the power and prestige of England.[18] As an essential element of these schemes, Petty urged repeatedly the collection of statistical data on population, trade, manufacture, education, diseases, revenue and many other topics. The breadth of his approach is strikingly illuminated by his "Method of enquiring into the state of any country." This memorandum outlined a complete scheme for a political, economic, social and health survey. Among the topics listed are not only a census of the population, and the nature of the public revenue, but even such questions as "What are the bookes that do sell most."[19]

Within this broad frame of reference Petty was able to grasp clearly the social relations and implications of a number of health problems. Thus, he recognized that it was not enough simply to acknowledge natural fertility and population as major conditions of national prosperity. The acceptance of this premise went hand in hand with the responsibility for removing impediments to the full development of these resources. A major aspect of this responsibility was the creation of conditions and facilities which would promote health, prevent disease and render medical care easily accessible to those who should have it. The achievement of these aims required that medical knowledge be advanced to the greatest degree possible, and Petty pointed out that it is the duty of the state to foster medical progress. "Now suppose," he said, in a lecture given at Dublin in 1676, "that in the King's Dominions there be 9 millions of people, of which 360,000 dye every year, and from whom 440,000 are borne. And suppose that by the advancement of the art of Medicine, a quarter part fewer dye. Then the King will gain and save 200,000 subjects per annum, which valued at 20£ per head, the lowest price of slaves, will make 4 million per annum benefit to the Commonwealth. Now I consider that the thorough and profound search into the naturall and entire state of animals by anatomy, and into their depraved and vitiated estate by the comparitive and contrasted observations in hospitalls, may in 100 years advance the art of medicine as above said. Wherefore it is not the Interest of the State to leave Phisitians and Patients (as now) to their own shifts."[20]

Almost thirty years earlier, Petty had recognized the crucial importance of the hospital in the training of physicians and in the furthering of medical research, and to this point he returned again and again. In various connections, he urged the establishment of hospitals. In the lecture cited above, he commented that "Another cause of defect in the art of medicine and consequently of its contempt is that there have not been Hospitalls for the accommodation of sick people, Rich as well as Poor, so instituted and fitted as to encourage all sick persons to resort unto them —Every sort of such hospitalls to differ only in splendor, but not at all in the Sufficiency for the means and remedy for the Patients health. For by such means the most able understandings might be encouraged, equally with the best of the professions, to spend and to dedicate themselves wholly to this faculty; and a man shall learn in a well regulated hospitall, where he may halfe a hower's time observe his choice of 1000 patients, more in one yeare then in ten without it, even by reading the best Books that can be written. For, as one may learn to know and distinguish a face better by one minut's Inspection then by reading ten sheets of paper in the description of it, So wee may learn more of sick people by the Joynt assistance of all our sences together than by the lame descriptions of words alone."[21]

Petty supplemented these general recommendations by specific proposals. These dealt particularly with health problems where he felt that the state by establishing hospitals would derive the greatest gain. Thus, in 1687, in "An Essay for the Emprovement of London," Petty proposed "That there bee a Council of Health viz. for the Plague, acute and epidemicall diseases, aged foundlings, as also for persons and houses of correction, and all sorts of hospitalls and women in childbed."[22] Another memorandum composed in the same year suggests a hospital of 1000 beds for London. For Petty, the basic political and economic importance of population was axiomatic. Consequently, any measures to prevent impairment of population by disease and death were matters of high concern. Control of communicable disease, especially plague, and the saving of infant life would, Petty felt, contribute most toward this end. This conviction is reflected in his various suggestions for combating plague, and advocating maternity hospitals. In dealing with the plague, he suggested that the government should consider carefully "what sum of money, and Meanes ought to be prudently ventured for the probable cutting off 3 fifths of this Calamity."[23] Petty recommended the establishment of isolation hospitals, to which plague patients would be removed and where they would receive medical care. To buttress this recommendation, and in general the usefulness of any measures undertaken to combat the ravages of the plague, he undertook to calculate the economic loss due the disease.[24] Similarly, he advocated the creation of maternity hospitals, having in mind particularly unmarried pregnant women. Petty contemplated that in return for such provision provided by government, the children would become wards of the state and serve it for twenty-five years, thus adding to the labor resources of the country.[25] He also believed that certain other groups in the population were of direct concern to government. These elements comprised the occupational groups esteemed as most productive—farmers, manufacturers, merchants, seamen and soldiers. In his opinion, these occupations "are the very pillars of any commonwealth."[26] In keeping with this point of view are suggestions by Petty that studies be made of occupational morbidity and mortality.[27]

Finally, Petty realized that to achieve these ends an adequate supply of medical personnel would be required. Consequently, he proposed that an analysis be made of the medical need, using methods such as those of Graunt, and then on this basis to calculate the numbers of physicians, surgeons and others necessary to meet this need. In short, Petty proposed that the number of medical personnel be planned and adjusted to meet the actual need for medical care. "As for Physicians," he wrote, "it is not hard by the help of the observations which have been lately made upon the Bills of Mortality,[28] to know how many are sick in *London* by the numbers of them that dye, and by the proportions of the City to finde out the same of the Country; and by both by the advice of the learned Colledge of that Faculty to calculate how many Physicians were requisite for the whole Nation; and consequently, how many students in that art to permit and encourage; and lastly, having calculated these numbers, to adoptate a proportion of Chyrurgeons, Apothecaries, and Nurses to them, and so by the whole to cut off and extinguish that infinite swarm of vain pretenders unto, and abusers of that God-like Faculty, which of all Secular Employments our Saviour himself after he began to preach engaged himself upon."[29]

Petty's views on the social and economic implications of health problems are beyond all comparison the most significant English contribution to this area of social thought prior to the nineteenth century. To get a clear picture of Petty's position it is necessary to piece together numerous separate statements. When this is done, however, there emerges a relatively coherent and logical structure. Essentially a disciple of Hobbes in his political theory, Petty accepted the thesis that government is justified in carrying out any policy or instituting measures by which national power and wealth would be increased. At the same time, he recognized that while individuals or groups might be harnessed to the needs of the state, public policy should also aim at improving their living standards. Populousness was exceedingly desirable, but the people should also be healthy and happy.

Petty was not alone in dealing with the social aspects of health problems, or in attempting to study them quantitatively. Among his contemporaries and followers these interests were expressed in varying degree and some were keenly alive to the importance of a healthy population as a factor in national opulence. Closest to Petty, perhaps, was his younger contemporary Nehemiah Grew (1641–1712), also a physician, but best known today for his work in plant anatomy. Sometime in 1707 apparently, Grew prepared for Queen Anne a memorandum entitled *The Meanes of a Most Ample Encrease of the Wealth and Strength of England in a Few Years Humbly represented to her Majestie In the Fifth Year of Her Reign.*[30] As the title indicates, this document outlined an economic program to enhance the prosperity and power of England. Grew's focus of interest was the same as Petty's, and his handling of health problems occurs within a similar context. He knew Petty, to whom he refers as "my late Honoured Friend," and frequently mentions Petty's calculations, though he does not always accept them. Like Petty in the *Political Anatomy of Ireland,* Grew couched his discussion in terms of anatomy and physiology. In his opinion the four basic elements in the economic anatomy of England are land, manufactures, foreign trade, and population. Ultimately, however, Grew's program depended on the size and quality of the population, and to this subject he devoted the fourth section of his memorandum. Grew assumed as axiomatic the need for increasing population to provide the necessary labor power. Among his recommendations toward this end, he urged that the state do all in its power to maintain health and prevent disease. Grew emphasized the economic burden of disease, commenting that in economic terms the sick are worse than dead because they become either public or private charges. To make medical care available to all, Grew proposed that the government regulate physicians' fees according to their experience. If this were done the cost of medical care could be reduced and thus made accessible to those who needed it.

Despite their bold and penetrating character, the ideas of Petty and Grew had no immediately tangible results. Their proposals did not lead to a satisfaction of human needs in relation to health, because they were implicitly premised on a type of governmental structure which was even then being discarded. Effective implementation would have required the existence of a well-developed local administrative mechanism operating under strongly centralized control, in a manner comparable to the organizations of France or Prussia. But it was precisely these organs of administration which were then disappearing. After 1660 there was no planned effort to use local officials as efficient organs of a consistent policy.

Cunningham, the economic historian, employed the term "parliamentary Colbertism" to describe this period and its continuation in the eighteenth centry.[31] Although this designation is only partly correct, it calls attention to contemporary French developments, and by inviting comparison makes it possible to focus more sharply the characteristic features of English evolution. Colbert created a whole system of administrative regulation under central control, and built up a bureaucracy to keep the machinery in operation. In England, on the other hand, the administrative apparatus which had been developed under the first Stuarts had collapsed and was not being replaced. To a considerable degree this was due to a shift of emphasis in the interest of the state. Following the Restoration, and particularly after the revolution of 1688, the focus of governmental interest shifted more and more to commercial and colonial policy, and regulation in relation to these areas of activity. This had important results on the development of social policy, and on the evolution of ideas concerning the social relations of health.

As the control of the Crown relaxed, local government in the course of the eighteenth century became increasingly a matter of local initiative. In England, local government was carried on by the counties, and by the parishes into which the counties were divided. As a result, the county officials, especially the justices of the peace, gained in power and prestige. It was to the justices that the parish authorities were accountable.[32] There was very little explicit theorizing about this trend of development, but it is clearly reflected in the treatment of social problems, and provides the frame of reference within which thought and actions in matters of health must be viewed. Indeed, the outstanding feature of internal English administration during the period from the Act of

Settlement and Removal, passed in 1662, to the Poor Law Amendment Act of 1834 is its intensely parochial character. As a result, England was deprived of any uniform social policy, since there was no machinery to subordinate the interests of the parish to the welfare of the larger community.

During the earlier part of this period, ideas, proposals and programs relating to the social aspects of health took as points of departure either the responsibility of the parish in relieving the needs of the poor, or the desire to increase national wealth by employing the destitute in manufacture. The Elizabethan Poor Law had provided that the parish would carry out the "necessary Relief of the lame, impotent, old, blind and such other among them . . . not able to work," and in time the scope of this provision came to include medical care. Such provision for the sick meant that the parish had to assume considerable responsibilities. However, the parish officers generally had neither training nor desire to engage in such activities. This situation gave rise in parochial administration to the common practice of contracting with private persons to perform public tasks. This system of "contracting" or "farming out the poor" became a typical feature of English Poor Law administration in the eighteenth century. Following this general pattern, parish officers often contracted with a local practitioner for medical treatment of their poor.[33] These contracts varied from parish to parish. Sometimes, the medical practitioner contracted to attend all the poor living in the parish, or only those for whom the parish was legally responsible, and to supply medicine as well. Occasionally, a separate agreement was made with an apothecary. Other contracts exempted such items as smallpox inoculation or epidemic diseases. Some parishes paid per-head, others on a fee for service basis. The practice of farming out public functions such as poor relief became popular because it was regarded as offering an opportunity for reducing taxes. A system of this kind was bound to lead to abuses. Nevertheless, it must be recognized that medical care of a sort was provided, and that the pattern of administration developed in this area had an influence in shaping later schemes for the provision of medical care.

Nonetheless, little attention was given to this subject by contemporary writers and theorists. Such ideas as were developed concerning social problems of health arose rather out of another aspect of the problem of the poor, namely, the desire to put the poor to work. The problem of the laboring poor, concretely symbolized in the figure of the pauper, occupied a strategic position in the social logic of the eighteenth century. It must be recognized, however, that the category of the "poor" was a broad one, practically synonymous with the "common people." Generally speaking, the "poor" meant all the people who were actually in need, as well as all those potentially eligible for this unenviable distinction.

Behind this concern with the laboring poor were several distinctive motivations. Each parish was responsible for the maintenance of its own poor, and consequently was concerned to reduce this burden as far as possible. It was felt that this might be accomplished by making arrangements to employ the poor. At the same time, this approach was in keeping with the contemporary desire to stimulate national prosperity by using the unemployed poor in manufactures. England at this time was entering upon the path toward industrialism, and the proponents of this view believed that the poor could provide an easily available labor force for the expansion of industry. Between the Restoration and the end of the eighteenth century scores of books and pamphlets were written on this subject, and many projects were suggested to deal with the problem. These proposals, as well as the optimism and eagerness with which they were put forth are characteristic of the tendency of the period to indulge in projects. This tendency is perhaps best described in the words of Daniel Defoe. "Necessity, which is allowed to be the mother of invention," he wrote in 1697, "has so violently agitated the wits of men at this time, that it seems not at all improper, by way of distinction, to call it the Projecting Age. For though in times of war and public confusions the like humour of invention has seemed to stir, yet, without being partial to the present, it is, I think, no injury to say the past ages have never come up to the degree of projecting and inventing, as it refers to matters of negoce, and methods of civil polity, which we see this age arrived to."[34]

The avowed aim of the projectors was to create centers of manufacture in the form of workhouses where the poor could learn to support themselves. This idea did not actually become popular until the end of the seventeenth century, when a corporation for the relief and employment of the poor was established by act of Parliament at Bristol in 1696. Here all the parishes of the town were combined into a single unit. This experiment developed out of a frank recognition that the individual parish was too small a unit to provide remunerative employment for the poor.[35] The example set by Bristol was soon followed by other towns, and during the earlier eighteenth century there was a steady increase in the number of workhouses. It is of interest to note that while the Board of Trade was considering the problem of pauperism, John Locke, the philosopher, then a member of the Board, proposed a nation-wide system of workhouses.[36] The Bristol experiment probably influenced Locke, particularly since he was a friend of John Cary, its leading proponet.

While the enthusiastic belief in the efficacy of workhouses to deal with poverty was never realized, plans and programs for coping with the health problems of the poor were developed and some of these were even put into practice. Closest to the prevailing parochial pattern was the mode of providing medical care for the sick poor at Bristol. "To such as were sick," stated Carey, "we gave warrants to our physician to visit them; such as wanted the assistance of our surgeons were directed to them, and all were relieved till they were able to work; by which means the Poor, having been well attended, were set at work again, who by neglect might with their families, have been chargeable to the corporation."[37]

More imaginative, immeasurably broader in scope, and based on considerable insight into the socio-economic aspects of health was the plan proposed by John Bellers in 1714.[38] Bellers (1654 – 1725) was a Quaker cloth merchant of London who around 1679 began to carry on philanthropic work to improve the lives of the poor. Toward this end, he put forward a number of proposals, verbally and in books. Best known of these is his *Proposals for Raising a Colledge of Industry of all useful Trades and Husbandry* . . . which first appeared in 1695. In 1710, Bellers published *Some Reasons for an European State* . . ., presenting in essence a plan for a supranational organization like the League of Nations or the United Nations.

In 1714, Bellers published a treatise in which he set forth a plan for a national health service. This is the substance of his *Essay Towards the Improvement of Physick. In Twelve Proposals. By which the Lives of many Thousands of the Rich, as well as of the Poor, may be Saved Yearly. With an Essay for Imploying the Able Poor, by which the Riches of the Kingdom may be greatly Increased; Humbly Dedicated to the Parliament of Great Britain.*

The substance of Beller's argument and proposals may be summed up as follows: Illness and untimely death are a waste of human life. The health of the people is extremely important to the community so that it cannot be left to the uncertainty of individual initiative, which the high incidence of curable disease shows to be inadequate to the task of dealing with this social problem. On these grounds Bellers proposed the establishment of hospitals and laboratories to be used as teaching and research centers, the erection of a national health institute, and the provision of medical care to the sick poor.

While the full potentialities of this remarkable plan were to remain unrealized for over two centuries, there was an increasing recognition in Britain during the eighteenth century of the need for medical assistance to certain groups in the population. It was this period, particularly the years from 1714 to 1790, which witnessed the creation of dispensaries, general hospitals in London and the provinces, and hospitals for special groups of patients. The dispensary movement as well as the hospital movement found their impetus chiefly in private initiative and contributions, although there was some governmental assistance in the form of legislative action. This development of private initiative coupled with cooperative action is characteristic of Britain in the eighteenth century. To a very considerable degree this phenomenon is related to the limited character of local governmental activity. In many ways, this very aspect of the governmental system gave increasingly greater scope to private initiative, making it necessary and possible to deal on an empirical basis with new problems as they presented themselves. Indeed, throughout this period Parliamentary action was generally undertaken on the basis of previously established local programs and projects. Out of such activities there gradually emerged a theory of social action in relation to health. This "New Philosophy," as it was called by Sir Thomas Bernard, may be considered the British counterpart of the continental concept of medical police.[39] While not as systematically developed, it was an accurate reflection of the activities carried on by physicians and laymen. In fact, the "New Philosophy" did for the area of health and social welfare what Adam Smith achieved contemporaneously for economic organization. It provided a theoretical formulation of the consequences which men had already drawn practically from the new social order. But it was during the seventeenth century that the basis of this order was created. In retrospect, it is clear that English social policy in relation to medical care first began to take modern form in the seminal seventeenth century.

REFERENCES

1. a. de Schweinitz, K. *England's road to social security.* Philadelphia, Univ. of Pennsylvania Press, 1950, pp. 20 – 29.
   b. Marshall, D. *The English poor in the Eighteenth Century.* London, George Routledge & Sons, 1926, pp. 1 – 6; 15 – 18.
   c. James, M. *Social problems and policy during the Puritan revolution 1640* – 1660. London, George Routledge & Sons, 1930, pp. 241 – 243.
2. a. Firth, C. H. *Cromwell's army.* New York, James Pott & Co., 1902, pp. 266 – 270.
   b. James, M. Reference 1c. pp. 254 – 256.
3. Merton, R. K. Science, technology and society in Seventeenth Century England, *Osiris* *4*:360 – 632, 1938 (see page 422).

4. a. Hartlib, S. *A description of the famous Kingdome of Macaria*, 1641; reprinted in *Harleian Miscallany 4*:382, 1808 – 1811.
   b. James, M. Reference 1c, pp. 307 – 308.
   c. Stimson D. Hartlib, Haak and Oldenburg: Intelligencers, *Isis 31*:309 – 26, 1940.
   d. Turnbull, G. H. *Samuel Hartlib*. Oxford, 1920.
5. a. Mathew, D. *The social structure of Caroline England*. Oxford, Clarendon Press, 1948, pp. 59 – 62.
   b. Gretton, R. H. *The English middle class*. London, G. Bell & Sons, 1919, pp. 146–149.
6. Tate, W. E. *The parish chest. A study of the records of parochial administration in England*. Cambridge, England, University Press, 1946, pp. 79; 279.
7. a. James, M. Reference 1c, pp. 273 – 274.
   b. Woodhouse, A. S. P., editor. *Puritanism and liberty. Being the Army Debates (1647 – 9) from the Clarke manuscripts with supplementary documents*. London, J. M. Dent & Son, 1938, p. 48.
8. a. Gooch, G. P. *English democratic ideas in the Seventeenth Century*. 2. ed. Cambridge, England, University Press, 1927.
   b. Bernstein, E. *Cromwell and communism. Socialism and democracy in the great English revolution*. London, G. Allen & Unwin, 1930.
   c. Winstanley, G. *The Works of Gerard Winstanley*, edited with an introduction by G. H. Sabine. Ithaca, N.Y., Cornell University Press, 1941.
   d. Rosen, G. Left-wing Puritanism and science, *Bull. Hist. Med. 15*:375 – 80, 1944.
9. James, M. Reference 1c, pp. 311–313.
10. Fitzmaurice, E. G. *Life of Sir William Petty, 1623 –1687*. London, J. Murray 1895, p. 12.
11. a. James, M. Reference 1c, pp. 314 – 326.
   b. Jones, R. F. Puritanism, science and Christ Church, *Isis 31*:65 – 67, 1939.
   c. Simon, J. Educational policies and programmes, *Mod. Quart. 4*:154 – 68, 1949.
   d. Jones, R. F. *Ancients and moderns. A Study of the background of the Battle of the books*. (Washington University Studies. New series. Language and literature, No. 6). St. Louis, 1936, pp. 91 – 123.
12. Houghton, W. E., Jr. History of trades: its relation to Seventeenth-Century thought, *J. Hist. Ideas 2*:33 – 60, 1941.
13. Petty, W. *Economic writings*, edited by C. H. Hull. Cambridge, England, University Press, 1899, vol. 1, p. 129.
14. Petty, W. Reference 13, p. 244.
15. Clark, G. N. *Science and social welfare in the age of Newton*. Oxford, Clarendon Press, 1937, pp. 121 – 132.
16. Graunt, J. *Natural and political observations upon the Bills of Mortality*, in Petty, W. *Economic writings* (Reference 13), vol. 2, p. 352.
17. Petty, W. *Economic writings* (Reference 13), vol. 1, pp. *XIX, IXXII*.
18. Petty, W. *The Petty papers. Some unpublished writings of Sir William Petty*, edited from the Bowood papers by the Marquis of Lansdowne. London, Constable & Co., 1927, vol. 1, pp. 255 – 258; 263 – 276.
19. Petty, W. *The Petty papers* (Reference 18), vol. 1, p. 176.
20. Petty, W. Reference 18, vol. 2, p. 176.
21. Petty, W. Reference 18, vol. 2.
22. Petty, W. Reference 18, vol. 1, p. 35.
23. Petty, W. Reference 18, vol. 1, p. 274.
24. a. Petty, W. *Economic writings* (Reference 13), pp. 109 – 110; 151; 303; 463; 536.
   b. Petty, W. *The Petty papers*. (Reference 18), vol. 1, pp. 33; 36 – 40; 256 – 257.
   c. Fitzmaurice, E. G. *Life of Sir William Petty* (Reference 10), p. 121.

25. Petty, W. *The Petty papers* (Reference 18), vol. 1, p. 267; vol. 2, p. 55.
26. Petty, W. *Economic writings* (Reference 13), p. 259.
27. Petty, W. *The Petty papers* (Reference 18), vol. 1, p. 195; vol. 2, p. 170.
28. Graunt, J. *Observations* (Reference 16).
29. Petty, W. *Economic writings* (Reference 13), p. 27.
30. Johnson, E. A. *Predecessors of Adam Smith. The growth of British economic thought.* New York, Prentice-Hall, 1937, pp. 117 – 138.
31. Cunningham, W. *The growth of English industry and commerce in modern times.* Cambridge, England, University Press, 1912, vol. 1, pp. 403 ff.
32. Brown, W. *Astraeae abdicata restauratio or Advice to the Justices of the Peace.* London, 1695.
33. a. Marshall, D. *The English poor in the Eighteenth Century* (Reference 1b), pp. 115–118; 120–122.
    b. Tate, W. E. *The parish chest.* (Reference 6), pp. 165 – 166.
    c. Fessler, A. A medical contract from the Eighteenth Century, *Brit. med. J. 2:* 1112 – 13, 1950.
34. a. Defoe, D. *An essay upon projects, 1697,* in *The Earlier Life and the Chief Earlier Works of Daniel Defoe,* edited by Henry Morley, London, George Routledge & Sons, 1889, p. 31.
    b. Sombart, W. *Der Bourgeois. Zur Geistesgeschichte des modernen Wirtschaftsmenschen.* Munich and Leipzig, Duncker & Humbolt, 1920, pp. 54 – 55; 66 – 67.
35. a. Marshall, D. *The English poor in the Eighteenth Century* (Reference 1b), pp. 127 – 128.
    b. de Schweinitz, K. *England's road to social security* (Reference 1a), pp. 53 – 55.
36. Fox-Bourne, H. R. *The life of John Locke.* New York, Harper, 1876, vol. 2, pp. 376 – 392.
37. de Schweinitz, K. *England's road to social security* (Reference 1a), p. 53.
38. Bellers, J. *John Bellers, 1654–1725. Quaker, economist and social reformer. His writings reprinted, with a Memoir by A. Ruth Fry.* London, Cassell & Co., 1935, pp. 5 – 28.
39. *Reports of the Society for Bettering the Condition and Increasing the Comforts of the Poor.* London, W. Bulmer & Co., 1802, vol. 3, p. 2.

ECONOMIC AND SOCIAL POLICY IN THE DEVELOPMENT OF PUBLIC HEALTH

An Essay in Interpretation*

I

PUBLIC health as an area of human interest and activity owes its existence to the biological and social nature of man. As a biological organism, man is subject to fundamental needs, such as alimentation and excretion, and to vital processes whose varying manifestations are summed up in the concepts of health and disease. Throughout history, men have lived in larger or smaller social units and have had to reckon with the consequences of these biological facts for the welfare of the group. The ways in which this has been accomplished have been determined chiefly by the social and economic organization of the group and by the scientific and technical means available to it.

For this reason the history of public health must deal with two components. In one aspect it reflects the development of medical science and technology. Understanding of the nature and cause of disease provides a basis for preventive action and control. But the effective application of such knowledge depends on a variety of non-medical elements, basically on economic and social factors. This is the other major strand in the fabric of public health, and it is with this component that we are presently concerned.

The various elements of society are related to each other as parts of a total structural configuration. At any given time and place the dynamic or functional aspect of society is revealed in the circumstance that the social structure as a whole, and its constituent elements in varying degree, are directed toward definite goals in terms of implied or explicitly accepted values. The implementation and realization of these values require the formulation, statement, and application of demands and expectations concerning the future. The term *policy* is generally employed for such a projected program of goals and practices. Therefore, as used here, economic and social policy refers to the principles of

* An address delivered before the Osler Society of the University of Western Ontario Medical School on March 11, 1953.

societal action or inaction, most often exercised through the agency of government—the *agenda* or *non agenda* of the state as Bentham called them—in regard to economic and social problems.

The foregoing considerations lead directly to the thesis of this study, namely, that economic and social policy has been a fundamental factor in the development of public health. The historical significance of this factor has been profound and broad. In innumerable ways of which we are often unaware, earlier policy continues to affect us. Directly or indirectly, many far-reaching legislative and administrative developments in public health have emerged on the basis of economic and social policy. Indeed, it is no exaggeration to say that it is impossible to understand fully the evolution and meaning of public health, especially in the modern period, without recognition and comprehension of the rôle of economic and social policy. Here it will not be possible to explore this thesis in all its historical ramifications. Instead, we shall endeavor to see how it applies in one case, namely, in some developments of public health in Great Britain from the seventeenth century to the present. Where it appears relevant, attention will also be directed to appropriate points in the evolution of public health in other countries.

II

Mercantilist ideas and practices were as characteristic of England in the seventeenth and earlier eighteenth centuries as of the contemporary continental states.[1] For policy makers in all these countries the important question was: What policy must the government pursue in order to increase the national wealth and the national power? In each country, however, the answer given to the question was an answer in terms of its historical experience, its political structure, and its economic and social circumstances.

That industry was one of the chief means by which a country could attain productivity and wealth appeared clear to public officials, men of affairs, and writers on economics and politics. With the growth of industry in seventeenth century England, production came to be regarded as a matter of central importance in economic activity, and labor, one of the most important factors of production, as an essential element in the generation of national

[1] E. Lipson, England in the age of mercantilism. *Journal of Business History* 1932, 4, 691-707. Leo Gershoy, *From despotism to revolution 1763-1789*. New York and London, Harper and Bros., 1944, pp. 39-43; Maurice Dobb, *Studies in the development of capitalism*. London, George Routledge and Sons, 1946, p. 209.

wealth. Obviously, any loss of labor productivity due to illness and death was a significant economic problem.

It was in the interest of the state to have the largest possible number of healthy productive subjects. Moreover, since population was a factor of production it was essential to know the number and the "value of people,"[2] especially of those occupational groups esteemed most productive. It was the recognition of this need in England in the seventeenth century that led to the first significant attempts to apply statistical methods to the public health.

Another aspect of the larger question of population and productivity concerned the poor. To increase population was eminently desirable, but, unless employed, people were only potential sources of wealth. The problem of poverty was thus inextricably linked with that of employment, so that the poor occupied a strategic position in the logic of English social and economic policy. Numerous schemes for dealing with this question were proposed, and in this connection various individuals began to explore the problem of social action in matters of health, inclusive of medical care.

No one perhaps is more significantly representative of these trends than William Petty, physician, wealthy landowner, scientist, and above all, social projector. He personifies that combination of utilitarianism, commercial drive, and experimental philosophy which characterized the approach to social, economic, and health problems in the period following the Commonwealth.[3] Petty's proposals for the advancement of knowledge and educational reform stem in a straight line from Bacon's *New Atlantis* by way of Hartlib's *Macaria* and point to the enthusiastic promulgation of elaborate projects for commercial undertaking, technological innovation, and social reform during the later seventeenth and early eighteenth centuries. Petty is representative, however, not only as a projector, but equally as a pioneer in the quantitative study of social phenomena. The application of the numerical method to the analysis of social problems was an event of first-rate importance and was destined to prove extraordinarily fruitful for the study and development of public health. Petty was convinced that such problems could be dealt with most effectively in terms of func-

2 The phrase "value of people" is used repeatedly by William Petty. See *The economic writings of Sir William Petty. . . .* edited by C. H. Hull. Cambridge, at the University Press, 1899, 2 vols., pp. 108, 152, 267, 454.

3 W. E. Houghton, Jr., The history of trades: its relations to seventeenth century thought. *J. Hist. Ideas,* 1941, 2, 33-60.

tional analysis and measurement, what he called *political arithmetic*. "The method I take," he wrote, "is . . . to express myself in terms of number, weight, or measure; to use only arguments of sense, and to consider only such causes, as have visible foundations in nature. . . ."[4]

While Petty coined the term political arithmetic and outlined the significance of a quantitative study of social fact, the first important demonstration of the usefulness of the statistical approach was undertaken by his friend John Graunt. His classic contribution appeared in 1662 under the title *Natural and Political Observations . . . upon the Bills of Mortality*. While Graunt's work was not without antecedents, he blazed a new trail and brought to light a number of important facts.[5] In the first place, he demonstrated the regularity of certain social and vital phenomena. Thus he noted "that among the several casualties some bear a constant proportion unto the whole number of burials; such are chronical diseases, and the diseases whereunto the city is most subject; as for example, consumptions, dropsies, jaundice, gout, stone, palsie, scurvy, rising of the lights or mother, rickets, aged, agues, fevers, bloody flux, and scowring; nay, some accidents, as grief, drowning, men's making away themselves, and being kill'd by several accidents, & c. do the like; whereas epidemical and malignant diseases, as the plague, purples, spotted fever, smallpox and measles do not keep that equality: so as in some years, or months there died ten times as many as in others."[6] Secondly, Graunt was the first to note the excess of male over female births as well as the eventual approximate numerical equality of the sexes. Thirdly, he called attention to the excess of the urban over the rural death rate.

Although Graunt seems to have been aware of the social significance of his studies, he did not pursue further this aspect of the matter. It was precisely in this area, however, that Petty made his most pregnant contribution. In line with mercantilist thought and practice, he approached problems of health and disease in terms of

[4] Petty, *Economic writings*, vol. 1, p. 129.

[5] Jakob Burckhardt, *The civilization of the Renaissance in Italy*. London and New York, Phaidon Press, 1944, pp. 45-47, 50-52; Alfred von Martin, *Soziologie der Renaissance*. Stuttgart, Ferdinand Enke Verlag, 1932, pp. 26-31; G. N. Clark, *Science and social welfare in the age of Newton*. Oxford, Clarendon Press, 1937, pp. 121-132.

[6] Petty, *Economic writings*, p. 352. A good deal has been written about the possible authorship of the Graunt treatise by Petty. Those interested may consult the following: Petty, *Economic writings*, pp. XXXIX-LIV; *The Petty Papers*, 1927, vol. II, pp. 273-284; Major Greenwood, *Medical statistics from Graunt to Farr*. Cambridge, At the University Press, 1948, pp. 36-39.

their significance for the political and economic strength of the state. This characteristic orientation is clearly revealed whenever he deals with matters of health, in his discussion of population, and in his various statistical proposals. Throughout his numerous published and unpublished writings occur schemes to increase the power and prestige of England.[7] As an essential element of these schemes, Petty urged repeatedly the collection of statistical data on population, trade, manufacture, education, diseases, revenue, and many other topics. The breadth of his approach is strikingly illuminated by his "Method of enquiring into the state of any country." This memorandum outlined a complete scheme for a political, economic, social, and health survey. Among the topics listed are not only a census of the population and the nature of the public revenue, but even such questions as "What are the bookes that do sell most. . . ."[8]

Within this broad frame of reference Petty was able to grasp clearly the relations and implications of a number of public health problems. Thus, he saw that it was not enough simply to recognize natural fertility and population as major conditions of national prosperity. The acceptance of this premise went hand in hand with the responsibility for removing impediments to the full development of these resources. A major aspect of this responsibility was the creation of conditions and facilities which would promote health, prevent disease, and render medical care easily accessible to those who should have it. The achievement of these aims required that medical knowledge be advanced to the greatest degree possible, and Petty pointed out that it is the duty of the state to foster medical progress.[9] In 1648, Petty had published in London a small book entitled *The Advice of W. P. to Mr. S. Hartlib for the Advancement of Some Particular Parts of Learning.* In it he had recognized the crucial importance of the hospital in the training of physicians and in the furtherance of medical research, and to this point he returned again and again. In various connections Petty urged the establishment of hospitals, not only as a general recommendation, but also in specific proposals. Thus, in 1687, in "An Essay for the Emprovement of London," Petty proposed "That there bee a Councill of Health viz. for the Plague, acute

[7] *The Petty Papers. Some unpublished writings of Sir William Petty,* edited from the Bowood Papers by the Marquis of Lansdowne. London, Constable & Co., 1927, 2 vols., vol. I, pp. 255-258, 263-276.

[8] *Ibid.,* vol. I, p. 176.

[9] *Ibid.,* vol. II, p. 176.

and epidemicall diseases, aged foundlings, as also for persons and houses of correction, and all sorts of hospitalls and women in child-bed."[10] Another memorandum composed in the same year suggests a hospital of a thousand beds for London. For Petty, the basic political and economic importance of population was axiomatic. Consequently, any measures to prevent impairment of population by disease and death were matters of great concern. Control of communicable disease, especially plague, and the saving of infant life would, Petty felt, contribute most toward this end. This conviction is reflected in his various suggestions for combating plague and establishing maternity hospitals. He recommended the establishment of isolation hospitals to which plague patients would be removed and where they would receive medical care. To buttress this recommendation, and in general the usefulness of any measures intended to combat the ravages of the plague, he undertook to calculate the economic loss due to the disease.[11] Similarly, he advocated the creation of maternity hospitals, having in mind particularly unmarried women. Petty contemplated that in return for such provision by government, the children would become wards of the state and serve it for twenty-five years, thus adding to the labor resources of the country. He also believed that certain occupational groups in the population were of direct concern to the state. In keeping with this point of view, are his suggestions that studies be made of occupational morbidity and mortality.[12]

Finally, Petty realized that to achieve these aims an adequate supply of medical personnel would be required. Consequently, he proposed that an analysis be made of health needs, using the methods that Graunt had employed and then on this basis to calculate the numbers of physicians, surgeons, and others necessary to meet these needs. In short, Petty proposed that the number of medical personnel be planned and adjusted to meet the actual need for medical care.[13]

Petty was not alone in dealing with health problems, or in attempting to study them quantitatively. Among his contemporaries and successors, these interests were expressed in varying degree, and some were keenly alive to the importance of a healthy population as a factor in national opulence. One might mention

[10] *Ibid.*, vol. I, p. 35.

[11] For Petty's recommendations concerning the plague, and his various estimates of the economic loss due to the disease, see his *Economic writings*, pp. 109-110, 151, 303, 463, 536; also *The Petty Papers*, I, pp. 33, 36-40, 256-257.

[12] *Petty Papers*, I, pp. 195, 267; II, 55, 170; Petty, *Economic writings*, p. 259.

[13] Petty, *Economic writings*, p. 27.

Samuel Hartlib, Gerrard Winstanley, or Peter Cornelius Plockhoy, but perhaps closest to Petty was his younger contemporary Nehemiah Grew, also a physician, who is best known today for his work in plant anatomy. Sometime in 1707 apparently, Grew prepared for Queen Anne a memorandum entitled, *The Meanes of a Most Ample Encrease of the Wealth and Strength of England in a Few Years Humbly represented to her Majestie In the Fifth Year of Her Reign.*[14] As the title indicates, this document outlined an economic program to enhance the prosperity and power of England. Grew's focus of interest was the same as Petty's, and his handling of health problems occurs within a similar context. He knew Petty, to whom he refers as "my late Honoured Friend," and frequently mentions Petty's calculations, though he does not always accept them. In his opinion the four basic elements in the economic anatomy of England are land, manufactures, foreign trade, and population. Ultimately, however, Grew's program depended on the size and quality of the population, and to this subject he devoted the fourth section of his memorandum. Grew assumed as axiomatic the need for increasing population to provide the necessary labor power. Among his recommendations toward this end he urged that the state do all in its power to maintain health and prevent disease. Grew emphasized the economic burden of disease, commenting that in economic terms the sick are worse than dead because they become either public or private charges. To make medical care available to all, Grew proposed that the government regulate physicians' fees according to their experience. He felt that if this were done the cost of medical care could be reduced and thus made accessible to those who needed it.

Despite their bold and penetrating character, the ideas of Petty and Grew had no immediately tangible results. Their proposals did not lead to concrete action because they ran contrary to two major interrelated trends, one political and administrative, the other economic and social. Effective implementation would have required the existence of a well-developed local administrative mechanism operating under centralized control, in a manner comparable to the organizations of Prussia or France. But it was precisely this network of administration which had disappeared after the Revolution. Cunningham, the economic historian, employed the term "parliamentary Colbertism" to describe this period and its con-

14 E. A. Johnson, *Predecessors of Adam Smith. The growth of British economic thought.* New York, Prentice-Hall, 1937, pp. 117-138.

tinuation in the eighteenth century.[15] Although this designation is only partly correct, it calls attention to contemporary French developments, and by inviting comparison makes it possible to focus more sharply the characteristic features of English evolution. Colbert created a whole system of administrative regulation under central control, and built up a bureaucracy to keep the machinery in operation. In England, on the other hand, the state took on a form during the seventeenth century in which local government was carried on largely by local officials, among whom the justices of the peace were most important. The local officials were in theory representatives of the central government, and a centralized administrative apparatus had been developed under the first Stuarts; but the Civil War broke the bond between the local authorities and the Crown, and neither the Commonwealth nor the restored monarchy was able to re-establish the old system. Furthermore, for reasons to be presented shortly, the focus of governmental interest following the Restoration and particularly after the revolution in 1688 shifted more and more to commercial and colonial policy, and to governmental action in these areas.

As the control of the Crown relaxed, local government in the course of the eighteenth century became increasingly a matter of local initiative. Local government was carried on by the counties, and by the parishes into which the counties were divided. As a result, the county officials, especially the justices of the peace, gained in power and prestige. It was to the justices that the parish authorities were accountable.[16] There was little explicit theorizing about this trend of development, but it was clearly reflected in the treatment of social problems, and provided the frame of reference within which thought and action in matters of health must be viewed. Indeed, the outstanding feature of internal English administration during the period from the Act of Settlement and Removal, passed in 1662, to the Poor Law Amendment Act of 1834 is its intensely parochial character. This had important results on the development of public health, since there was no machinery to subordinate the interests of the parish to the welfare of the larger community.

These political and administrative developments coincided with and were reinforced by economic and social trends. The

15 W. Cunningham, *The growth of English industry and commerce in modern times.* Cambridge, University Press, 1912, vol. I, pp. 403 ff.

16 On the duties of the justices of the peace, see William Brown, *Astraeae abdicatae restauratio or Advice to the justices of the peace. . . .* London, 1695.

Elizabethan Poor Law had laid upon the parish the duty of providing relief for the indigent. Each parish was responsible for the maintenance of its own poor, and consequently was concerned to reduce this burden as far as possible. It was believed that this could be accomplished by arranging to employ the poor. This approach was in keeping with the contemporary desire to stimulate national prosperity by using the unemployed poor in manufactures. A favorable balance of trade was a prime desideratum of mercantilist economic policy. This came to be interpreted in the late seventeenth century as a favorable balance of employment created by trade. In other words, trade should be regulated so that only finished products would be exported and raw materials imported. Furthermore, attention should also be given to expanding the volume of trade. Increased export meant a greater employment of labor, and consequently more opportunity for investment in industry. While the central government turned its attention to questions of commercial and colonial policy, proponents of this view turned to the parish poor as an easily available labor force for the expansion of industry. Between the Restoration and the end of the eighteenth century scores of books and pamphlets were written on this subject, and many projects were suggested to deal with the problem. These proposals, as well as the optimism and eagerness with which they were put forth, are characteristic of the tendency of the period to indulge in projects. The avowed aim of the projectors was to create centers of manufacture in the form of workhouses where the poor could learn to support themselves. The first of these establishments was created at Bristol in 1696, and during the earlier eighteenth century there was a steady increase in the number of workhouses.[17]

While the enthusiastic belief in the efficacy of workhouses to deal with poverty was never realized, many of the plans and programs developed in this connection also turned attention to health problems, particularly the provision of medical care.[18] As a result of these developments there was an increasing recognition in

[17] Dorothy Marshall, *The English poor in the eighteenth century*. London, George Routledge & Sons, 1926, pp. 127-128; Karl de Schweinitz, *England's road to social security*. Philadelphia, University of Pennsylvania Press, 1943, pp. 53-55; H. R. Fox Bourne, *The life of John Locke*. New York, Harper & Brothers, 1876. 2 vols., vol. II, pp. 376-392.

[18] De Schweinitz, *op. cit.*, p. 53; A. Ruth Fry, *John Bellers, 1654-1725, Quaker, economist and social reformer*. London, Cassell and Company, 1935, pp. 5-28; John Bellers, *An essay towards the improvement of physick. . . .* London, J. Sowle, 1714; George Rosen, An eighteenth century plan for a national health service. *Bull. Hist. Med.*, 1944, *16*, 429-436; Bernard Mandeville, *The fable of the bees: or, Private vices, public benefits. With an essay on charity and charity schools:. . . .* Edinburgh, J. Wood, 1772, 2 vols., p. 220.

Britain during the eighteenth century of the need for medical assistance to certain groups in the population. It was this period, particularly the years from 1714 to 1760, which witnessed the creation, in London and the provinces, of dispensaries and general hospitals as well as hospitals for special groups of patients. The dispensary movement as well as the hospital movement found impetus chiefly in private initiative and contributions, although there was some governmental assistance in the form of legislative action. This development of private initiative coupled with cooperative action is characteristic of Britain in the eighteenth century and is to a very considerable degree related to the character of local governmental activity. While the parish officers had to assume considerable responsibilities, generally they had neither the training nor desire to perform their functions. In many ways, this very aspect of the governmental system gave increasingly greater scope to private initiative, making it necessary and possible to deal on an empirical basis with new problems as they presented themselves. Indeed, throughout this period Parliamentary action was generally undertaken on the basis of previously initiated local programs and projects.

The first institutions to provide medical care for the sick poor appeared in London. The metropolis was growing, wages were high, and workers were attracted to the city. Many of them, however, unable to establish the needed residence requirement, were ineligible for parochial relief when sick.[19] Furthermore, the two older hospitals, St. Bartholomew's and St. Thomas's, were overcrowded and unable to care for all those in need. Recognizing the problem, a group of London laymen and physicians in 1719 organized the Charitable Society in Westminster to provide for such sick persons as were unable to obtain proper care. This was the beginning of the Westminster Hospital, which was soon followed by the establishment of other institutions: Guy's (1724), St. George's (1733), London Hospital (1740).[20] About the middle of the century special hospitals were created. The influence of this

19 The Act of Settlement of 1662 gave the parish authorities the right to remove within forty days any newcomer unable to rent a dwelling worth £10 if they believed that such a person was likely to be a burden to the parish.

20 B. Kirkman Gray, *A history of English philanthropy*. London, P. S. King and Son, 1905, pp. 126-131. For Guy's Hospital see Samuel Wilks and G. T. Bettany, *A biographical history of Guy's Hospital*. London, Ward, Lock, Bowden and Co., 1892, pp. 52-53, 56-73. Discussion of analogous developments in Scotland and Ireland may be found in Thomas Ferguson, *The dawn of Scottish social welfare*. London, Edinburgh, Thomas Nelson and Sons, 1948, pp. 255-284, and K. H. Connell, *The population of Ireland 1750-1845*. Oxford, Clarendon Press, 1950, pp. 198-207.

trend was soon felt and paralleled outside London. By the end of the century, hospitals were to be found in most of the larger cities and towns of England, Scotland, and Ireland.[21]

But even while hospitals were being founded, it was realized that these institutions would have to be supplemented by some other kind of establishment. To fill this need the dispensary was developed. The dispensary idea may be traced to the seventeenth century, but it was not until 1769 that the first establishment of this type came into being. This was the Dispensary for the Infant Poor, opened by Dr. George Armstrong at a house in Red Lion Square, Holborn, London.[22] The opening of Armstrong's dispensary was followed in 1770 by the founding of the General Dispensary by John Coakley Lettsom, a Quaker physician, and a group of associates.[23] Following the example set by Lettsom, dispensaries sprang up in London and the provinces. From 1770 through 1792, fifteen were founded in London, and from 1775 through 1798, thirteen in the provinces.

The causes of this expansive growth were varied, but they may be considered in two major categories: socio-economic and medical-scientific. These two elements are interdependent, but as some of the social and economic factors have already been mentioned, attention will be turned briefly to the changes in medicine that made knowledge available for use. The great scientific outburst of the sixteenth and seventeenth centuries had laid the foundation for the application of science to medicine. A basis for an accurate knowledge of the structure of the human body was created through simple, critical observation by Vesalius, his contemporaries, and his successors. From this knowledge both obstetrics and surgery were already able to benefit in the eighteenth century. Equally basic, though on a more complex level, was Harvey's discovery of the circulation, which provided a firm basis for consideration of the body as a functional system. Observation and classification also

21 M. C. Buer, *Health, wealth and population in the early days of the Industrial Revolution.* London, George Routledge & Sons, 1926, pp. 257-258; Connell, *op. cit.*, pp. 274-275.

22 Ernest Caulfield, *The infant welfare movement in the eighteenth century.* New York, Paul B. Hoeber, 1931, pp. 55-58, 146-176; Gray, *op. cit.*, pp. 132-134; A. M. Carr-Saunders and P. A. Wilson, *The professions.* Oxford, Clarendon Press, 1933, pp. 72-73; Harvey Cushing, Dr. Garth: The Kit-Kat Poet. *Bull. Johns Hopk. Hosp. 1906, 17,* 1-17. G. F. Still, *The history of pediatrics.* London, Oxford University Press, 1931, pp. 417-421.

23 James Johnston Abraham, *Lettsom, his life, times, friends and descendants.* London, William Heinemann, 1933, pp. 109-110; Thomas Joseph Pettigrew, *Memoirs of the life and writings of the late John Coakley Lettsom . . . with a selection from his correspondence.* London, 1817, 3 vols., vol. I, pp. 36-38; J. C. Trent, John Coakley Lettsom. *Bull Hist. Med.,* 1948, *22,* pp. 528-542.

made possible the more precise recognition of diseases. At the same time, the possibility and importance of applying scientific knowledge for the improvement of human health and welfare were given philosophical form by Francis Bacon. These trends are already evident in the ideas and proposals of Hartlib, Winstanley, Petty, Grew, Bellers, and Mandeville, but they assumed a concrete form in the hospital and dispensary movement of the eighteenth century.

The mere accretion of medical ideas and knowledge cannot of itself assure application. Social environment and intellectual milieu must provide favorable conditions and patterns of behavior in terms of which knowledge can be put to use. Precisely this, however, characterized England during the eighteenth century, particularly during the latter part of the period. The tempo and character of economic life had been changing in England before the middle of the eighteenth century, but by comparison the industrial and agricultural changes during the latter half of the century were both rapid and revolutionary. Not without reason have these developments been designated as the Industrial and Agricultural Revolutions. These profound alterations in the economic life of the country necessarily disturbed its social structure and gave rise to a new attitude of mind toward problems of community life. Representing essentially the views of the middle classes, this distinctive ethos was characterized by two dominant facets: an insistence on order, efficiency, and social discipline, and a concern with the conditions of men. Appreciation of the social aspects and effects of disease led merchants, physicians, clergymen, and other public-spirited citizens to undertake ameliorative efforts. It is significant that the hospital and dispensary movement, the infant welfare movement, and others originated in urban centers, first in London, then in other cities and towns. Wealth, commerce, and industry were largely centered there, and at the same time it was much easier for the middle class, many of whose members were Dissenters, to make themselves felt. They fostered the growing social conscience, but it was a humanitarianism coupled with a firm belief in the sober and practical virtues of efficiency, simplicity, and cheapness.

Despite various ameliorative activities, however, the problem of the laboring poor as a fundamental social and economic question remained unsolved. By the end of the eighteenth century, augmented by agricultural and industrial change, poverty and social distress were more widespread than ever. Nevertheless, the situation remained basically unchanged until 1834, when the drastic and revolutionary Poor Law Amendment Act was passed, ushering in a new period of thought and practice in relation to public health and social welfare. The existing Poor Law System affected the economic and administrative fabric of the state. It regulated the migration of labor and limited its mobility. While there was a widespread awareness that the existing Poor Law had to be replaced, there was little agreement on what to put in its stead. The problem of the poor remained a heavy burden for local administrators, and a subject for polemics among social reformers. But out of this ferment of thought came a new and radical approach to the treatment of the poor which was to give a uniform direction to British social and health policy throughout most of the nineteenth century.

The revolutionary changes in governmental structure and policy brought about by the Poor Law Amendment Act of 1834 were rooted in specific practical and theoretical considerations. The foremost social problem facing England during the first quarter of the nineteenth century was the organization and financing of poor relief. Assistance to the destitute was administered by 15,000 separate parishes, varying widely in size, population, and financial resources. Furthermore, to all intents and purposes, each parish was autonomous. Within this patchwork system of local authorities, annual expenditures for relief of the poor mounted steadily. From £2,000,000 in 1784 the cost climbed steadily to £8,000,000 in 1818, and still amounted to £7,000,000 in 1832 even though the price of bread had decreased by one-third since 1818. Furthermore, the leaders of the new industrialism, which was gaining momentum at the end of the eighteenth century, felt themselves hampered by the irrational restrictions of a system handed down from a pre-industrial period. Mobility of the laboring population was an essential requirement for the burgeoning industrial civilization. The labor force had to be available in adequate quantity in the places where it was most needed, and consequently the industrialists demanded a labor market open to the free play of supply and demand. This condition already existed to a considerable extent in the north of England. In the agricultural south, however, while the enclosure movement was driving the peasantry off the land, various obstacles still prevented the achievement of the desired goal. The rationalization of agriculture uprooted the peasant laborer and undermined whatever traditional social security he had. At the same time the settlement laws tied him to his parish, so that some form of social assistance was required to relieve the unemployed or underemployed rural worker. The various forms of poor relief employed for this purpose helped to maintain a reserve of rural labor and to prevent it from moving into the towns.

Naturally, such stagnant pools of labor and the system that produced them were anathema to the new industrial middle class and to those who voiced its interests and ideals. Since the system of poor relief was alleged to be the chief obstacle to the attainment of a perfectly elastic supply of labor for industry, the remedy proposed was to do away with assistance to the able-bodied poor, and thus to free labor for the play of economic self-interest. This approach was firmly rooted in specific theoretical tenets, namely, the doctrine of philosophical necessity, the political economy of Smith, Malthus, and Ricardo, and the Benthamite philosophy of administration.

The doctrine of philosophical necessity was based on faith in a natural order of society. The world of man was believed to be as ordered and regular as the Newtonian universe. Consequently, any effort to tamper with social processes was contrary to nature. The sharpest formulation of this doctrine in relation to the poor is to be found in the social ideas of Joseph Priestley. In his opinion, "individuals when left to themselves are, in general, sufficiently provident and will daily better their circumstances."[24] Poverty and idleness ought to be governed by reason and necessity, and not by any legal provision for the poor which could act only as an incitement to idleness. If government held aloof and permitted necessity to operate unchecked, material progress would result in decreased poverty and increased education, which in turn would lead to moral improvement. Consequently, any attempt to provide relief through the Poor Law was actually an obstacle to self-help, a sin against philosophical necessity, and an impediment to progress. Instead, the poor should be compelled to fend for themselves and stimulated to help themselves by being provident.

The second strain of doctrine derived from the economic theoreticians of the new order. Political economy developed with the industrial age as the science that established and expounded the laws by which the new economic system operated. According

24 Joseph Priestley, *Lectures on history and general policy*, p. 305, cited in Anthony Lincoln, *Some political and social ideas of English dissent 1763-1800*. Cambridge, University Press, 1938, p. 175.

to the political economists, the motive for economic activity was the powerful and pervasive force of self-interest. This motive, it was held, was guided by the force of competition and the mechanism of the market. Given free play the interests of different individuals would thus be harmonized and would lead to a system of spontaneous co-operation. This would mean more productivity, and more productivity meant more well-being. In short, as a basic principle, it was accepted that unfettered private enterprise was the mainspring of social progress. It was in this context that the Poor Laws were regarded as hampering, anti-social impediments to be removed so as to liberate the immense potential of individual initiative. Maximum self-help by individuals would do more to improve the condition of the poor than any legal assistance.

Nevertheless, this was not an ideal of freedom in a vacuum.[25] It was recognized that desirable economic ends and harmonious relations between individuals were not likely to come into being without a firm framework of law and order. In other words, if things were just left to take their course, chaos and not ordered economic activity would result. Consequently, it was necessary consciously to create the environment within which such factors as competition and the market could properly function. This leads to a recognition that the hand of the law-giver and the administrator is the invisible hand that guides men in their economic and social action. This concept is at the heart of Jeremy Bentham's legal and administrative philosophy. The problem is to devise means whereby private interests can be brought to coincide with the public interest.

These ideas found their most potent and practical expression among the group known as the Philosophic Radicals, whose great teacher and prophet was Bentham. They were a small band of intellectuals who proposed to deal with public problems on a rational, scientific basis. Their approach to specific political, economic, or social questions was rather hard-boiled, but curiously admixed with a considerable degree of naïveté. They contributed greatly to the development of the social sciences in their day, and on the basis of these researches called for a whole series of reforms. The schemes for which this group of highbrows labored so mightily included parliamentary reform, free trade, law reforms, educational reforms,

[25] For a lucid exposition of these positions see Lionel Robbins, *The theory of social policy in English classical political economy.* London, Macmillan and Co., 1952; also *Jeremy Bentham's economic writings.* Critical edition . . . by W. Stark. New York, Burt Franklin, 1952, vol. I, pp. 223-273.

and birth control. Even though they were a small group with little emotional appeal (in fact some of the group were heartily disliked by their contemporaries), they managed to put through a large part of their program. Directly or indirectly, the Philosophic Radicals exercised a profound influence on their contemporaries; and many of the far-reaching changes in the English constitution as well as in economic and social legislation between the 1820's and the 1870's were reforms of the kind for which they had argued and fought.

Their opportunity came in 1832. Almost the first action of the reformed Parliament was the appointment of a Royal Commission to inquire into the operation and administration of the Poor Laws. Through the appointment of Edwin Chadwick, an ardent Radical and favorite disciple of the master, first as Assistant to the Commission and later as a Commissioner, Benthamite thought was brought to bear directly on the Poor Law inquiry. In Chadwick's mind, Benthamism and classical political economy were fused to produce a dynamic social philosophy ready to be urged to action by propitious circumstances. That Chadwick did not shirk his opportunities is evident even from a superficial examination of the history of nineteenth century England. As *The Times* put it ironically in 1854:

> Future historians who want to know what a Commission, a Board whether working or Parliamentary, a Report, a Secretary of State or almost any other member of our system was in the nineteenth century, will find the name of Chadwick inextricably mixed up with his inquiries. Should he want to know what a job was in those days he will find a clue to his researches in this ubiquitous name . . . Ask—Who did this? Who wrote that? Who made this index or that dietary? Who managed that appointment, or ordered that sewer, and the answer is the same—Mr. Edwin Chadwick.[26]

The Report of the Commission appeared early in 1834, having been written by Chadwick and his friend Nassau Senior, the economist.[27] The Poor Law Amendment Act which became law on August 14, 1834 incorporated the principles of the Report and implemented them. The provisions of the Act may be divided into two parts, those concerning the principles on which relief was to be administered, and those dealing with the new administrative ma-

26 *The Times,* 8 July 1854, cited in S. E. Finer, *The life and times of Sir Edwin Chadwick.* London, Methuen & Co. Ltd., 1952, pp. 1-2.

27 Sidney and Beatrice Webb, *English poor law history*: Part II: *The last hundred years,* 1929, 2 vols., vol. I, pp. 47-103, Finer, *op. cit.,* pp. 39-49, 69-95; Marian Bowley, *Nassau Senior and classical economics.* New York, Augustus M. Kelley, Inc., 1949, pp. 282-334. Thomas Mackay, *A history of the English poor law, Volume III. A.D. 1834-1898.* London, P. S. King & Son, 1904, pp. 37-46, 52-156.

chinery it created. The principles on which relief was to be granted were openly deterrent. No able-bodied persons and their families were to be given assistance except in a well-regulated workhouse. In addition, the lot of the able-bodied pauper was to be made "less eligible" or, in other words, more miserable than that of the worst situated laborer outside the workhouse. On the administrative side the outstanding feature was the endeavor to secure centralization, uniformity, and efficiency. In place of the parish officers, the Act provided for three paid Government Commissioners and a paid secretary who would constitute a central Poor Law Commission. This body would issue orders and regulations to guide local poor law officials in the administration of the law. The unit of local administration was to be the union of parishes, and in each union the law would be carried out by an elective Board of Guardians.

The significance of the New Poor Law as a focal point of social change can hardly be overestimated. The immediate objective of the Act was to reduce the poor rates, but its broader aim was the creation of a free labor market as a precondition for investment. The market economy was asserting itself and clamoring for human labor to be made a commodity. This end was achieved, and it is no exaggeration to say that the social history of the nineteenth century was determined by the logic of the market system after it was established by the poor law reform of 1834. It was no accident that men began to explore the problems of community life with a new anguish of concern in the following decades. For the fact is that the setting up of the labor market simultaneously broached the larger question of how to organize life in a complex industrial and urban society.

A major aspect of this question was the organization of the community to protect its health. The problem of the public health was inherent in the new industrial civilization. The same process that created the market economy, the factory, and the modern urban environment also brought into being the health problems which made necessary new means of health protection and disease prevention. It is significant that public attention was first attracted to these problems at Manchester, the first industrial city.[28] Beginning in 1784, a series of epidemic fevers brought sharply to the notice of

[28] B. L. Hutchins and A. Harrison, *A history of factory legislation.* 2d ed. London, P. S. King and Son, 1911, pp. 7-13; M. W. Thomas, *The early factory legislation.* Leigh-on-Sea, Essex Thames Bank Publishing Co., Ltd., 1948, pp. 8-9; Leon S. Marshall, The emergence of the first industrial city. Manchester, 1780-1850, in *The cultural approach to history* edited by Caroline F. Ware. New York, Columbia University Press, 1940, pp. 140-161. George Rosen, John Ferriar's "Advice to the Poor," *Bull. Hist. Med.,* 1942, *11,* 222-227.

the community the significance of factories and congested dwellings as providing conditions in which such diseases could flourish and spread. During the winter of 1795 the spread of typhus alarmed and terrified the inhabitants and led a group of wealthy townsmen, magistrates, and physicians, among them Thomas Percival and John Ferriar, to form a voluntary Board of Health. Despite its multifarious activities and recommendations, however, opposition to and neglect of its program rendered the Board ineffectual. At the same time, as the nineteenth century progressed, the growth of unhealthy conditions far outran attempts at improvement.

This situation was generally true throughout the country. More and more England lived in towns and worked in factories, and as this new way of life spread, health conditions deteriorated, leaving far behind any voluntary, piecemeal efforts to cope with the problem. Thus, between 1801 and 1841 the population of London leaped from 958,000 to 1,948,000; between 1801 and 1831 that of Leeds expanded from 53,000 to 123,000, and of Huddersfield from 15,000 to 34,000. This rapid growth was soon reflected in mounting death rates. Between 1831 and 1844, the mortality rate per thousand population of Birmingham rose sharply from 14.6 to 27.2, of Bristol from 16.9 to 31, of Liverpool from 21 to 34.8, and of Manchester from 30.2 to 33.8.[29]

Unconsciously, the creation of the Poor Law Commission in 1834 also brought into being the instrument which was to open up fully the question of the health of the population and to provide the means for dealing with this problem. Chadwick was appointed Secretary to the Commission, and while his interests and activities were directed at first to the limited goal of reducing the poor rates, he had a much deeper sense of the causes of pauperism. Among the members of the Royal Commission of Enquiry into the Poor Laws, he was the only one to investigate the health of the pauper population.[30] Furthermore, he had a concept of preventive social action applicable to the problems of poverty and disease. Around 1824 Chadwick had become acquainted with Southwood Smith and Neil Arnott, two medical men who were also friends and disciples of Bentham.[31] "From Arnott and Smith," he wrote in 1844, "I derived a strong conviction of the superior importance of the

29 G. T. Griffith, *Population problems of the age of Malthus.* Cambridge University Press, 1826, p. 186.

30 Finer, *op. cit.*, p. 69.

31 *Ibid.*, p. 10.

study (as a science) of the means of *preventing* disease, and I was the better enabled to perceive some of the important relations of the facts expressed by vital statistics which were brought before me in my public investigations."[32] Recognizing that pauperism was in numerous instances the consequence of disease for which the individual could not be held responsible, and that disease was an important factor in increasing the burden of the poor rates, Chadwick concluded that it would be good economy to undertake measures for the prevention of disease. In a letter to Southwood Smith around 1848, Chadwick stated his position frankly.

> The sanitary measures, [he wrote], had strictly and exclusively an official origin . . . . they arose as a consequence, though an indirect and perhaps an accidental one of measures directed by Government in 1832, viz. the Enquiry into the administration of the Poor Laws; in the course of some investigations with the view to discriminate the causes of pauperism, excessive sickness, and its preventible causes were suggested by circumstances which appeared in the course of that enquiry and are noticed as one of the topics of examination in my report, laid before Parliament with others . . . . afterwards, under the Administrative Commission, in 1838 when a heavy amount of claims appeared as a consequence of the prevalence of an epidemic, I felt it my duty to call the attention of the Commissioners to the preventible nature of the causes of a large proportion of these cases, and recommended a special investigation of them . . . .[33]

This approach to the problem of poverty and disease was reinforced by Chadwick's deep-rooted conviction that health was affected for better or worse by the state of the physical and social environment. In fact, before the crucial study of the sanitary condition of the population was undertaken, he circulated a letter of instruction to medical officers pointing out the need "to ascertain the existence and extent of the visible and removable agencies promoting the prevalence of such disease as are commonly found connected with defects in the situation and the structure or internal economy or the residences of the labouring classes."[34] Furthermore, Chadwick saw clearly that accurate statistical information could be exceedingly important in disease prevention. He tried to set up a Bureau of Medical Statistics in the Poor Law Office, and when the Registration of Births and Deaths Act was passed in 1836, he saw immediately and listed the uses to which it could be put. This list illustrates how, even at this early date, problems of pecuniary

[32] *Ibid.*, p. 158.

[33] *Ibid.*, p. 157.

[34] *Report to Her Majesty's Principal Secretary of State for the Home Department, from the Poor Law Commissioners, on an inquiry into the sanitary condition of the labouring population of Great Britain; with appendices.* London, W. Clowes, 1842, p. XIV.

profit, disease prevention, environmental causation, and governmental action were all intimately interwined in his thought. Thus, he thought the Act could make possible:

(a) The registration of the causes of disease, with a view to devising remedies or means of prevention.

(b) The determination of the salubrity of places in different situations with a view to individual settlements and public establishments.

(c) The determination of comparative degrees of salubrity, as between occupation itself and occupation in places differently circumstanced, in order that persons willing to engage in insalubrious occupations may be the more effectually enabled to obtain adequate provision for their loss of health.

(d) The collection of data for calculating the rate of mortality, and giving safety to the immense mass of property insured, so as to enable every one to employ his money to the best advantage for his own behalf, or for the benefit of persons dear to him; and that without the impression of loss to anyone else.

(e) The obtainment of a means of ascertaining the progress of population at different periods, and under differing circumstances.

(f) The direction of the mind of Government and of the people to the extent and effects of calamities and casualties; the prevention of undue interments; concealed murder; and deaths from culpable heedlessness or negligence.[35]

It is within this context that the fundamental document of modern public health, the *Report . . . on an inquiry into the Sanitary Condition of the Labouring Population of Great Britain,* appeared in 1842. The report proved beyond any doubt that disease was related to filthy environmental conditions, due to lack of drainage, water supply, and means for removing refuse from houses and streets. Attention was further focused on these problems by Chadwick's adherence to the theory that epidemic fevers were due to miasmas arising from decaying animal and vegetable matter. "The defects which are the most important," wrote Chadwick, "and which come most immediately within practical legislative and administrative control, are those chiefly external to the dwellings of the population and principally arise from the neglect of drainage."[36] Thus, the problem of the public health was reoriented by definition. It was declared to be an engineering rather than a medical problem. As Chadwick saw it, what was needed was an administrative organ to undertake a preventive program by

[35] Edwin Chadwick, *The health of nations. A review of the works of Edwin Chadwick. With a biographical dissertation, by Benjamin Ward Richardson.* London, Longmans, Green and Co., 1887, 2 vols., vol. I, pp. XLIII-XLVI, 77-78.

[36] *Report . . . on an inquiry into the sanitary condition of the labouring population. . .*, p. 25.

applying engineering knowledge and techniques in an efficient and consistent manner. In the *Sanitary Report,* he stated his position bluntly and without qualification. "The great preventives," he wrote, "drainage, street and house cleansing by means of supplies of water and improved sewerage, and especially the introduction of cheaper and more efficient modes of removing all noxious refuse from the towns, are operations for which aid must be sought from the science of the Civil Engineer, not from the physician, who has done his work when he has pointed out the disease that results from the neglect of proper administrative measures, and has alleviated the sufferings of the victims."[37] It is clear, however, that Chadwick recognized the need for a physician to point out the location, nature, and course of infection in a given area, and in line with this idea suggested in the *Report* the appointment of "a district medical officer independent of private practice, and with the securities of special qualifications and responsibilities to initiate sanitary measures, and reclaim the execution of the law."

Chadwick's *Report* led to the Royal Commision on the Health of Towns, appointed by Sir Robert Peel in 1843. Its report was to public health what the Poor Law Report of 1834 was to public assistance, and, as in the earlier instance, Chadwick played the leading rôle in the work of the Commission. He drafted the major part of the report issued by the Health of Towns Commission, and the administrative and operational proposals were his own. In view of Chadwick's Benthamite orientation and his experience with the Poor Law Commission, it is not surprising that when the first central health department, the General Board of Health, was created in 1848, it followed the model of the Poor Law Commission.

The creation of the General Board of Health is a major landmark in the history of public health. Despite its brief existence and the handicaps under which it operated, the Board achieved much. However, it is not our intention to examine in detail the activities of the Board or the further immediate development of public health in England. The changes initiated in the 'thirties and 'forties were underlined and carried further during the following period from 1848 to the present. At the same time, there pushed into the foreground new currents of thought and practice, of which some were hitherto only latent, while others appeared in response to new problems. The two strains of *laissez-faire* and social regulation, which were present in Bentham's thinking and

37 *Ibid.,* p. 341.

were applied by Chadwick to public assistance and public health, persisted both in theory and practice throughout the century, but the relative emphasis and significance given to these approaches shifted more and more to social regulation.

"How quaint the ways of Paradox!" observed Sir William Gilbert, and nowhere is this comment more apposite than in the development of social action in relation to public health. The paradox has two aspects, one medical, the other social and political. The former concerns the rôle of medicine in the development of public health. Objective analysis of the beginnings of the public health movement in England around the middle of the last century leads to the conclusion that medicine played a secondary part in this process. The impulse to sanitary reform did not come from the medical profession, even though some physicians played a significant part in calling attention to the community problem of ill-health. Furthermore, medicine had little real knowledge to contribute toward a solution of the major problem, which concerned the transmission of communicable disease. Contagionists fought anti-contagionists, but the bitter medical controversy had little effect on the establishment of public health legislation and administration. Indeed, it is noteworthy that the early public health program was based on a structure of erroneous theories, and while it hit upon the right solution, it was mostly for the wrong reasons. (Parenthetically, the rôle of these theories in the evolution of public health illustrates strikingly what I have described as the rôle of negative factors in the development of positive advances, or what Galdston has characterized as the creative function of the erroneous idea.)[38] Broadly speaking, what happened was that the builders of modern public health, accepting certain postulates of economic and social policy, established institutional forms into which later more accurate and effective medical knowledge could be fitted. Significant instances of such forms are the supervision of local health services by a central authority, and the post of the health officer.

Consideration of these institutions, however, goes directly to the heart of the political and social paradox. It is indeed a striking paradox in modern English history that the introduction of economic freedom in the nineteenth century, far from doing away with the need for governmental intervention, control, and regula-

[38] George Rosen, Negative factors in medical history. A preliminary inquiry into their significance for the dynamics of medical progress. *Bull. Hist. Med.*, 1938, *6*, 1015-1019. Iago Galdston, Mesmer and animal magnetism, *Ciba Symposia*, 1948, *9*, 832-837 (see p. 833).

tion, eventually led to an enormous increase in the administrative functions of the state. The 'thirties and 'forties saw an outburst of legislative activity abolishing restrictive regulations and social obligations prevalent before the industrial revolution; but even while certain forms of social regulation were being discarded, others were replacing them. While the industrial revolution was still in its infancy, Robert Owen had foreseen the need for state action to curb some of the consequences of economic freedom. "The general diffusion of manufactures throughout a country," he wrote in 1815, "generates a new character in its inhabitants; and as this character is formed upon a principle quite unfavorable to individual or general happiness, it will produce the most lamentable and permanent evils, unless its tendency be counteracted by legislative interference and direction."[39] Owen's warning was soon realized and while the New Poor Law created a system of labor incentives for the new class of factory workers, factory laws and health laws were laying the foundation for centralized authority to promote human health and welfare.

In fact, the question of health serves as a focal point around which the doctrines of economic freedom and political liberalism can be seen in various stages of modification. This transformation did not arise simply from the growth of humanitarian sentiment or of social conscience. Legislation on health and sanitation resulted from a variety of forces within the social and economic order. It resulted less from a concern for the welfare of the poor than from a growing realization after 1850 that epidemic disease caused by defective sewerage or infected food was a problem of the entire community. Furthermore, there was an increasing awareness that the cost involved was a form of social waste that could be eliminated. Thus, by 1859, Edwin Chadwick, the architect of the New Poor Law, which had been created in order to bring into being a highly competitive labor market and to enforce competition, was advocating that governmental authorities go into business, and that such enterprises be organized on a monopolistic rather than a competitive basis.

> The earlier politico-economical doctrines as to competition [he said] must now receive considerable modifications. The waste and possible saving of capital indeed admit of as little dispute as do cases of the waste of mechanical power, or the direction of the means of economy. To the questions sometimes put to me, where I would stop in the application of my principle,

[39] Robert Owen, *A new view of society and other writings* (Everyman's Library Edition). London, J. M. Dent; New York, E. P. Dutton, 1927, p. 121.

I am at present only prepared to answer, 'where waste stops'; and that public intervention in whatever form for the prevention of waste may stay where it ceases to be charged upon the public, which must be a matter of inquiry in each case involving the question where the application of the principle needs authoritative intervention, or where it may be best left to voluntary means guided by an advanced intelligence.[40]

A decade later, in 1870, the Poor Law Board seriously considered the establishment of a system of free medical advice to all wage-earners in England and Wales.[41] The annual report for 1869-70 discussed "how far it may be advisable, in a sanitary or social point of view, to extend gratuitous medical relief beyond the actual pauper class . . . to the poorer classes generally." In the early 'eighties, Joseph Chamberlain described health progress in Birmingham in a letter to Morley. "Putting aside personal compliments," he wrote, "what are the facts? A saving of seven per thousand in the deathrate—2,800 lives per annum in the town. And as five people are ill for everyone who dies, there must be a diminution of 14,000 cases of sickness, with all the loss of money, pain, and grief they involve."[42] At the same time, while the organization of the labor market established by the New Poor Law was maintained relatively intact, protective legislative action improved working conditions in mines and factories and mitigated the harshness of the early *laissez-faire* system. This legislation was not extensive enough to throw the system out of gear. In fact, as compared with the stigma of the poor law and its workhouse, factory life was a lesser evil. Nevertheless, these laws helped to undermine the prevailing social philosophy. Furthermore, the new class of industrial workers, taking seriously the democratic implications of liberalism in terms of human rights and human dignity, and recognizing the effectiveness of group solidarity, organized themselves in trade unions and political parties, refused to compete against one another, and took action to secure for themselves various kinds of social services, including medical care.

These have been some of the factors significantly involved in the process by which since the beginning of this century the health of the English people has become a major concern of government,

40 Edwin Chadwick, Economical results of different principles of legislation and administration in Europe . . . *Journal of the Statistical Society of London,* September, 1859, p. 408.

41 Sidney and Beatrice Webb, *The state and the doctor.* New York and London, Longmans, Green and Co., 1910, p. 7; *Twenty-second Annual Report of the Poor Law Board,* 1869-70, p. III ff.

42 J. L. Garvin, *The life of Joseph Chamberlain.* London, Macmillan, 1932, vol. 1, p. 385.

and the provision of services for the promotion and maintenance of health a fundamental part of an impressive edifice of social services. This summary presentation is enough to indicate, however, how the contemporary state of public health has been and is being influenced by changing economic and social policy.

This brings me back to the point from which I started: the influence of economic and social policy on the development of public health. If my interpretation of the history of public health is sound, and I want to emphasize that this is an essay in interpretation, then certain consequences follow. First, there can be no real comprehension of the history of public health at any period without a thorough understanding of the political, economic, and social history of that period in its relation to the contemporary public health situation. This is not to disparage the medical and scientific elements in the historical process, but simply to indicate the great, and in many cases overriding, importance of the nonmedical factors in creating the structure and the channels within which the former may operate. Secondly, the task of the historian must be to investigate and to demonstrate how economic, social, medical, and scientific events intertwine and interact to create specific public health developments. I have tried to demonstrate this process of interaction at different periods in English history, and to show how success or failure in achieving public health aims was related to conditions under which such activity was pursued. It must be emphasized that the same approach will be found equally applicable to the history of public health in other countries and other parts of the world.[43] At the same time, while certain general trends may be found, for example, to apply to all of Europe and North America, the historian in dealing with public health in a specific country will have to discover and show how and under what circumstances the general trend manifests itself, and wherein there are differences.

It has not been possible to do more here than to present and illustrate a problem. But if this analysis should happen to make those interested in the development of public health more conscious of the problem and what it involves, it will have achieved its purpose.

43 See, for example, George Rosen, Cameralism and the concept of medical police. *Bull. Hist. Med.,* 1953, 27, 21-42.

MERCANTILISM AND HEALTH POLICY IN EIGHTEENTH CENTURY FRENCH THOUGHT

THE way in which Frenchmen of the seventeenth and eighteenth centuries thought and acted in matters of health and social policy arose out of their orientation to the mercantilist position. As in Britain and other countries, French mercantilist theory and practice dealt with such matters as self-sufficiency, population policy, productivity and public assistance; and it is to these areas that one must look for theoretical or practical awareness of the connection between health problems and social conditions.

The era of personal or bureaucratic autocracy, which began in France under Henri IV, developed in the age of Richelieu and Mazarin, and reached its apogee in the monarchy of Louis XIV. French mercantilism represented the economic counterpart of this political development. The men who endeavoured to bring all phases of economic life under royal control were more concerned with practical situations and conditions than with theory. Neither Richelieu nor Colbert was an economic theorist, yet implicit in their actions is a complex of ideas, a pervasive set of premises on which to reason and to act. For the most part, abstract statements reveal only in a small degree their thinking on social policy in relation to health. It is chiefly in their practical efforts that this is to be found.

Among mercantilist ideas, the concept of self-sufficiency was one of the most basic. To be dependent on foreigners for anything at all was a cause for deep concern. As early as the sixteenth century, there was an awareness that increased productivity was necessary if France was to be made independent of foreign lands. Increased productivity, however, required a large and growing population. But while increase of population might be a ground for deep satisfaction, the full benefits of this resource could be attained only by having as many of the people as possible productively engaged. Consequently, as in Britain, a special

This article is one of a series of studies on the history of social medicine. Earlier papers in this series to which the reader may wish to refer are: What is Social Medicine? A Genetic Analysis of the Concept, *Bull. Hist. Med.* **21**, 674–733, 1947; The Idea of Social Medicine in America, *Canadian Medical Association Journal* **61**, 316–23, 1949; Political Order and Human Health in Jeffersonian Thought, *Bull. Hist. Med.* **26**, 32–44, 1952; Cameralism and the Concept of Medical Police, *Bull. Hist. Med.* **27**, 21–42, 1953; Medical Care and Social Policy in Seventeenth Century England, *Bull. N.Y. Acad. Med.* (2nd ser.) **29**, 420–37, 1953; Economic and Social Policy in the Development of Public Health, *Jour. Hist. Med.* **8**, 407–30, 1953; Hospitals, Medical Care and Social Policy in the French Revolution, *Bull. Hist. Med.* **30**, 124–49, 1956; The Fate of the Concept of Medical Police 1780–1890, *Centauru* **5**, 97–113, 1957.

In part these studies have been supported financially by the Milbank Memorial Fund, and I wish to express to the officers of the Fund my appreciation of their generosity.

problem of the larger question of productivity concerned the poor, especially those who were unemployed. All those capable of productive labour should contribute to the wealth and power of the state. Those in need because of infirmity or ill-health should receive assistance, including medical care.

As early as the reign of Henri IV, plans had been made to establish institutions for the care of the poor, but little had been accomplished. Until well into the seventeenth century, medical relief was provided by local authorities along uncentralized lines. Thus, in 1649, among the activities of the Commissioners in charge of poor relief at Paris was the examination and treatment of those suffering from venereal diseases and scurvy.[1] Under Cardinal Mazarin a determined effort was made to cope with the problem of the poor by establishing *hôpitaux généraux*. The creation of these institutions reflects the increasing role of the state in dealing with economic and social problems. This trend was carried further under Colbert in various undertakings intended to provide care for the sick, and in general to improve the health of the nation.[2] Among these was the practice of sending remedies to various parts of France for distribution to the needy. Another phase of Colbert's interest in health problems was his encouragement of the search for medicinal springs, and of the study and use of those already known.

Theoretical approaches to the social relations of health began to appear at the end of the seventeenth century. These views were often incidental to considerations of pressing economic and political problems, and represented the reaction of conscientious men to the shocking effects of bad government. The last years of the reign of Louis XIV were years of increasing impoverishment for France, and thinking men began to grow critical of autocracy. This criticism came from various sources—from a clergyman and poet like Fénelon, a military engineer like Vauban, or a magistrate like Boisguillebert.

It came in the first instance in the name of political reform. In 1699, François de la Mothe-Fénelon, archbishop of Cambrai, published a didactic poem entitled *Les Aventures de Télémaque*.[3] Ten years earlier, in 1689, he had been appointed tutor to the Duke of Burgundy, grandson and successor to Louis XIV, a position which Fénelon occupied until 1697 when he was compelled to retire to the diocese of Cambrai where he spent the rest of his life. Based on his experience at the court, and in the hope that his pupil would some day occupy the throne, Fénelon developed what he believed to be principles of proper government. These ideas, particularly on the ethics of governing, are presented in *Télémaque*, and their practical consequences are drawn in the *Tables de Chaulnes* (1711). Like his contemporaries, Fénelon believed in the supreme importance of an increasing population. But it was clear to him that the population question was not a simple matter of mere numbers, but a more complex problem whose solution was a function of diverse conditions. The people should not only be numerous but also happy, and this aim required attention to their welfare. In short, the achievement of social happiness required consideration and solution of problems of social welfare. Fénelon saw that poverty, due to a variety of circumstances, was a major hindrance to an increasing population and proposed governmental action to relieve the masses. He had in mind a system of public assistance in a broad sense, including the unemployed, the aged, the sick and the disabled. In his theoretical views and practical proposals, Fénelon explicitly recognized the obligation of the state for positive action in questions of social policy, including health.

While the views of Fénelon were in no small degree inspired by religious ideals, the ideas and proposals of his contemporary, Vauban, grew out of quite a different context.[4] Sebastien Le Prestre de Vauban was a military engineer who served in almost all the wars of Louis XIV. In the course of his long and active career, he became interested in the social and economic conditions of various localities, especially as these related to military problems, and eventually broadened his perspective to consider such matters in terms of national policy and welfare. Seriously concerned with the condition of the mass of the French people, Vauban looked with alarm at the growing economic deterioration of France during the last decades of the seventeenth century. He believed that this situation was due in large measure to fiscal inequities, and that if France were to prosper and its population to grow, tax reforms would have to be instituted. To this end, Vauban outlined in his *Projet d'une dixme royale* (1707) a comprehensive plan of fiscal reorganization.[5] Convinced of the importance of a large and growing population of workers, Vauban pointed out that the adoption of his plan would lead to an increase of population and provide the monarch with greater resources. To buttress this point he calculated on a statistical basis the revenues to be derived from certain specified localities.

Vauban is in many respects reminiscent of William Petty, but in none more so than in his emphasis on 'political arithmetic'. In this connection, he insisted on the need for population surveys to provide the necessary demographic and fiscal information on which to base political and social policies. The idea of collecting quantitative information for such purposes was not new. The importance of statistical knowledge had been recognized in the Italian cities during the Renaissance, and, in France, Jean Bodin had devoted a chapter in his work, *Les six Livres de la République* (1577), to the advantages to be derived from an enumeration of the population of a state.[6] It was not, however, until the end of the seventeenth century, in 1693, that a general survey of the population of France was undertaken.[7] A few years later, in 1697, the royal officials in the provinces, the *Intendants*, were ordered to draw up descriptions of the districts for which they were responsible. These detailed historical, political, economic and demographic accounts were to be used for the education of the Duke of Burgundy, grandson of Louis XIV. Vauban, who in the preceding year had prepared a *Description géographique de l'election de Vézelay*, containing a detailed census of the parishes comprising this area, helped to draw up the questionnaire which was sent to the *Intendants*. The information received in answer to the questionnaire was used by Vauban for the calculations published in the *Dixme royale*. Furthermore, he devoted one chapter of the *Dixme royale* to the usefulness of demographic surveys, going into considerable practical detail as to their organization, and urged that they be undertaken annually. In this way, Vauban pointed out, it would be possible to learn whether the population was increasing or declining, which diseases and accidents affected the people, and how these were connected with the social conditions of the people. It is clear that Vauban considered the protection of the productive classes a major pillar of social policy, and regarded statistical investigations a major instrument toward that end.

The same general position was taken by Pierre Le Pesant de Boisguillebert, who served as lieutenant-general of Rouen from 1690 to his death in 1714. From his writings it is clear that he was acutely aware of the economic misery of France.[8] In the first of his major works, *Le Detail de la France*, which appeared in 1697, Boisguillebert recommended fiscal reforms and emphasized the importance of the working classes. Later, in his *Traité des Grains*, which appeared sometime between 1697 and 1707, he showed that the condition of the working classes, primarily rural, improved or deteriorated as prices of commodities were high or low. Finally, in the *Dissertion sur la Nature des Richesses . . .*, published during this same decade, he emphasized that man is a social being who must work to live, and since labour is a necessary condition for the existence of society, it follows that every worker should be able to obtain the necessaries of life. For if the workers, particularly the poor, cannot easily get what they need, they will not contribute so much to the nation's strength or to the national treasury as they otherwise could.

The ideas put forth by Fénelon, Vauban and Boisguillebert did not directly affect government policy, but they were seminal in their influence. While this influence was at first limited to a small circle, in the course of the eighteenth century it expanded in various directions. Early in the century, for example, the Abbé Claude Fleury, one of the tutors to the Dukes of Burgundy, Anjou, and Berry, the grandsons of Louis XIV, prepared some notes for the guidance of his pupils.

> The aim of politics [he said], is to make the people happy. . . . Extreme poverty and great riches are almost equally bad in their effects; the ideal should be a large number of people with comfortable means living as far as possible on terms of equality . . . It is the number of men and not the extent of land which determines the strength of the State . . . The most essential function of Government: to preserve health and morals, increase the population, prevent disease, lawsuits and crime.[9]

Directly inspired by the ideas previously discussed was Henri, Comte de Boulainvilliers, historian and student of politics. His numerous works appeared after his death in 1722. Among these was a volume published in 1727, addressed to the Duke of Orleans, outlining a plan for fiscal reform. In it Boulainvilliers proposed a system of social security based on wage deductions.[10]

Singularly influenced by these currents of thought was the Abbé de Saint Pierre, moralist and political reformer. Imbued with a passionate desire to promote the welfare of mankind, Saint-Pierre became a prolific author of projects, some of which were naïve and fantastic, while others were more closely tied to reality. In the latter group were his proposals for the collection and utilization of statistical data, including vital statistics. Furthermore, in relation to the problem of poverty he insisted on the right of the poor to social assistance by the state.[11]

Somewhat the same position, although in a more qualified form, was taken by Montesquieu.[12] In his famous book, *De l'Espirit des Lois*, which appeared in 1748, he commented that:

> alms given to a naked man in the street do not fulfil the obligations of the state, which owes all its citizens an assured existence, food, proper clothing, and a mode of life not incompatible with health.

Montesquieu was aware that in countries predominantly commercial,

> where many people have only their craft, the state is often obliged to provide for the needs of the aged, the sick and the orphans.

Acknowledging that workers might be thrown into need by rapid shifts in economic conditions, Montesquieu felt that such situations were only temporary. Consequently, while the state ought to provide assistance promptly and to prevent suffering, such action should aim only at tiding over the urgent, immediate need.

Ideas and proposals which had been broached by various social thinkers and critics from Fénelon to Montesquieu were placed in the dominant social and intellectual context of the eighteenth century when they began to appear in the volumes of the *Encylopédie* after 1751. The *Encyclopédie* was not only the most important literary enterprise of the period, but also the consummate ideological expression achieved in France by the Enlightenment. At its height, the Enlightenment was an international movement, but there is no doubt that its intellectual leadership was French. Furthermore, scrutiny of the social context of the Enlightenment reveals it as essentially a middle-class movement. Its leaders were recruited from among the middle classes of town and country. Voltaire was the son of a notary; Montesquieu's father was a titled judge of middle-class origins; Diderot's was a prosperous cutler; Rousseau and Beaumarchais were the sons of watchmakers; and Grimm was the son of a pastor.

The leaders of the Enlightenment believed that their activities would redound to the greater benefit of humanity, that their ideas coincided with the truest interests of mankind. In keeping with this approach they tested the existing edifice of social relations and advanced an endless variety of projects and plans for reconstruction of social institutions. Nevertheless, it is clear that the critical thought and humanitarian idealism of the *philosophes* were associated with the elaboration of an ideological and programmatic basis in terms of which the advancing middle classes and later the workers would assert their respective claims to power. The transitional character of the thought of the Enlightenment is clearly revealed in the *Encyclopédie*.

Brunétière aptly characterized the *Encyclopédie* as the *noeud vital*, the vital centre into which were gathered the political, social and intellectual threads of

French life in the eighteenth century.[13] But this characterization does not go far enough. Diderot declared that the aim of the *Encyclopédie* was to collect scattered knowledge, explain it to the contemporary reader and 'hand it down to those who follow us, so that the labour of centuries past may not become lost labour for the centuries which follow'.[14] It was a crucible where thinking men tried to fuse theory and practice, so that knowledge might become more readily available for the betterment of man's condition.

As a result, the theoretical ideas and practical proposals of the Encyclopedists on the social relations of health and disease are not to be found in any single systematic presentation, but rather scattered in various articles on such subjects as *Arithmétique politique*, *Enfants exposé*, *Homme*, *Hôpital*, *Hôtel-Dieu*, *Population*, and *Durée de la vie*.[15] They are most clearly expressed in relation to policies and measures intended to foster the growth of population. For example, in his article on *Man*, Diderot emphasized the importance of infant mortality for growth or decline of population, and pointed out that a sovereign who was seriously interested in increasing the number of his subjects must take measures to reduce the number of infant deaths. Such measures should go hand in hand with a policy of encouraging marriages. Furthermore, in his article on the *Hospital*, Diderot took up the ideas put forth by Boulainvilliers, developing them more precisely and in greater detail. He outlined a public assistance scheme including old-age insurance, and medical assistance provided by the various hospitals of Paris. In general, Diderot stressed the need for reforming and improving the hospitals, especially the Hôtel-Dieu where mortality was exceedingly high. Generally, the Encyclopedists favoured social assistance to families, improvement in hospital facilities, and a more equitable fiscal system—all measures intended to prevent poverty or to ameliorate its effects.

Basic to the thought and action of the Enlightenment was an acceptance of the supreme social value of intelligence, and as a corollary, a belief in the great utility of intelligence or reason as a force in social progress. At the same time, the intellectual climate was shot through with utopian elements. During the Enlightenment, when the philosophy of history was imbued with and dominated by the idea of progress, and the history of mankind was considered to be an unbroken ascent from barbarism to civilization, the concept that the rational ideals of the present are the realities of the future was entirely acceptable and logical. If to this sense of the inevitability of progress is added an expectation of human salvation from a revolution in social morality based on a rational way of life, as well as a desire to persuade others of the necessity and reasonableness of such a change, one begins to understand why utopia flourished in the eighteenth century. Simply to demonstrate how to better conditions, and to convince others of this, would in time be sufficient to improve them.

The desire to influence social action was directed, however, not so much at realizing the utopian ideal somewhere on the globe, but rather at confronting contemporary society with an ideal counterpart, a standard or model, and thus appealing to it to improve itself. To be sure, this desire has played a role in a greater or lesser degree in all serious utopias. In the eighteenth century, however,

Zeitkritik, the critical dissection of contemporary social evil, became the predominant or even exclusive purpose of Utopia. During the eighteenth century, forty utopias appeared in France. French literature of the Age of Enlightenment, even strictly scientific books, exhibits a marked critical character. It is an oppositional, even revolutionary literature, and this is true also of the French utopias of this period.

Utopian social thought and policy in relation to health and welfare are characteristically represented by the writings and ideas of Morelly,[16] an otherwise unknown philosophe, and Sebastien Mercier, a writer and politician. In 1751, the year in which the publication of the Encyclopedia was started, there appeared at Amsterdam a work in two volumes entitled *Le Prince. Les Délices des coeurs, ou Traité des qualités d'un Grand Roi, et Sistême général d'un sage Gouvernement.* The author was indicated as Mr. M***; internal evidence, however, clearly shows that it was written by Morelly. Apparently intended as a critique of Montesquieu's *Esprit des Lois*, particularly his defence of obsolete feudal theories, Morelly set forth what he regarded the best form of political and social organization. Pointing out that the ruler must have accurate information concerning the human and other resources of his realm, Morelly took up again Vauban's project for a census. He also stressed the need for social assistance to the poor and to older people, proposing that the state assume this responsibility and that this function be financed by transferring all ecclesiastical wealth to the state. Morelly's ideas are better and more precisely stated, however, in his principal work, *Code de la Nature*, which appeared in 1755.

Morelly contended that nature was fundamentally communal. Starting from the premise that moral evil and depravity resulted from social conditions, he outlined and advocated an ideal society in which it would be 'impossible to be depraved'. In this utopian community, there would be no private property except what was needed for individual daily wants. Every citizen would be a public servant, contributing to the general welfare according to age and ability, and in return receiving at public expense everything necessary for his support. Morelly developed this scheme in an elaborate code which described to the smallest detail the organization and behaviour of the entire population. Each nation was to consist of families, organized in tribes and living in carefully planned garden cities.

The infirm and aged would be comfortably lodged and cared for in a public institution designed and constructed by each city for this purpose. Furthermore, all sick citizens, without exception, would be cared for in public hospitals. Here they would be cared for as accurately and as carefully as if they were in their own homes, nor would there be any kind of discrimination. The Senate of each city would take particular care in the administration of these institutions to see that nothing was lacking to speed the recovery and restore the health of the patient, and to render convalescence as pleasant as possible. While the organization of health services was not further specified, Morelly did indicate that he expected them to be advanced and improved by scientific research. His code gave complete freedom to speculative and experimental science whose object was to seek out the secrets of nature in order to improve the arts useful to society. Discoveries in physical, mathematical or mechanical science that had been confirmed by experience and reason would be recorded in a public repository of scientific knowledge. This would not include anything relating to metaphysics or morals.

To project ideal states into the future was a new thing in the eighteenth century, and when in 1770 Louis Sebastien Mercier described what Paris would be like in 2440 A.D., his method was a result of the rise of the idea of *Progress*. Mercier (1740–1814) wrote a number of plays, romances and essays, including the satiric *Tableau de Paris*. A follower of Rousseau, he became a member of the Convention, where he belonged to the Girondists. It seems likely that he was also an adherent of the group that gathered around Cabanis, Condorcet, and Destutt de Tracy at Auteuil, the home of Mme. Helvétius. Mercier's utopia *L'An deux mille quatre cent quarante* (The Year 2440) was published anonymously at Amsterdam in 1770.[17] Its circulation in France was rigorously forbidden, because it implied a severe criticism of the existing order. It was reprinted at London and Neuchâtel, and translated into English and German. As the motto of his book, Mercier took the saying of Leibnitz that 'the present is pregnant of the future'. His picture of Paris in 2440 is serious and naïve. Yet with all its sentimental rhetoric, it shows a sound common sense and contains a number of shrewd suggestions.

The world of 2440 A.D. in which a man born in the eighteenth century, who has slept an enchanted sleep, awakes to find himself, is composed of nations living in a state of concord rarely interrupted by war. Japan has been opened to the world, Italy united, Australia settled; serfdom has been abolished in Russia, and the British colonies on the Atlantic seaboard of North America have become independent. But in general, we hear little of the world at large. Mercier concentrates on France, and particularly on Paris. Changes in Paris are a sufficient index of the transformation.

The constitution of France is still monarchical. While the total population of the country has increased by one-half, that of the capital remains about the same. Paris has been rebuilt on a scientific plan, and every provision has been made for the public safety. There is no system of credit; everything is paid for in ready money, and this practice has led to a remarkable simplicity in dress. Marriages are contracted only through mutual inclination; dowries have been abolished. Education is governed by the ideas of Rousseau. The study of classical languages has disappeared, but the modern tongues, Italian, German, English and Spanish are taught in the schools.

Houses in the Paris of 2440 have running water laid on; and on each street corner is a beautiful fountain providing clear, cool water with which the passers-by may slake their thirst. This is in striking contrast to eighteenth century Paris, where itinerant vendors of beverages hawked their wares. Furthermore, the houses are no longer constructed with steep roofs and high chimneys, from which loose tiles and bricks so often descended upon the heads of unfortunate pedestrians.

Of the greatest interest for us are the attitudes toward health problems and the organization of health services. As might be expected the hospital service has been greatly improved. The Hôtel-Dieu is no longer in the centre of the city, and a patient is no longer 'imprisoned in some disgusting bed between a cadaver and a dying person, where he breathes the poisoned air of death, and where a simple ailment is transformed into a cruel malady'. The Hôtel-Dieu has been divided into twenty separate sections situated in different parts of the city. All citizens have a right to free treatment, and are not driven to the hospitals by extreme indigence. Characteristic is the emphatic statement that each patient has his own bed. In these hospitals, learned and kind-hearted physicians do not pronounce death sentences on the basis of a guess, but take the trouble to examine each patient thoroughly. Furthermore, the medical profession is highly respected. Surgery and medicine have united and buried forever their ancient feud. The statement that prominent physicians in Mercier's day did not make home visits to patients who resided higher than the first floor throws a harsh light on the medical profession of eighteenth century Paris. Thanks to active research the physicians of 2440 have learned to understand and to deal with diseases, such as pneumonia, phthisis and dropsy, which had baffled the medical contemporaries of Mercier. Anatomy is taught at the Sorbonne where learned anatomists study the structure of the body by dissection. Of particular interest is an inoculation institute. Smallpox inoculation is practised as it had been in China, Turkey and England during the eighteenth century. Furthermore, there is a research institute which investigates diseases and prepares remedies for them. These are some of the leading features in the health service of the ideal future to which Mercier's imagination reached. He did not present them as a final result. Later ages, he said, will go much further, for 'where can the perfectibility of man stop, armed with geometry and the mechanical arts and chemistry?'

Utopia being a man-made world cannot transcend the human instruments and materials of its construction. Its architects have not been wizards replete with esoteric lore and mantic wisdom, but men subject to the advantages and limitations of their own times. But because what is utopian is rooted in concrete existence, it has definite values for historical perspective. On the one hand, it appears in intimate connection with its own cultural background, thus presenting itself as a 'documentary' reflection of existing conditions; on the other, by rejecting the present and attempting to supersede it by comparing it with a fictitious *nowhere*, or with a prophetic future springing from the present, it is possible for Utopia to anticipate the realities of tomorrow.

Both facets are clearly evident in eighteenth-century France. Even though the passionate affirmation of an indefinite progress in enlightenment and social welfare was for the moment realized only in the imagination, the fact remains that the Utopian writers of the time were dealing on a speculative level with problems of social organization which were at the same time questions of practical debate and action. The basic problem related to health was the grinding poverty which oppressed a large part of the rural and urban population.

Exact data are lacking, but contemporary opinions and estimates help to define the character and dimensions of the problem. Observations gathered over more than forty years led Vauban in his *Dixme royale* to estimate that a tenth of the French population was reduced to beggary, while another five-tenths lived in dire poverty, continually on the verge of destitution.[18] Baudeau in 1765 stated that out of eighteen million Frenchmen, three million were paupers.[19] According to the census of 1791, Paris had 118,884 indigents in a total population of 650,000.[20] In the same year, the Committee on Mendicity of the National Assembly reported that even in normal times about one-twentieth of the population of France were destitute and required some kind of relief, while in periods of distress, this proportion increased to one-tenth or one-ninth of the population.[21] In fact, indigence was so widespread that the very idea of the 'people' was part and parcel of the concept of poverty. Thus, Necker, in 1775, seeking to define the term, 'the people', wrote that it was impossible either 'to fix the limits of the word or the degree of indigence which characterized it'. It could be defined, he concluded, only as 'the most numerous and most miserable class' in society.[22]

At the root of this problem were economic and social conditions, frequently aggravated by natural catastrophes such as floods or severe winters. But whatever, the cause, the hard fact remained that a large part of the French people needed assistance of some sort. Employment, food, medical care and shelter are the needs that stand out most sharply. The problem of relief to the needy was further exacerbated by the failure of existing private and public agencies.[23] Down to the time of the Revolution, the basic principle of social assistance in France was that relief to the needy should be provided locally as far as possible. Each community was supposed to care for its own indigent, sick and afflicted. The provincial or royal government stepped in only when problems of relief were too large for the local community to handle. Relief to the indigent was also provided by the church, charitable organizations and individuals.

Within this structure, aid was provided to those afflicted with disease and infirmity. In line with practices started during the reign of Louis XIV, the royal government contribution to the maintenance of hospitals and the provision of medical care in cities and rural districts.[24] At periodic intervals medicines were sent to the provinces for free distribution to the needy. To cope with the widespread epidemics, medical personnel (physicians and surgeons) as well as medicaments might be dispatched to the ravaged district. The problem of medical personnel, however, was not limited to periods of epidemic outbreak. In fact, throughout the century there was a great shortage of physicians, surgeons and midwives. Efforts to deal with this problem were made in almost all instances by local communities. One of the most common methods was to contract annually with a physician or surgeon to provide medical care to the needy. In some instances, private charitable organizations, religious or secular, arranged for domiciliary medical care to the poor. Thus, in Paris, the parish of Saint-Eustache had three physicians and two surgeons who attended the sick poor in their homes. However, if the illness lasted more than three weeks the patient was sent to the Hôtel-Dieu.[25] Various mutual aid organizations also provided medical care for their members.[26] The gravediggers guild of Paris provided hospitalization for its sick members. In the French glass industry, benefits to the workers in some cases included medical attention, monetary assistance during sickness and old age pensions. An association of domestics organized at Paris in 1789 provided medical attention for its members when sick. Governmental authorities also endeavoured to improve conditions by providing free instruction in surgery and midwifery. Sometimes they published or purchased for distribution books intended to enlighten the public on health matters. Perhaps the most popular of these was Tissot's *Avis au peuple sur sa santé*, which went through ten editions in six years.

All efforts failed, however, to meet the problem of the poor. Public-spirited Frenchmen saw the need for profound change and set forth measures calculated to relieve the situation. One of the most interesting of the proposals concerned with health and medical care was that devised by Claude Humbert Piarron de Chamousset (1717–73), a wealthy Parisian philanthropist, who dedicated his life to the public welfare. He was interested in such matters as a postal service for Paris, a registry for servants and workmen, the organization of fire insurance, and the care of the sick. For a time he served as Inspector-General of military hospitals. In 1754, Chamousset's *Plan d'une maison d'association*, outlining a scheme for medical care and hospitalization insurance, appeared anonymously at Paris.[27] It was reprinted in 1757 in a collection of his writings issued under the title *Vues d'un citoyen*. This volume makes it abundantly clear that Chamousset was interested in developing a system of social protection, in which sickness insurance would be an integral part. The purpose of such a system was to prevent destitution, and where this was not possible to provide means of mitigating it.

> Of the two main scourges of humanity, disease and poverty [Chamousset wrote], the first is inherent in our nature, a physical evil which calls for alleviation. The second is an alien force, the fruit of neglect, and calls for preventive measures . . . Destitution among the productive classes which live by their labour and industry . . . arises from a combination of two effects of illness, the expenditure of savings on the necessary relief and the loss of working time incurred.[28]

In his plan for sickness insurance, Chamousset developed these ideas more fully.

> Men are the most valuable possession of a state [he pointed out], and their health is their most valuable possession. But it is not enough that they have the means of preserving it. An object of more importance to them is that in case of sickness they may count on all the aid necessary to their recovery . . .
>
> There are asylums available to the destitute, and that is a resource useful to those to whom it is not humiliating to accept the free assistance which charity offers.
>
> But between these two extremes is the class of the greatest number of citizens, who not being rich enough to procure sufficient aid at home or poor enough to be taken to an almshouse, languish and often perish miserably, victims of the propriety to which they are subjected by their class of society. Such are the industrious artisans, merchants whose trade is limited, and in general all those valuable men who live daily by the fruits of their labour, and who often for that reason have no recourse to treatment when a disease becomes incurable. The start of a disease exhausts all their resources, the more they deserve help, the less can they bring themselves to profit by the only resources that remain to them, and they find themselves in public asylums.

In this plan, however, human dignity and self-respect would be maintained.

The establishment having no funds other than the quotas of the members, it would not be discreditable to receive assistance already paid for. No one could pity anyone else, since each will have his own interest in it. All establish the funds together, for no one can be assured of continual health, and if those who are fortunate enough not to be compelled to seek recourse there, furnish the association with more than the association renders to them, they at least enjoy the benefit of knowing there is such an asylum for them whenever it becomes necessary to take advantage of it; and by that they are exempt from anxiety. If when I am well, I pay a modest sum to my association for someone else who is suffering, then the same thing is done for me when I am sick . . .

In a word, this association, as in all those which it is an honor to join, is a community of funds established for the needs of all members. Can there be any dishonour in enjoying advantages one has procured for himself?'

Finally, the efficacy of the medical care provided

will shorten the duration of the diseases and even prevent them from becoming more serious, because one will not have to wait for an emergency before having recourse to the proper remedies, but on the contrary, be cared for from the moment he feels ill. Thus services owed to the country will not be interrupted for such a long period. One will no longer see the families of artisans ruined by the length and excessive expense of illnesses or citizens a burden to their government when they should be its mainstay.[29]

Specifically, Chamousset proposed an organization which in return for a monthly payment would, in case of illness, provide its members with medical care in a hospital or at home. Treatment would be the same for all, but

in order to allow for different conditions and means, there will be established five classes of members who will pay more or less . . . for optional accommodations which vary according to conditions and which are necessary only to those who habitually enjoy them.[30]

Chamousset envisaged group enrolment at reduced rates and suggested that apprentices, workmen or servants might collectively be enrolled by their employers. Such groups would also be represented on the board of administration. As a measure of prudence, Chamousset suggested certain limitations on admission of members and provision of service to them. In general, he proposed:

that there be an interval of a month between the date of membership and the date of admittance to the hospital, for the first time only.[31]

For pregnant women the only qualification would be membership for at least nine months. Persons with venereal diseases or incurable diseases would be excluded.

Physicians and surgeons would be selected with all possible care, and appointed on a salaried basis. Patients who preferred a medical attendant not associated with organization could have his services but would have to pay the fee themselves. The hospital would have extramural consultants in addition to the resident staff. A well-managed, well-stocked pharmacy would provide the necessary medicaments. Careful records would be kept on all patients, and the doctors would prescribe diets and drugs in writing.

Chamousset also saw that such an institution might serve an important educational purpose.

> A fixed number of young physicians [he wrote], will be received, lodged and fed, for a modest fee, who doubtless will be eager to train there and who will at the same time be of great help at the bedside of the sick, reporting to the physicians of their prescriptions and an infirmity of enlightening observations to render the treatment more certain . . .
>
> Surgery will be cultivated with no less care, and there will be added to the number of surgeons, aides and boys admitted and boarded in the hospital, other pupils paying also a very modest sum for their food and lodging. These will be trained under the eyes of the masters and will be inspired by the hope and desire of winning in the competition, the only way by which any of the positions in the hospital may be obtained.[32]

Chamousset's ideas and proposals aroused some interest, but not enough to lead to their realization. While his views and goals were shared by various contemporaries, they looked to the state for positive action in dealing with social problems and their health aspects. Throughout the century it became increasingly evident that private charitable organizations and local authorities were unable to deal adequately with poverty and its associated problems. More and more the opinion became prevalent that care of the needy, including the provision of medical attention, was an obligation of society to be carried out through the agency of the state.

The physiocrat Baudeau in 1765 stated as a fundamental axiom 'that the true poor have a real right to demand basic necessities'.[33] Turgot, in a similar vein, declared in an article in the *Encyclopédie* that 'the poor man has an incontestable claim upon the wealth of the rich'.[34] In 1770, while still governor of Limousin, he said: 'The relief of men who suffer is the duty of all, and all the authorities will co-operate toward this end.'[35]

This position was formulated even more explicitly by Montyon, the author of the *Recherches et considérations sur la population de la France*, published in Paris in 1778.[36] With a lively awareness of the relations between social conditions and health, he directed attention to the inimical effect of poverty on duration of life, commenting that poverty was 'a slow poison which destroys the person attacked by it'. High infant mortality among the poor, diseases resulting from the trades by which men are compelled to support themselves and their families, ill-health produced by malnutrition—these were some of the health problems among the poor classes of the community. In view of the significance of population for the State, it behoves the sovereign to deal with these problems, particularly since the poor people are the largest population group. Such a programme must deal equally with the economic, social and medical aspects of the problem.

Fully aware of the inadequacies of medical practice, Montyon nevertheless urged that more attention be paid to making available the services of competent physicians and surgeons.[37] It was still a question, he said, whether medicine destroyed more people than it saved. However, in large cities where there were better trained and more experienced physicians the results of the care provided clearly outweighed any defects. This was not the case in small towns and in rural areas where there were few trained physicians, with the result that many resorted to quacks. Montyon had a higher opinion of surgery and its practitioners, and he felt it was fortunate for France that the art of surgery had reached a state of perfection there unknown in other countries.

Moreover, he indicated, beside curative medicine there was a preventive medicine, connected with general administration (*police générale*) which was essential for the preservation of the public health. While this branch of medicine had been recognized and applied with beneficial results in France, much still remained to be done.[38] This was particularly the case with regard to environmental sanitation, the provision of better housing and improved nutrition for the poorer classes.

Furthermore, Montyon proposed the establishment of an institution for the study of the problems of occupational health. This establishment, he wrote:

> would occupy itself within the field of the mechanical arts with an object to which no one has paid any attention because it has been foreign to all special interests, namely, the conservation of men. The field is vast, the subject practically untouched, the aim noble, and perhaps success will not be too difficult.[39]

In the last analysis, however, these proposals and activities would have to be related to the fundamental constitution of the State. Commenting on conditions in hospitals and related institution, Montyon pointed out that men who had given much thought to the problem of social assistance felt it would be better to suppress completely all asylums for the poor, for infants and old people, and to retain only those intended for the sick.

> In a well-organized state [he wrote], there are no paupers, except for invalids or loafers; in extraordinary cases the poor should receive aid at home, and the best charity is assurance of work.[40]

This position may be compared with Necker's statement in his *Administration des finances*.

> It devolves upon the government [he wrote], to do everything that order and justice will permit for the numerous class of unfortunates. The government will determine the duties of society toward the unfortunates, in the establishment of public works, and in all provisions calculated to prevent misery and mendicity which follows in its wake.[41]

Similar ideas appeared in the provincial assemblies of 1787–9. A specific example is Lavoisier's proposal in 1787 to the Assembly of Orléanais of a scheme for insurance against poverty and old age.[42]

> We propose, therefore [he said], to institute at Orleans, under the title of the People's Savings Bank (*Caisse d'épargne du peuple*), an establishment to receive sums contributed by persons of every age and condition who wish to insure for themselves, their widows, or their children, an annuity determined according to the tables that have been drawn up for this purpose. The whole province will be the guarantor of the commitments undertaken by the bank and of all the actions that are carried out in conformity with the regulations that will be prescribed for it.

Imbued, likewise with this spirit, was the commission of which Lavoisier was a member, appointed in 1786 to study the hospitals of Paris, particularly the

Hôtel-Dieu. The commission had been appointed by the Academy of Sciences at the request of the government. Besides Lavoisier, its members were the outstanding physical scientists, Laplace, Coulomb and Darcet; Lassone, first physician to the king; Daubenton, the eminent anatomist; Bailly, the astronomer and later president of the National Assembly; and Tenon, surgeon and oculist. The last-named was actually the most important member of the commission. Jacques René Tenon (1724–1816) was a pioneer in ophthalmic surgery, and is still remembered for his studies of the capsule of the eye which is named after him. Furthermore, he had long been interested in problems of hospital organization, and had visited hospitals in England where he had collected statistics, particularly on sanitary and health conditions in these institutions.

The commissioners made a thorough study of the problem. Conditions at the Hôtel-Dieu were appalling. The mortality exceeded that of any other hospital in Europe, and small wonder. Wards were overcrowded, with many patients in one bed. Patients with communicable diseases were mixed with those suffering from other conditions. Ventilation was totally inadequate, and the wards were often made to serve several functions that were mutually inappropriate. Under such conditions, how could patients recover? Furthermore, they examined the other hospitals in Paris, noting their defects and within the year completed their reports. The commission proposed that the Hôtel-Dieu be abandoned and its patients moved to four new hospitals to be established in widely separated suburbs of Paris.

The government and the general public received this proposal with interest and approval. In fact the government issued orders for the execution of the project. Unfortunately, however, all this came on the very eve of the Revolution, and in the ensuing upheaval was abandoned. Nonetheless, the commission and its work have a significance transcending the immediate problem with which it dealt. For one thing, through Tenon, its guiding spirit, it exerted a continuing influence on future developments. In 1788, based on his earlier studies and the work of the commission, Tenon published his remarkable volume, *Mémoires sur les hôpitaux de Paris*, which had a tremendous influence on the reconstruction of the French hospital system during and after the Revolution. A hospital in Paris today bears his name, in tribute to his contribution toward the reorganization of the French hospital system. Secondly, the work of the commission focused ideas and proposals expressed earlier by thinkers and reformers as diverse as Diderot, Morelly, Mercier, Chamousset and Montyon.[43], [44]

By the last decade of the eighteenth century it was obviously clear to many Frenchmen that profound changes were needed in social organization in order to deal effectively with community problems of health and welfare. This position was intimately interlocked with and reinforced by contemporary views on scientific and technological advance, the social utility of reason and enlightenment, and the nature of man as a being destined to achieve happiness in this life. Invention and scientific knowledge were required as indispensable for the improvement of man's living conditions.

Throughout his writings, Voltaire expressed his enthusiastic recognition of the value of science; and D'Alembert's introduction to the *Encyclopédie* is a veritable paean to scientific knowledge. As a part of the field of science, medicine was regarded as capable, through increased knowledge and improved techniques, of contributing mightily to social betterment. Voltaire in his *Age of Louis XIV* referred approvingly to Boerhaave's role in teaching the physicians of Europe.[45] Diderot's opinion of Daviel, the ophthalmic surgeon, is reflected in his rhetorical question: 'Who does not know or has never heard of the famous Daviel?'[46] Montyon felt that advances in preventive medicine and public health practice had in his time led to the control of 'a multitude of fatal diseases that had afflicted preceding centuries, some of which have disappeared, while others have become less frequent.'[47] This fervent affirmation of the value of scientific and medical knowledge reached its apogee in Condorcet's *Esquisse*, with its chiliastic conjectures that preventive medicine, once improved, would lead to the disappearance not only of communicable diseases, but to those diseases due to climate, nutrition and occupation.

Coupled with this faith in science was a belief in the great utility of intelligence or reason as a force in social progress. The theoretical underpinning for this eighteenth century confidence in the capacity of human reason came from John Locke's epoch-making *Essay Concerning Human Understanding*, and its denial of innate ideas. As the mind owed everything to environment, to sensations from the outer world, the shaping of the mind and the practical expression of this process in education became matters of profound social significance. It was realized that social intelligence could be made most effective through an informed public opinion. Characteristic of the period, therefore, was an eager didactic impulse to make the results of science and medicine available to the public, and in line with this trend efforts were made to enlighten the people in matters of health and hygiene. Illustrative of the many books and pamphlets written to further health education are S. A. Tissot's *Avis au peuple sur sa santé*, which appeared in France in 1762, went through ten editions in six years, and was translated into several languages; and an anonymous book that appeared in the same year under the title, *De la santé. Ouvrage utile a tout le monde.*[48] The advocates of health education addressed themselves to the upper and middle classes, not to the peasants and labourers. Illuminating are the comments of Tissot.

> The title 'Advice to the People' [he says] is not the result of an illusion which has convinced me that this book is going to become a household fixture in the home of every peasant. Nineteen-twentieths of them undoubtedly will never know that it exists; many will never know how to read it; much greater numbers will not understand it, no matter how simple it is; but I address it to intelligent and charitable persons who live in the country, and who, by a kind of providential vocation, are called upon to help through their counsel all the people around them.[49]

The earnest conviction, humanitarian devotion and enthusiasm that these apostles of health brought to their enterprise was related to the conviction widespread in the eighteenth century that man was destined to be happy in this world.[50] This can be seen in Pope's apostrophe to 'Happiness! Our being's end and aim!' Or in Montesquieu's remark that throughout life one should seek to have as many moments of happiness as possible.[51] Throughout the century, it is reflected also in the spate of publications on public happiness.[52] And for happiness, health was necessary; but how to attain this desired condition. Most people who recognized the need for political and social change believed that education, increased knowledge and social invention could further the process greatly, but significant differences of opinion prevailed over the steps to be taken and the rate at which changes should be made. This was the problem that faced France on the eve of the Great Revolution, and the context within which the revolutionary governments would undertake to deal with problems of health and welfare.

REFERENCES

1. COLE, C. W., *Colbert and a Century of French Mercantilism*, New York, Columbia University Press, 1939 (2 vols.), I, 263.
2. *Ibid*, II, 467–72.
3. For Fénelon and his views see Albert Bertolini: *Esplorazioni nella Storia del Pensiero Economico*, Firenze, La Nuova Italia, 1950, pp. 145–218; Paul Hazard: *La Crise de la Conscience Européenne (1680–1715)*, (3 vols.), Paris, Boivin et Cie, 1935, II, 65–9, C. E. Stangeland: *Pre-Malthusian Doctrines of Population: A Study in the History of Economic Theory* (Studies in History, Economics and Public Law, XXI, No. 3), New York, Columbia University Press, 1904, pp. 176–8.
4. LAZARD, P. *Vauban 1633–1707*, Paris, Felix Alcan, 1934: Henry Guerlac: Vauban. The Impact of Science on War, in E. M. Earle (editor): *Makers of Modern Strategy*, Princeton, Princeton University Press, 1943, pp. 26–48.
5. VAUBAN, *Projet d'une dime royale*, in Eugène Daire (Editor): *Économistes-Financiers du XVIIIe Siècle*, Paris, Chez Guillaumin, 1843, pp. 26–48.
6. BURCKHARDT, JACOB., *The Civilization of the Renaissance in Italy*, London and New York, Phaidon Press, 1944, pp. 45–6, 50–2: Jean Bodin: *Les six Livres de la Republique*, Paris, 1577, Lib. VI, Chap. I, pp. 581 ff.
7. VINCENT, PAUL E., French Demography in the Eighteenth Century, *Population Studies* I : 44–71, 1947–8.
8. BOISGUILLEBERT; *Le Detail de la France, Factum de la France, et opuscules divers*, in Daire, *op. cit.*, pp. 157–431.
9. SAND, RENÉ, *The Advance to Social Medicine*, London, St. Martin's Press, 1952, pp. 187–8.
10. DE BOULAINVILLIERS, HENRI, *Mémoires presentés à Monseigneur le duc d'Orléans, contenant les moyens de rendre ce royaume tous puissant et d'augmenter considerablement les revenue du roi et du peuple*, La Haye, 1927, cited in, Helene Bergues: La Population vue par les utopistes *Population* 6: 261–6, 1951. See also Bertolini, *op. cit.*, pp. 200–1.
11. GOUMY, EDOUARD, *Étude sur la vie et les écrits de l'Abbé de Saint-Pierre*, Paris, L. Hachette et Cie, 1859, pp. 273–7; Bertolini, *op. cit.*, pp. 202–3.
12. MONTESQUIEU, *Oeuvres Complètes* (2 vols.) Paris, Bibliothèque de la Pléiade, 1951, II, 712–13.
13. BRUNÉTIÈRE, FERDINAND, *Histoire de la littérature française*, Paris, Delagrave, 1931, III, 321.
14. DIDEROT, DENIS, Encyclopédie, *Oeuvres complètes* (ed. Assezat), Paris, Garnier Frères, 1876, XIV, 415.
15. FAGE, ANITA, Les doctrines de population des Encyclopédistes, *Population*, 6; 609–24, 1951.

16. MORELLY, *Code de la Nature ou le veritable esprit de ses lois*, publié avec une introduction et des notes par Gilbert Chinard, Paris, Raymond Clavreuil, 1950, pp. 7–11; Maxime Leroy: *Histoire des Idées sociales en France*, t. 1. (*de Montesquieu à Robespierre*), Paris, Gallimard, 1946, pp. 243–5; Hans Girsberger; *Der utopische Socialismus des 18. Jahrhunderts in Frankreich und seine philosophischen und materiellen Grundlagen*, Zürich, Rascher & Cie. A.-G., 1924, pp. 130–57.
17. I have used the edition published at London in 1773.
18. VAUBAN, *op. cit.*, pp. 31–5.
19. LEROY, *op. cit.*, p. 54.
20. LEVASSEUR, E., *Histoire des classes ouvrières en France depuis 1789 jusqu'à nos jours* (2 vols.), Paris, L. Hachette et Cie, 1867, 1, 85, Note 2. It should be noted that these figures are only approximate. For a discussion of the population problem see A. Landry: 'La démographie de l'ancien Paris', *Journal de la Société statistique de Paris* 76: 34–45, 1935.
21. MCCLOY, SHELBY T., *Government Assistance in Eighteenth-Century France*, Durham, N.C., Duke University Press, 1946, p. 262.
22. NECKER, *Sur la legislation et le commerce des grains*, Paris, 1775, pp. 165ff., cited by Leroy, *op. cit.*, pp. 54–5.
23. SEE, HENRI, *Economic and Social Conditions in France during the Eighteenth Century*, New York, Alfred A. Knopf, 1927, pp. 214–20; Georges Lefebre: *La Revolution Française*, Paris, Presses Universitaires de France, 1951, p. 58; McCloy, *op. cit.*, pp. 463–5.
24. MCCLOY, *op. cit.*, pp. 158–73, 181–98.
25. DELAUNAY, PAUL, *Le Monde médical parisien au dix-huitième siècle*, Paris, Jules Rousset, 1906, p. 90: Alfred Franklin: *La Vie privée d'autrefois. Variétés chirurgicales*, Paris, E. Plon, Nourrit et Cie, 1894, pp. 297–8.
26. MCCLOY, *op. cit.*, pp. 456–7; Warren C. Scoville: Labour and Labour Conditions in the French Glass Industry, 1643–1789, *Journal of Modern History* 15: 287, 1943.
27. ANNAN, GERTRUDE L., A Plan for Hospitalization Insurance Devised by Piarron de Chamousset, 1754, *Bulletin of the New York Academy of Medicine*, February, 1944, pp. 113–28.
28. *Vues d'un citoyen*, Paris, Lambert, 1757, pp. 1, 2, 3, 7, cited by Sand, *op. cit.*, p. 191.
29. ANNAN, *op. cit.*, pp. 116, 117, 125–6, 128.
30. *Ibid.*, p. 120.
31. *Ibid.*, p. 122.
32. *Ibid.*, pp. 118–19.
33. BAUDEAU, *Idées d'un citoyen sur les droits et les devoir des vrais pauvres*, Paris-Amsterdam, 1765, 1, 169, cited by Leroy, *op. cit.*, 1, 320.
34. LEROY, *op. cit.*, 1, 247.
35. SEE, *op. cit.*, p. 217.
36. This book was originally published under the name of Moheau but it has now been proved to be the work of A. J.-B. Huget, Baron de Montyon (1733–1820). The main points are summarized by René Goddard in the introduction to his reprint of the *Recherches* (Collection des Economistes et des Reformateurs Sociaux de la France), Paris, 1912. Newer evidence is presented by Paul E. Vincent in his article cited above (footnote 7), pp. 57–8.
37. MOHEAU, *Recherches et Considerations sur la Population de la France*. Published with an introduction and analytical table by René Goddard, Paris, Paul Genthner, 1912, p. 285.
38. *Ibid.*, pp. 285–6.
39. *Ibid.*, p. 221.
40. *Ibid.*, p. 287.
41. SEE, *op. cit.*, p. 217.
42. *Mémoires presentées a l'Assemblée provinciale de l'Orléanais*, in *Oeuvres de Lavoisier* publiées par . . . le Ministère de l'Instruction publique et des Cultes, Paris, Imprimerie nationale, 1893, VI, 241–50: Douglas McKie: *Antoine Lavoisieur, Scientist, Economist, Social Reformer*, New York, Henry Schuman, 1952, pp. 244–7.

43. Franklin, *op. cit.*, pp. 36–7: McCloy, *op. cit.*, pp. 197–8; McKie, *op. cit.*, pp. 201–2.
44. Franklin, *op. cit.*, pp. 37–56.
45. Voltaire, *The Age of Louis XIV* (Everyman Library) London, J. M. Dent & Sons, 1926, p. 380.
46. Diderot, *Oeuvres* (Bibliothèque de la Pléiade), Paris, Gallimard, 1951, p. 893. See also p. 894.
47. Moheau, *op. cit.*, p. 286.
48. *De la santé. Ouvrage utile a tout le monde*, Paris, Chez Durand, 1762.
49. Tissot, S. A., *Avis au peuple sur sa santé, Traité des maladies les plus fréquentes*, Paris, 1762, p. xxxv.
50. Hazard, *op. cit.*, I, 17–33.
51. Pope, Alexander, *An Essay on Man*, 1733–34, Epistle IV; Montesquieu, *op. cit.*, I, p. 1267.
52. For example: de Chastellux, F.-J., *De la felicité publique*, 1772: Muratori, L.-A., *Della pubblica felicita*, 1749: Ferguson, Adam: *An Essay on the History of Civil Society*, *1782*. Sections IX and X. Of National Happiness.

HOSPITALS, MEDICAL CARE AND SOCIAL POLICY IN THE FRENCH REVOLUTION *

L'homme est le même dans tous les États, le riche n'a pas l'estomac plus grand que le pauvre ; les besoins naturels étant partout les mémes, les moyens d'y pouvoir doivent être partout égaux.

Rousseau, *Émile,* III

Il faut faire disparaître du sol de la République la servilité des premiers besoins, l'esclavage de la misère et cette trop hideuse inégalité parmi les hommes qui fait que l'un a toute l'intempérance de la fortune et l'autre toutes les angoisses du besoin.

Barère, Rapport du 22 Floréal an II.
(Buchez et Roux, *Histoire parlementaire de la révolution,* IX, 95.)

There were good reasons for the enthusiasm with which the French people welcomed the States-General in 1789. Here was an opportunity to air grievances which had accumulated during two centuries of arbitrary rule, and to deal with problems clamoring for solution. Prior to the meeting of the States-General every electoral assembly had been entitled to draw up an address to the crown (*cahier de doléances*) embodying its complaints and demands. These very human documents reveal a vivid and unique picture of a great country on the eve of a revolution. They reveal with equal clarity the deep discontents which provided the driving force for the Revolution, and the programs for reform popularized by the writers of the day.

The *cahiers* reveal as well how obvious it was to many Frenchmen by the last decade of the eighteenth century that profound changes in social organization were needed to deal effectively with problems of welfare and health. This recognition was intimately interlocked with and reinforced by contemporary views on the social utility of reason, enlightenment, and scientific and technological progress. In turn, these views were firmly grounded in the conviction widespread in the eighteenth century that man was destined to be happy in this life.[1] This attitude is evident in Pope's

* Paper read at the twenty-eighth annual meeting of the American Association of the History of Medicine, Detroit, May 12, 1955.

[1] Paul Hazard: *La pensée européenne au XVIIIème siècle* (3 vols.), Paris, Boivin et Cie, 1946, vol. 1, pp. 17-33.

apostrophe to " Happiness! Our being's end and aim! "; or in Montesquieu's remark that throughout life one should seek to have as many moments of happiness as possible.[2] It is reflected as well in the spate of publications on public felicity that appeared throughout the century.[3] There was also general agreement that for happiness, health was necessary. But how to attain this desired state?

Whatever their differences, the *cahiers* show that all orders of society were at one in accepting poverty and mendicity as the major problems to which other social problems were related. Any consideration of questions of health had to take account of the grinding poverty which oppressed a large part of the rural and urban population. Exact information is lacking, but contemporary opinions and estimates help to define the character and dimensions of the problem. Observations gathered over more than forty years led Vauban in his *Dixme royale* (1707) to estimate that a tenth of the French population was reduced to beggary, while another five-tenths lived in dire poverty, continually on the verge of destitution.[4] Baudeau, in 1765, stated that out of eighteen million Frenchmen, three million were paupers.[5] According to the census of 1791, Paris had 118,884 indigents in a population of 650,000.[6] In the same year the Committee on Mendicity of the Constituent Assembly reported that even in normal times about one-twentieth of the population of France were destitute and required some kind of relief, while in periods of distress, this proportion increased to one-tenth or one-ninth of the population.[7] In fact, indigence was so widespread that the very idea of the " people " was part and parcel of the concept of poverty. Thus, Necker, in 1775, seeking to define the term, " the people," wrote that it was impossible either " to

[2] Alexander Pope: *An Essay on Man*, New Haven, Yale University Press, 1950, p. 128; Montesquieu: *Oeuvres complètes* (Bibliothèque de la Pleiade, 2 vols.), Paris, 1951, vol. 1, p. 1267.

[3] See for example, L.-A. Muratori: *Della pubblica felicità*, 1749; F.-J. de Chastellux: *De la felicité publique*, 1772; Adam Ferguson: *An Essay on the History of Civil Society*, 1782 (Sections IX and X: Of National Happiness).

[4] Vauban: Projet d'une dixme royale, in Eugène Daire (ed.): *Economistes-financiers du XVIIIe siècle*, Paris, Guillaumin, 1843, pp. 31-154.

[5] Maxim Leroy: *Histoire des idées sociales en France*, t. I (*de Montesquieu à Robespierre*), Paris, Gallimard, 1946, p. 54.

[6] E. Levasseur: *Histoire des classes ouvrières en France depuis 1789 jusqu'à nos jours* (2 vols.), Paris, L. Hachette et Cie., 1867, vol. 1, p. 85, note 2. It should be noted that these figures are only approximate. For a discussion of the population problem see A. Landry: La démographie de l'ancien Paris, *Journal de la Societé Statistique de Paris* 76: 34-45, 1935.

[7] Shelby T. McCloy: *Government Assistance in Eighteenth Century France*, Durham, N. C., Duke University Press, 1946, p. 262.

fix the limits of the word or the degree of indigence which characterized it." It could be defined, he concluded, only as "the most numerous and most miserable class" in society.[8]

At the root of the problem of poverty were economic and social conditions, frequently aggravated by natural catastrophes such as floods or severe winters. But whatever the cause, the hard fact remained that a large part of the French people needed assistance of some sort. Employment, food, medical care, and shelter are the needs that stand out most sharply. The problem of relief to the needy was further exacerbated by the failure of existing private and public agencies.[9] Down to the time of the Revolution, the basic principle of social assistance in France was that relief to the needy should be provided locally as far as possible. Each community was supposed to care for its own indigent, sick, and afflicted. Relief was also provided by the church, charitable organizations, and individuals. The provincial or royal government stepped in only when problems of relief were too large for the local community to handle.

In line with practices started during the reign of Louis XIV, the royal government contributed to the maintenance of hospitals and the provision of medical care in cities and rural districts.[10] At periodic intervals medicines were sent to the provinces for free distribution to the needy. To cope with widespread epidemics, medical personnel (physicians and surgeons) as well as medicaments might be dispatched to the ravaged district. The problem of medical personnel, however, was not limited to periods of epidemic outbreak. In fact, throughout the century there was a great shortage of physicians, surgeons, and midwives. Efforts to deal with this problem were made in almost all instances by local communities. One of the most common methods was to contract annually with a physician or surgeon to provide medical care to the needy. In some instances, private charitable organizations, religious or secular, arranged for domiciliary medical care to the poor. Thus, in Paris, the parish of Saint-Eustache had three physicians and two surgeons who attended the sick poor in their homes. However, if the illness lasted more than three weeks

[8] Necker: *Sur la législation et le commerce des grains,* Paris, 1775, pp. 165 ff., cited by Leroy, *op. cit.*, pp. 54-55.

[9] Henri Sée: *Economic and Social Conditions in France during the Eighteenth Century,* New York, Alfred A. Knopf, 1927, pp. 214-220; Philippe Sagnac: *La formation de la société Française moderne,* Paris, Presses Universitaires de France, 1946, vol. 2, pp. 72, 74; Georges Lefebvre: *La Révolution Française,* Paris, Presses Universitaires de France, 1951, p. 58, McCloy, *op. cit.*, pp. 463-465.

[10] McCloy, *op. cit.*, pp. 158-173, 181-198.

the patient was sent to the Hôtel-Dieu.[11] Various mutual aid organizations also provided medical care for their members.[12] In the French glass industry, benefits to the workers in some cases included medical attention, monetary assistance during sickness, and old age pensions. The gravediggers guild of Paris provided hospitalization for its sick members. An association of domestics organized at Paris in 1789 provided medical attention for its members when sick. Governmental authorities also endeavored to improve conditions by providing free instruction in surgery and midwifery. Sometimes they published or purchased for distribution books intended to enlighten the public on health matters. Perhaps the most popular of these was Tissot's *Avis au peuple sur sa santé,* which went through ten editions in six years.

Throughout the century it became increasingly evident, however, that private charitable organizations and local authorities were unable to deal adequately with poverty and its associated health problems. More and more the opinion became prevalent that care of the needy, including the provision of medical attention, was an obligation of society to be carried out through the agency of the state. The physiocrat Baudeau, in 1765, stated as a fundamental axiom "that the true poor have a real right to demand basic necessities." [13] This position was formulated even more explicitly by Montyon, the author of the *Recherches et considérations sur la population de la France,* published at Paris in 1778.[14] With a lively awareness of the relations between social conditions and health, he directed attention to the inimical effect of poverty on duration of life, commenting that poverty was "a slow poison which destroys the person attacked by it." High infant mortality among the poor, diseases resulting from the trades by which men are compelled to support themselves and their families, ill health produced by malnutrition—these were some of the health problems among the poor classes of the community. In view of the sig-

[11] Paul Delaunay: *Le monde médical parisien au dix-huitième siècle,* Paris, Jules Rousset, 1906, p. 90; Alfred Franklin: *La vie privée d'autrefois: Variétés chirurgicales,* Paris, E. Plon, Nourrit et Cie., 1894, pp. 297-298.

[12] Warren C. Scoville: Labor and Labor Conditions in the French Glass Industry, 1643-1789, *Journal of Modern History* 15: 287, 1943; McCloy, *op. cit.,* pp. 456-457.

[13] Baudeau: *Idées d'un citoyen sur les droits et les devoirs des vrais pauvres,* Paris-Amsterdam, 1765, vol. 1, p. 169, cited by Leroy, *op. cit.,* vol. 1, p. 320.

[14] Moheau: *Recherches et considérations sur la population de la France.* Published with an introduction and analytical table by René Gonnard, Paris, Paul Geuthner, 1912. This book was originally published under the name of Moheau, but it has now been proven to be the work of A. J.-B. Auget, Baron de Montyon (1733-1820). The main points are summarized by Gonnard, and newer evidence is presented by Paul E. Vincent: French Demography in the Eighteenth Century, *Population Studies* 1: 44-71, 1947-48.

nificance of population for the state, it behooves the government to deal with these problems, particularly since the poor people are the largest population group. Such a program must deal equally with the economic, social, and medical aspects of these problems. Furthermore, commenting on conditions in hospitals and related institutions, Montyon pointed out that men who had given much thought to the problem of social assistance felt it would be better to suppress completely all asylums for the poor, for infants, and old people and to retain only those intended for the sick. " In a well-organized state," he wrote, " there are no paupers, except for invalids or loafers; in extraordinary cases the poor should receive aid at home and the best charity is assurance of work." [15]

Similar ideas appeared in the provincial assemblies of 1787-1789. A specific example is Lavoisier's proposal, in 1787, to the Assembly of Orléanais of a scheme for insurance against poverty and old age.[16] Imbued likewise with this spirit was the commission of which Lavoisier was a member, appointed in 1786 to study the hospitals of Paris, particularly the Hôtel-Dieu. One of the most important members of the commission was Jacques René Tenon (1724-1816), surgeon and oculist. The commission made a thorough study of the problem and proposed that the Hôtel-Dieu should be abandoned. Its patients would be moved to four new hospitals to be established in widely separated suburbs of Paris. All this, however, came on the very eve of the Revolution, and in the ensuing upheaval the idea was abandoned. Nonetheless, the commission and its work have a significance transcending the immediate problem with which it dealt. For one thing, through Tenon, its guiding spirit, it exerted a continuing influence on future developments. Secondly, the work of the commission focused ideas and proposals expressed earlier by thinkers and reformers as diverse as Diderot, Morelly, Chamousset, and Montyon.[17]

[15] *Ibid.*, p. 287.

[16] Mémoires presentées à l'assemblée provinciale de l'Orléanais, in *Oeuvres de Lavoisier* publiées par . . . le Ministère de l'Instruction Publique et des Cultes, Paris, Imprimerie Nationale, 1893, vol. VI, pp. 241-250; Douglas McKie: *Antoine Lavoisier: Scientist, Economist, Social Reformer*, New York, Henry Schuman, 1952, pp. 244-247.

[17] Morelly, an otherwise unknown *philosophe*, who stressed the need for social assistance to the poor and to older people, proposing that the state assume this responsibility and that this function be financed by transferring all ecclesiastical wealth to the state. Morelly's ideas are most precisely stated in his principal work, *Code de la nature*, which appeared in 1755.

Louis Sebastien Mercier (1740-1814) was a writer and politician, who is best known today for his satiric *Tableau de Paris*. A follower of Rousseau, he became a member of the Convention, where he belonged to the Girondists. His utopia, *L'an deux mille quatre cent quarante*, describing Paris as it would be in 2440 A. D., was published in 1770.

Claude Humbert Piarron de Chamousset (1717-1773), a wealthy Parisian philanthropist,

But while a recognition of the need for change was present in all orders of society, significant differences prevailed over the precise steps to be taken and over the tempo at which social change should take place. This was the situation that faced France on the eve of the Great Revolution, and the context within which the revolutionary governments would undertake to deal with questions of health and welfare.

II.

The States-General assembled on May 4, 1789. Not until the end of January, 1790, however, did the Constituent Assembly turn to an investigation of the serious social problems demanding attention. The solicitude of the Assembly for the cause of the poor and the unfortunate was not spontaneous, but owed its origin rather to the initiative of the Paris commune. For the workers of Paris 1789 was a bad year. An exorbitant increase in food prices coincided with the aftermath of a hard winter, a bad harvest, and unemployment resulting from political unrest.[18] The cruel distress that prevailed led to unrest among the workers and aroused demands for assistance to the poor. In December 1789, Boncerf,[19] a municipal official at Paris, and Lambert, supervisor of apprentices at the Hôpital Général, addressed pamphlets to the Assembly calling attention to the pressing problem of the poor. The latter, who had already published numerous philanthropic brochures,[20] demanded a committee "to apply especially for the protection and preservation of the unpropertied class the great principles of justice decreed in the Declaration of the Rights of Man and in the Constitution."[21] The Paris commune vigorously sup-

dedicated his life to the public welfare. He was interested in such matters as a postal service for Paris, a registry for servants and workmen, the organization of fire insurance, and the care of the sick. For a time he served as Inspector-General of military hospitals. In 1754, Chamousset's *Plan d'une maison d'association*, outlining a scheme for medical care and hospitalization insurance, appeared anonymously at Paris.

For Montyon see footnote 14 above.

[18] Grace M. Jaffé: *Le mouvement ouvrier à Paris pendant la Révolution Française (1789-1791)*, Paris, Presses Universitaires de France, 1924, pp. 41-61.

[19] Pierre-François Boncerf (1745-1794), engineer and administrator, in 1776 had published a pamphlet entitled *Les inconvénients des droits féodaux* which was condemned to be burned. In 1789 he was employed by the municipality. During the Revolution (1792-1793) he was arrested and tried before the Revolutionary Tribunal. He escaped death by one vote.

[20] C. Chassin: *Les élections et les cahiers de Paris en 1789*, Paris, Jouaust et Sigaux, 1888, vol. 2, pp. 579-581.

[21] Camille Bloch and Alexandre Tuetey: *Procès-verbaux et rapports du Comité de Mendicité de la Constituante 1790-1791* (Collections de documents inédits sur l'histoire

ported this proposal, but it was not until the end of January, 1790, that the procrastinating Assembly finally appointed a committee to seek ways and means of destroying mendicity and relieving the sick, the infirm, and the aged poor.

Initially, the Committee on Mendicity consisted of four appointees, but by April 1790 eighteen members were participating in its work, and a nineteenth member was added in July of that year. It was a diverse group comprising clergymen, lawyers, officials and administrators, physicians, and soldiers. Several years later, two of the lawyers, Bertrand Barère and Pierre-Louis Prieur (of the Marne), would occupy the center of the revolutionary stage as members of the Committee of Public Safety.[22] Of the two physicians, one, Joseph Ignace Guillotin, is remembered today chiefly in connection with the beheading machine known as the guillotine; the other, Michel-Augustin Thouret, in 1794, became the director of the reorganized Paris medical school, the École de Santé, and later dean of the medical faculty of Paris. The leading spirit of the Committee, however, was its chairman, the Duc de la Rochefoucauld-Liancourt, one of the great noblemen of France, who even before the Revolution had turned his attention and given thought to problems of pauperism and social assistance, of hospitals and health.[23]

Setting to work without delay, the Committee undertook to investigate and to deal with all questions relating to pauperism, mendicity, charity, and assistance in all forms, whether in institutions or at home. By April 30, 1790, Liancourt had prepared a plan of action which was adopted by the Committee and which provided the basis for its further work.[24] In order to carry out its broad program as efficiently as possible, the Committee organized itself into several sections to deal with specific problem areas such as aid to the urban and rural poor, aid to foundlings, administration and finances, and repression of mendicity.

From February 2, 1790, to September 25, 1791, the Committee held seventy sessions. During these eighteen months the commissioners labored sedulously at their task. Casting their nets as widely as possible, they endeavored to collect whatever information appeared pertinent to the

économique de la Révolution Française publiés par le Ministère de l'Instruction Publique), Paris, Imprimerie Nationale, 1911, p. 1.

[22] R. R. Palmer: *Twelve Who Ruled. The Committee of Public Safety during the Terror,* Princeton, Princeton University Press, 1941, pp. 8-9, 14.

[23] Ferdinand Dreyfus: *Un philanthrope d'autrefois: La Rochefoucauld-Liancourt 1747-1827*, Paris, Plon-Nourrit et Cie., 1903, pp. 34-35, 44-46.

[24] Bloch and Tuetey: *op. cit.*, pp. 23, 309-327.

problem of public assistance.[25] Advice and information on many topics were solicited and obtained from various departments of the central government, from provincial municipalities, from other committees of the Constituent Assembly, from hospital administrators and from members of learned societies such as the Academy of Science and the Royal Society of Medicine. Throughout its existence the Committee corresponded actively with public bodies, administrative officials and private persons both in France and in foreign countries. For example, on April 23, 1790, Liancourt wrote on behalf of the Committee to Dr. Alexander Hunter of York for information on the mental hospital in that city.[26] On November 1, 1790, having received no reply, he addressed himself to Richard Price, the famous dissenting minister, for information on the treatment of the mentally ill, as well as on the handling of bastard children.[27] Not content with information obtained by correspondence, the Committee held hearings for all who might have information, ideas, or proposals bearing on the question of public assistance. Finally, the commissioners recognized the need to visit the hospitals and other institutions for the poor in Paris, and as far as possible to learn at first hand the actual conditions in these establishments.[28]

The term " hospital " in eighteenth century France carried a broader connotation than it does today. It covered a variety of charitable institutions established for the benefit of the needy, whether sick, disabled, or dependent. Thus, while a number of establishments were hospitals in our sense of the word, others were asylums housing unfortunates of different kinds.

Paris, in 1789, had two classes of hospitals. Those concerned primarily with the care of the sick were administered by the Bureau of the Hôtel-Dieu. In this group for example, were the Santé hospital, the hospital for Incurables, the Hôtel-Dieu and the Hôpital Saint-Louis. The head of

[25] Alexander Tuetey: *L'assistance publique à Paris pendant la Revolution*, vol. I. Les *hôpitaux et hospices 1789-1791*, Paris, Imprimerie Nationale, 1895, pp. II-VIII; Bloch and Tuetey, *op. cit.*, pp. XXVIII-XXXIX.

[26] Bloch and Tuetey, *op. cit.*, p. 19; Alexander Hunter (1733-1809) was a Scottish physician who helped found the hospital for mental patients at York. In 1792, he published a book entitled *Observations on the Nature and Method of Cure of the Phthisis Pulmonalis . . . with the Origin, Progress and Design of the York Lunatic Asylum.*

[27] Bloch and Tuetey, *op. cit.*, pp. 163-164; For Richard Price see Carl B. Cone: *Torchbearer of Freedom. The Influence of Richard Price on 18th Century Thought*, Lexington, University of Kentucky Press, 1952.

[28] Dreyfus, *op. cit.*, pp. 153-160; Bloch and Tuetey, *op. cit.*, pp. 32, 38, 57, 54, 127, 226; Michel Bouchet: *L'assistance publique en France pendant la Révolution*, Paris, Imprimerie Henri Jouve, 1908, pp. 146-150.

3

the Bureau was the Archbishop of Paris and it comprised a number of municipal administrators and legal officials as well as ten laymen. The Bureau of the Hôpital Général administered the institutions for the aged and the indigent, among them the Bicêtre, the Salpêtrière, the Pitié, and the Foundling Hospital. Administrative responsibility for these establishments rested with the same officials who looked after the Bureau of the Hôtel-Dieu, and to whom were added eighteen laymen. The sole agency for domiciliary assistance was the Grand Bureau des Pauvres which also had two hospitals, the Trinité for children and the Petites-Maisons for the aged.[29]

Various members of the Committee took part in the survey of these institutions, but Liancourt was the driving force. Between May and September 1790, he alone or together with several colleagues investigated some nine hospitals. Furthermore, he was responsible for the preparation of the reports embodying the results of all the visits made by the commissioners.[30] These reports contain a mass of information on conditions in the Paris hospitals, and more generally on the state of public assistance to the sick, the disabled, and the aged. In the main the reports confirm the findings of pre-revolutionary investigators and underline the need for reform. Based on this survey as well as on information gathered from a wide variety of other sources, the Committee concluded that a new organization of public assistance was needed. On December 1, 1790, Liancourt presented to his colleagues a plan for a complete national system of assistance to all in need through no fault of their own.[31] Later, as a pendant to this plan, he prepared a proposal for the reform of public assistance at Paris.[32]

Before turning to the proposals, however, it is necessary to glance briefly at the environment within which the Committee on Mendicity carried out its appointed task, and to which Liancourt's plans were clearly related. The Constituent Assembly faced a twofold task, to liquidate the old regime and, at the same time, to construct the new France. The Declaration of the Rights of Man promulgated by the Assembly abolished

[29] Léon Lallemand: *Histoire de la charité*, vol. 4, part i, Paris, Alphonse Picard et Fils, 1940, p. 331; Dreyfus, *op. cit.*, p. 154.

[30] Bloch and Tuetey, *op. cit.*, pp. 575-693.

[31] Quatrième rapport du Comité de Mendicité. Secours à donner à la classe indigente dans les différents âges et dans les différentes circonstances de la vie, par M. de La Rochefoucauld-Liancourt, in: Bloch and Tuetey, *op. cit.*, pp. 383-464. See also subsequent reports.

[32] Rapport sur la nouvelle distribution des secours proposés dans le départment de Paris, par le Comité de Mendicité, in: Bloch and Tuetey, *op. cit.*, pp. 758-777.

the privileges of the *Ancien Régime.* The paragraphs dealing with the freedom and equality of the individual, and with the sovereignty of the nation and the law provided the pillars upon which the constitution prepared by the Assembly was intended to rest. But how to turn these general principles into specific acts? This was the problem that the Assembly had to face. It was the more difficult because there was no accepted design for the new France, and the new structure as it evolved had to be erected on ground encumbered by the debris of the old.

The Paris of the first years of the Revolution was hardly the place to discuss calmly and judiciously how best to apply the lofty principles of the Revolution to specific problems. All Paris was in a ferment, and an atmosphere of tension, suspicion, and suppressed anger pervaded the city. The political problem was complicated by economic crisis. Fear of famine, anger provoked by hoarding, and resentment of the high cost of living mingled and alternated in the popular consciousness with revolutionary idealism and patriotic confidence in the future of France.[33] In that dawn of human freedom it was bliss to be alive, but the deputies could hardly go out of the Assembly without being reminded of urgent problems pressing for immediate solution. Food riots began at Versailles in January, 1790, and recurred during the following months. Expedients had to be devised to deal with the exigencies of the moment.

This was the situation faced by the Committee on Mendicity and the atmosphere in which it endeavored to carry out its task. The hospital problem is a case in point. The economic storm which had been gathering ominously for several years before the Revolution broke in all its fury in 1789. As a result, hospital revenues fell heavily. According to the Committee, the income of 1,438 hospitals fell from 20,874,665 livres in 1788 to 13,987,778 livres in 1790. In Paris there was a drop in hospital revenue from 7,958,799 livres to 4,129,206 livres. Hospital income was derived from rentals on real estate belonging to the institutions; from taxes, fines, lotteries, and occasional grants by the central or local governments; and from private charity in the form of legacies and gifts. The political and economic crisis affected all these sources. Fear, emigration, and economic depression diminished private charities. Furthermore, inability to pay taxes and a decrease in revenues from hospital investments intensified the financial plight of the institutions. Finally, in March 1791,

[33] Georges Lefebvre: *La grande peur de 1789*, Paris, Librairie Armand Colin, 1932; *idem: Études sur la Révolution Française*, Paris, Presses Universitaires de France, 1954, pp. 271-387; *idem: La Révolution Française*, Paris, Presses Universitaires de France, 1951, pp. 131-133.

all indirect taxes were suppressed, and on May 1, 1791, the *octroi*, the chief tax for hospital revenue, was abolished. As a result, hospital revenue from taxes disappeared, and the hospitals became completely dependent on the government. To deal with the immediate need, grants were made to the hospitals by the state in 1791 and 1792.[34] But the larger question still remained, how to organize the hospitals and their functions and how to finance them?

In the light of these problems, it is not surprising that there are two parts to the work of the Committee. The first comprises those measures proposed to deal with immediate problems; the second involves the preparation of a national and systematic plan for the reconstruction of public assistance which would be a part of the order of the new France. In the former category fall the efforts of the Committee to deal with the *ateliers de charité*, charity workshops set up to provide work relief for the unemployed. Much more significant in the long view, however, is the plan developed by Liancourt for a national system of assistance to the needy.

This plan is important not because it was ever realized, but rather because of its seminal ideas and breadth of view. The influence of the pre-revolutionary reform movement is clearly evident, and the mark of Rousseau's ideas on Liancourt is inescapable. The plan, however, developed the implications of the earlier ideas and proposals, and carried them forward to a level at which their significance transcended the immediate situation and the limits of the period.

After pointing out that no government had yet given constitutional recognition to the problem of assistance, Liancourt proclaimed the right of every man to existence.[35] "It appeared to the Committee," he asserted, "that this fundamental truth of all society, which imperiously demands a place in the Declaration of the Rights of Man, should be the basis of every law and every political institution which proposes to wipe out mendicity. . . . No state has yet considered the poor in its constitution. . . . The idea has always been to give charity to the poor, but never of asserting the claims of the poor on society, or those of society on them. There is the great task for the French constitution to achieve, since no other has yet recognized and respected the rights of man in this way. . . . The duty of society, then, is to seek to prevent distress and misery, to provide assistance in these circumstances by offering work to those who need it to live, by forcing them to work if they refuse, and finally by assist-

[34] McCloy, *op. cit.*, p. 199.
[35] Bloch and Tuetey, *op. cit.*, p. 310.

ing without work those who because of age or infirmity lack all means of providing for themselves." [36] In short, while accepting poverty as an evil inherent in human society, it was felt that "where there existed a class of men without means of support, at that point there existed a violation of the rights of humanity, there the equilibrium of society was disturbed," and action had to be taken to restore the balance.

Consequently, if public assistance is an obligation of society, it must be governed by principles other than those of charity.[37] It is no longer a concern only of an individual or of a community, but rather of the nation as a whole, and must be organized and financed on a national basis. Furthermore, if assistance is a national charge, all resources intended for this purpose should be nationalized. All wealth and possessions from which revenue is derived to support hospitals and other charitable institutions should be declared the property of the nation (*biens nationaux*). The financial resources allocated by the state for public assistance would be divided into two funds. The first would provide for the indigent sick, foundlings, the aged, the disabled, and for houses of correction, and the financial allocations would be distributed by departments, districts, and municipalities. Administrative machinery would be set up to administer and to supervise the work. The second would be a reserve fund to deal with extraordinary situations and unforeseen catastrophes.

Liancourt recognized full well the important role of sickness as a cause of indigency, and the first section of the plan deals with assistance to the sick poor in country and city.[38] These unfortunates should receive free and complete medical care promptly. As far as possible the sick poor should be attended at home, where they would remain in familiar surroundings. Each rural district (*canton*) would have a physician or surgeon appointed by the department, who would care for the indigent and supervise the health of children receiving assistance. These practitioners would render care when called. At stipulated times they would inoculate the children and adults on their panels. In the event of serious or epidemic disease, they would report to the welfare bureau of the district or department and request consultation from physicians attached to these bodies. Each year these practitioners would be required to report to the district office their observations and reflections on the climate and the soil, on the epidemics that had occurred, on the treatment of these diseases, and

[36] *Ibid.*, pp. 310, 328, 317.
[37] *Ibid.*, pp. 380-385.
[38] *Ibid.*, pp. 399-426.

to make a comparison of births, marriages, and deaths. The position of cantonal physician or surgeon would carry a remuneration of 500 livres. Midwives approved by the health agency of the canton would be paid out of public funds for delivering indigent women. Medicaments would be provided by a centrally located depot in the canton, in such a manner in each locality that the service would be as efficient, convenient, and economical as possible.

As in the country, the indigent town dweller would, insofar as possible, receive free medical attention at home. Towns of less than 4000 inhabitants would share provision for medical care with the rural areas of their canton. Towns of 4000 to 12,000 people would have one physician or surgeon to care for the sick poor. Municipalities with more than 12,000 people would have one practitioner for each administrative district (*arrondissement*). Liancourt saw that in large cities particularly domiciliary medical care would not be enough. He proposed, therefore, that cities of more than 4,000 population have general hospitals to receive those indigents who could not be attended at home. These establishments would not contain more than 150 beds. In addition to these, large cities would have special hospitals for obstetrics, major surgical procedures, for contagious diseases, venereal diseases, and curable mental illness.

The proposals advanced by the Committee also included assistance to foundlings, aid to large families, workshops for the unemployed, punishment of recurrent beggary, aid to the aged—in short, projects dealing with all the social problems of eighteenth century France. The budget for this program of social assistance was calculated at 51.5 million livres per year. Of this sum, 12 million livres were estimated for the indigent sick, 27.5 million for children, the aged and the disabled, 5 million for work relief, 3 million for repression of beggary and vagabondage, and 4 million for reserves and administration.[39] In addition, the Committee explored the possibility of creating a system of social insurance as a means of preventing indigency by promoting provident saving.[40] This was the plan developed by Liancourt and presented by the Committee on Mendicity to the Constituent Assembly. Basic to the plan was the premise that from the cradle to the tomb, man henceforth in the new France would be an integral member of a maternal and provident society.

These generous hopes, however, were not to be realized. The Assembly was concerned with other matters. The Constitution of September 3,

[39] *Ibid.*, pp. 551-552.
[40] *Ibid.*, pp. 454-464.

1791, stated simply that there "will be created and organized a general establishment for public assistance to provide for foundlings, care for the infirm poor, and provide work for the indigent who are unable to secure it themselves." [41] On September 26, Liancourt demanded that the proposals for organizing public assistance be placed on the agenda for discussion. Calling attention to the precarious financial situation of the hospitals, he pointed out that the abolition of the toll (*octroi*) had deprived them of their income, and that nothing had been done to solve the problem. The following day Liancourt returned to the subject, but to no avail. Prior to adjournment, however, the Assembly expressed the view "that the immensity of its labors had prevented it, in this session, from organizing the assistance which had been ordered to be established by the Constitution," and left to its successor "the honorable task of fulfilling this duty." [42] Nevertheless, the ideas had been sown; they would germinate in the future.

III.

The Legislative Assembly, the *corps législatif* set up under the constitution of 1791, met on October 1, 1791, unaware that its career would be short and stormy. It was imbued with a new spirit, the spirit of a nation in its third year of revolution and within six months of war. Among its members sat Carnot, the future architect of victory, the philosopher and mathematician Condorcet, and the surgeon Tenon. Most of the new deputies were lawyers, but among them were also 28 doctors. The Legislative Assembly was to have little time for social reform. It was convoked under ominous auspices. War threatened from without, and inside the country the opposition between the moderates and the radicals became more and more acute. Invasion, foreign war, the rising of August 10, the dethronement of the King, the September massacres—these are the events which characterize the problems faced by the Legislative Assembly. Compelled to devote its energy chiefly to a defense of the Revolution against internal and external foes, it was unable to transform into social reality the plan of assistance outlined by the Committee on Mendicity. Nonetheless, it gave some attention to this problem, took specific action as the occasion demanded, and developed a body of thought on the organization of public assistance, including medical care.

On October 13, 1791, Camus, the national archivist, reviewed for the

[41] J. M. Thompson: (editor): *French Revolution Documents 1789-94*, Oxford, Basil Blackwell, 1933, p. 113.

[42] Dreyfus, *op. cit.*, pp. 189-190.

Legislative Assembly the activities of the committees set up by the preceding Assembly, including those of the Health Committee and the Committee on Mendicity. The Health Committee (*comité de salubrité*) had been created by the Constituent Assembly on September 12, 1790, on a motion by Guillotin, and had been charged to look into all matters "relating to the art of healing and its teaching, to health establishments in city and country, such as hospitals, schools and the like, and in general to all subjects likely to be of interest for the public health." [43] Concerning itself with matters of professional practice and public health administration, it was consulted by the Committee on Mendicity on the provision of surgeons for rural areas. As part of the work of the Health Committee, Jean Gabriel Gallot, its secretary, in 1790 laid before the Constituent Assembly a plan for the complete reorganization of the medical system, as well as a plan for the erection of hospitals in the country.[44] Turning to the Committee on Mendicity, Camus reminded his audience that the Constituent Assembly had adjourned without acting on its proposals. Emphasizing the importance of the matter, he urged the deputies to take up and "to discharge the nation's debt to miserable and suffering humanity." [45]

The following day, on October 14, Tenon moved the creation of a new committee which would combine the areas of activity of the two earlier committees. After some discussion, the motion was adopted, and on October 27, 1791, the Committee of Public Assistance came into being. The name of the committee is worth noting as indicative of a change in public sentiment. The need for a coordinated program of public assistance was now an accepted axiom of public policy. Consisting of twenty-five members and eleven alternates, the Committee contained most of the twenty-eight physicians in the Assembly. Among them were Tenon, who became chairman of the Committee, Gastellier,[46] who received one of the two secretarial positions, and Bô, surgeon and apothecary, as well as one of the most radical members of the Mountain.[47] The Committee organized

[43] Bloch and Tuetey, *op. cit.*, p. XXIX.

[44] A. G. Chevalier: The Physicians in the Revolutionary Assemblies, *Ciba Symposia* 7: 245, 1946.

[45] Ferdinand Dreyfus: *L'Assistance sous la Législative et la Convention (1792-1795)*, Paris, 1905, p. 10.

[46] René Georges Gastellier (1741(?)-1821) did not play a prominent political rôle. He was so addicted to scientific polemics that his contemporaries called him "Guy Patin redivivus." His moderate political views almost brought him to the guillotine, and he was saved only by the fall of Robespierre. Chevalier, *op. cit.*, p. 247.

[47] Chevalier, *op. cit.*, p. 244.

itself into three sections concerned respectively with public assistance, health, and mendicity. From October 29, 1791, to September 19, 1792, it held 106 sessions.

At first sight, it might seem that the Committee's task was relatively simple. All it had to do was to discuss the reports and recommendations of the Committee on Mendicity and if these were found acceptable to submit them to the Assembly for a vote. *Aber die Verhältnisse die sind nicht so!* By the beginning of 1792, the Committee had not even begun its work. What was it doing during these two months? The answer is simple. It was fully occupied with specific requests and petitions for assistance. Created to study and to recommend legislative measures, the Committee soon found that through force of circumstances it was turning into an administrative agency concerned with proposals for action by the Legislative Assembly to relieve distressed individuals or localities.

Requests for relief came from all parts of the country, from individuals and from public officials, all calling attention to the distress of the poor, and to the calamitous position of the institutions intended for their relief, above all that of the hospitals. The reasons for the increasingly critical situation of the hospitals were known. Roland, Minister of the Interior, pointed them out to the Convention several months later. The hospitals, he said, " like all public establishments in France had delevoped in relation to a scheme of things which no longer exists in the present regime, that is to say, the obligations still exist but a part of the means of discharging them has vanished. The tithes and the feudal rights, so pernicious in themselves, were not exclusively the prey of the church and the nobles; they were also one of the main sources of income of the hospitals and colleges. . . ." [48] On November 2, 1789, the government had confiscated the property of the church and the religious orders, declaring euphemistically that " all church property is at the disposal (*disposition*) of the nation." [49] This decree also included hospital property. In support of this action it was argued that if the state takes over social services such as charity it can take as well the resources necessary to support them. Logically, therefore, the property of the secular hospitals could not long remain untouched, and in January, 1791, the Committee on Mendicity proposed its confiscation. The opposition was too powerful, however, and the measure was defeated. The defeat was temporary, however, for on July 11, 1794, all hospital property was taken over by the state.

48 Bouchet, *op. cit.*, p. 285.

49 J. M. Thompson: *The French Revolution*, Oxford, Basil Blackwell, 1944, p. 146.

The financial situation was further aggravated by increased demands for assistance.[50] Appeals for aid came from departments or municipalities suffering from the ravages of invasion or of natural calamities, such as floods or poor harvests. Individuals of all kinds who believed they had a claim on the beneficence of the nation appealed for assistance. The blind, the deaf-mute, the veteran crippled in the defense of the Revolution—all demanded relief. Public assistance began more and more to serve a dual purpose, to care for the needy and also to reward the patriot. (The latter purpose was to become increasingly prominent as the Republic fought for its life on many fronts.) The Committee examined all these appeals, decided what action to recommend, and then referred them to the appropriate executive department or agency. In large measure the report prepared by the Committee of Public Assistance for the Legislative Assembly was based on these petitions.

The report on the organization of public assistance was presented to the Assembly on June 13, 1792, by Bernard, deputy from the Yonne department. It was not received with any marked interest. The deputies were more concerned with other cares. This was the day on which the Brissotin ministry was dismissed. The Assembly and the people were preparing for a showdown with the King and his party. A week later the Tuileries were invaded by the " sovereign People." Involved with more pressing problems, the Legislative Assembly had no time to discuss Bernard's report. It was put on the shelf alongside that of the Committee on Mendicity.

What is the essence of Bernard's report? The ideas of Liancourt and his colleagues provided a point of departure for Bernard. This report, like that of the Committee on Mendicity, has as its *leitmotiv* a fundamental concept: the right of the indigent to public assistance. As Bernard clearly acknowledged, it derived from Rousseau's *contrat social.* " The object of the Revolution," he said, " is to protect those who have little against those who have much, the poor against the rich. It was made for the poor." [51] " The state owes each of its members security and protection; the property of the rich man and the existence of the poor man, which is his property, must receive equal protection as a public trust. Whence follows the principle still lacking in the Declaration of the Rights

[50] Raoul Mercier: *Le monde médical de Touraine sous la Révolution*, Tours, Arnault & Cie., 1936, pp. 300-374; Pauly Gargues: *Les hospices d'Angers: Précis historique et documentaire*, Angers, 1933, pp. 35-39; Dreyfus, *op. cit.*, pp. 16-19; Bouchet, *op. cit.*, pp. 286-287.

[51] Dreyfus, *op. cit.*, p. 25.

of Man, the principle worthy of being placed at the head of the Code of Humanity which you are going to issue: Every man is entitled to existence through work if he is able-bodied, through free assistance if he is unable to work."[52] The right to assistance is a counterpart of the obligation to work. Assistance at any age is therefore a compensation either for work performed or for work to be performed. Thus, aid either to the young or to the old, to the sick or the disabled, is no longer a matter of charity but a national obligation.

Based on these principles, medical care would be provided to the needy. Bernard was convinced of the superiority of domiciliary care and insisted on the danger and uselessness of increasing the number of hospitals. The plan of the Committee of Public Assistance, like that of its predecessor, ranged from the womb to the tomb.[53] Children would be protected even before birth. Trained midwives would be available in each canton to give free care to indigent expectant mothers. Not only foundlings would have a right to national assistance. Children of indigent parents would also be assisted. Efforts would be made to have foundlings adopted, preferably by childless couples. Pensions would be given to the aged, and they would be free to choose whether to remain with their families or to live in homes provided by the government. The sick poor would receive free medical attention at home from a health officer (*officier de santé*) serving the canton. This would suffice, in Bernard's opinion, for all indigents with homes and families. However, since many lacked any domicile, a certain number of "lazarettos" (*maladreries*) would have to be maintained in proportion to the population. Furthermore, it would be necessary to establish in each department a large hospital for special diseases, for major surgical operations, and for mental patients. Finally, the Committee felt that the prevention of indigency was an essential part of such a program. As one means to this end it suggested the extension of land-ownership, and proposed that the government assist rural laborers to become small proprietors. Another proposal was to encourage the formation of provident societies and savings establishments. Ideas of mutual aid societies were much in the air at this time. Condorcet advocated the organization of Assistance and Savings Societies (*Caisses de secours et d'accumulation*);[54] and a certain Marsillac proposed to replace hospitals

[52] *Ibid.*, p. 26.

[53] Bouchet, *op. cit.*, pp. 313-315.

[54] Léon Cahen: *Condorcet et la Révolution Française*, Paris, Felix Alcan, 1904, pp. 309-312.

by " civic societies, which would assure artisans of all physical or moral assistance in case of sickness or other human affliction." [55]

While the report of the Committee of Public Assistance was not discussed by the Legislative Assembly, its ideas were presented to the Convention several months later by Bô, one of its medical members, and helped to influence the action taken by that body in 1793. The Assembly did pass measures, however, which had serious consequences for hospitals and the provision of medical care. The Constituent Assembly in February 1790, had abolished the religious orders, except those devoted to nursing and teaching. Under the Legislative Assembly, relations between the revolutionary government and the religious orders worsened as part of the general religious crisis. By decrees of August 4 and 18, 1792, the religious orders were finally suppressed, although their members were asked to continue their work in the hospitals on an individual basis.[56] This action created a certain amount of confusion and disorder in the hospitals of the religious orders.

The situation was further confused by a decree of August 18, 1792, abolishing all " privileged associations," a category which included universities, medical schools, and scientific societies.[57] In this way the freedom of occupation proclaimed by the Revolution was to be secured. However, with the abolition of the teaching institutions and the disappearance of examinations, the quacks were given a free field. An act intended to remove discrimination and to enlarge the medical profession soon redounded to the great disadvantage both of the profession and the people it was supposed to benefit. This was the situation that faced the Convention.

IV.

On September 20, 1792, at Valmy in the Argonne, French revolutionary soldiers fought to a standstill the invading troops of Prussia and forced their withdrawal. Goethe, who was with the Duke of Brunswick, clearly grasped the significance of the Prussian reversal, when he wrote: " Here and today begins a new age in the history of the world. Some day you will be able to say—I was there." By one of those symbolic coincidences of history, it was on this day of victory that the National

[55] Dreyfus, *op. cit.*, p. 30.

[56] Bouchet, *op. cit.*, pp. 322-325.

[57] Chevalier, *op. cit.*, p. 247; Mercier, *op. cit.*, p. 40; A. Bordier: *La médecine à Grenoble: Notes pour servir à l'histoire de l'école de médecine et de pharmacie*, Grenoble, 1896, pp. 155-156.

Convention met to elect its officers. It was this body, the most radical of all the revolutionary assemblies, which abolished the monarchy, proclaimed the Republic, and executed Louis Capet. It was in the Convention and the government of revolutionary terror that the Republic concentrated all its energies and fought for its life. It was under the Convention that the Jacobins seized power and in a bitter internecine struggle established a dictatorship to save the state by overcoming foreign foes, internal anarchy, and civil war. It was the Convention that carried the revolutionary doctrines beyond the borders of France and left the Republic mistress of Belgium and Holland, at peace with Spain and Prussia, and a menace to Germany and Lombardy. And it was the Convention, which in the midst of the alarms of war and the turmoil of party strife, found the time to undertake the radical changes recommended by the Committee on Mendicity and the Committee of Public Assistance. It remained for the Convention to carry out the promise incorporated in the Constitution of '91 that all assistance would become a public service on a national footing.

The work of the Convention in the field of assistance was carried out through several bodies. Executive functions were divided among the Ministry of the Interior, the Committee of Public Assistance, and the Committee of Public Safety. The Committee of Public Assistance in the Convention was simply an extension of the committee of the same name in the preceding assembly. Originally set up on April 6, 1793, after the treachery of Dumouriez and the defeat of Nerwinden, the Committee of Public Safety passed through several phases before it finally became the organ of revolutionary government. On the 12 germinal, Year II (April 2, 1794), twelve executive commissions were created under the jurisdiction of the Committee of Public Safety. These were in essence departments of the Committee, and reported to certain of its members. The sixth of these commissions dealt with public assistance and was responsible to a group of three comprising Carnot, Prieur (of the Côte d'Or), and Lindet, who were charged with the organization of defense, control of commerce, agriculture and food, and internal administration.[58] As the role of the Committee of Public Safety increased in importance, that of the Committee of Public Assistance declined. The former made important executive decisions that were carried out by its sixth commission, while the latter was occupied with the theoretical discussion of general projects,

[58] Palmer, *op. cit.*, p. 307; Dreyfus, *op. cit.*, pp. 38-39; Marcel Reinhard: *Le Grand Carnot* (2 vols.), Paris, Hachette, 1950-1952, vol. II, p. 127.

technical aspects of administration, and the distribution of some minor forms of assistance. The Committee of Public Assistance also played a very important part in preparing the fundamental laws on assistance which were presented to the Convention by Bô and Barère.

The task which confronted the Convention in the midst of revolutionary turmoil was no simple one. It was not only a matter of creating a means of providing for the poor, the sick, the infirm, the unemployed, or any of the other classes of unfortunates who appealed to the government for aid. While the French troops fought to hurl back the foreign invader, what was to become of their families, of their wives and children if the state did not look after them? Thus, the trend initiated by the Legislative Assembly of employing assistance as a resource for the defense of the country became a policy under the Convention. Aid was given to the widows and orphans of soldiers, to the wounded and the maimed, and to invaded departments. As these obligations grew in magnitude and complexity, it was clear that a workable system of public assistance was essential, and this was accomplished by a series of laws passed in 1793 and 1794.

The fundamental basis of this legislation was laid down in the Constitution of 1793.[59] A constitutional committee had been set up by the Convention on September 29, 1792. Among its members were Danton, Barère, Condorcet, and Tom Paine. In reply to an invitation to "all friends of Liberty and Equality to present their plans and views," hundreds of communications were received. These amateur constitution makers all recognized public assistance as "a sacred debt of society." Carnot declared "that society should provide for the needs of those whose services it required; equally it owes assistance to those whom age or infirmity render unable to provide for themselves." In his *Project for a People's Constitution*, the deputy Poultier elaborated a complete plan of public assistance. Recognizing, he wrote, "the right of a citizen to existence and the security of his life, every citizen in a state of indigency will receive subsistance and support in proportion to his needs and services." Each department would have an establishment to provide aid to the aged, the disabled, and the orphan, work for the able-bodied poor, and medical care for the sick. Romme, a member of the Mountain, summed up the general principle underlying these projects and proposals in his statement that the Rights of Man are divided into political rights and social rights.

[59] For the Constitution of 1793 see Albert Mathiez: *Girondins et Montagnards*, Paris, Firmin-Didot et Cie., 1930, pp. 82-108.

The latter comprise "civil liberty, education, assistance, justice, public safety, and equality before the law." [60]

The draft of the new constitution based on the materials studied by the committee and prepared chiefly by Condorcet was presented to the Convention on February 15, 1793. As a preamble it contained a Declaration of the Rights of Man and the Citizen, which was discussed from April 17 to May 29, 1793. The debate was carried on in an atmosphere of increasing tension and hostility aroused by military reverses and by the bitter fight for power between Jacobin and Girondist. The social doctrine embodied in the constitutional draft entered into the power struggle of the parties. The Declaration of Rights prepared by Condorcet contained a statement that "public assistance is a sacred debt of society." For the Jacobins this formulation was inadequate, and they insisted on strengthening it. Oudot cried out: "The wealthy must cease to regard as generosity that which is a duty." More significant, however, were the principles expressed by Robespierre on April 24 in his speech on the limitations of property rights. "The right of property," he said, "is limited like all others by the obligation to respect the rights of others. It must not impair either the safety, or the liberty, or the existence, or the property of our fellowmen." [61] Following the defeat and expulsion from the Convention of the Girondist deputies, the Jacobins hurriedly redrafted the constitution to embody their principles. Introduced into the Convention on June 10, 1793, and adopted on June 24, its Article 21 states unequivocally: "Public assistance is a sacred debt. Society owes subsistance to unfortunate citizens, either by providing them with work, or by assuring the means of existence for those unable to work." [62]

Meanwhile, the legislative application of these principles had been initiated by a law passed on March 19, 1793, establishing a basis for a logically organized national system of social assistance.[63] All who needed assistance would receive it at state expense. Charity and begging were prohibited. Work relief would be provided for the able-bodied, while the infirm poor of whatever kind would receive assistance at home or in hospitals. The law also envisaged the creation of a national social insur-

[60] Dreyfus, *op. cit.*, pp. 55-57.

[61] Mathiez, *op. cit.*, pp. 94-95.

[62] J. M. Thompson (ed.): *French Revolution Documents 1789-94*, Oxford, Basil Blackwell, 1933, pp. 240-241.

[63] L. Cahen and R. Guyot: *L'Oeuvre législative de la Révolution*, Paris, Felix Alcan, 1931, pp. 434-436; Jacques Godechot: *Les Institutions de la France sous la Révolution et l'Empire*, Paris, Presses Universitaires, 1951, p. 379.

ance fund, based on voluntary contributions to be placed on the "altar of the nation" (*autel de la patrie*) on civic holidays. Offices of health would care for the poor receiving domiciliary assistance, for foundlings, and for the children of indigent parents.

Having set out the general scheme for a national system, the Convention proceeded to deal with special groups requiring assistance. A decree of June 28-July 8 provided for children, expectant mothers, and the aged. According to the first article of this law, "Fathers and mothers who have no other resource but the product of their labor have a claim to assistance by the nation whenever the result of their labor is inadequate for the needs of the family."[64] Large families were to be aided by granting allowances for every child after the second. Assistance to expectant mothers would begin with the sixth month of pregnancy. Unwed mothers, illegitimate children, and foundlings would have the same rights as other women and children. In each district, an institution, to be known as a *maternité* would be established for unwed mothers. If an unwed mother wished to nurse and keep her child, the state would provide financial assistance. Should such an arrangement be impossible or undesirable, the authorities would place the child with a wet-nurse or in an institution. All children supported by the state would have to be inoculated against smallpox. At the age of twelve, poor boys would be apprenticed at public expense. For the aged the law provided pensions and care at home or in an institution. Each district was to have a medical practitioner (officer of health), a midwife, and a store of medicaments.

Almost a year later, on the 22 floréal, Year II (May 11, 1794), the Convention passed another comprehensive law to assist the needy.[65] Its author was Barère who had been a member of the Committee on Mendicity. Prepared at the request of the Convention, it was intended to deal with other needs, financial and medical, of the poor.

This measure reflects the political and social circumstances out of which it grew. As the Jacobin dictatorship intensified its struggle against enemies on all sides, it was forced to lean for support more heavily on the masses of the towns and the countryside, *the true sansculottes*. For Saint-Just, as for Robespierre, society comprised two classes, "the good citizens, who are at the same time the poor, the Jacobins, the sansculottes, and the rich, the aristocrats, the corrupt."[66] In his important speech of

[64] Cahen and Guyot, *op. cit.*, p. 440.
[65] *Ibid.*, pp. 443-446.
[66] Dreyfus, *op. cit.*, p. 71.

19 vendémiaire (October 10, 1793), Saint-Just had indicated the line that Jacobin policy would take. " In a wisely ruled state," he said, " bread belongs to the people by right. . . ."[67] Then, on February 26, 1794, in presenting the first of the Laws of Ventôse, he went even further. " Abolish mendicity which dishonors a free state," he demanded of the Convention. " The property of patriots is sacred, but that of conspirators is at the disposal of the unfortunate, who are the masters of the earth. They have a right to dictate to governments that neglect their interests." [68] In this spirit the Jacobin government formulated its social policy, and appealed to the people. Price regulation by means of the law of the *maximum*, and the laws of Ventôse are aspects of this endeavor; Barère's law is still another.[69]

It dealt largely with pensions and medical care for the poor in country and town. Characteristic of its spirit is the statement that the words " alms " and " hospital " must be erased from the republican vocabulary.[70] There would be only domiciliary assistance in the country. Every department would draw up a Book of National Beneficence (*Livre de la bienfaisance nationale*) in which would be inscribed every tenth day (*décadi*) the names of needy agricultural laborers, artisans, and mothers and widows with children. Once a year in the capitol of each district there was to be held a festival of misfortune (*malheur*) at which the Book of Beneficence would be read aloud and the beneficiaries would receive their pensions. This festival would be dedicated to maternity and old age. As Barère saw the exalted scene with his mind's eye, he waxed eloquent. To the Convention, he said: " The two extremities of life will be united with the sex which is its source. Aged laborers and infirm artisans will be there, and beside them mothers and unfortunate widows with their children. This spectacle is the most beautiful one that politics can present to Nature and which a fertilized earth can offer to a consoling Heaven." [71] Each sick indigent was to receive 10 *sous* a day, and 6 *sous* for each dependent child. To obtain this support they would have to be inscribed in the Book of Beneficence. To care for the sick poor each district would have three medical practitioners. They would receive 1000 livres a year a

[67] *Oeuvres de Saint-Just, répresentant du peuple a la Convention Nationale*, Paris, Prevot, 1834, p. 173.

[68] *Ibid.*, p. 212; see also Albert Ollivier: *Saint-Just et la force des choses*, Paris, Gallimard, 1954, pp. 325-335.

[69] Mathiez, *op. cit.*, p. 129.

[70] Dreyfus, *op. cit.*, p. 73.

[71] *Ibid.*, p. 74.

piece, and would have at their disposal eight boxes of medicaments, valued at 30 livres, as well as a supply of rice, flour and potatoes.

Steps were taken to put the law into operation. Each district received a copy of the text, an explicatory circular, and a sample of the Book of National Beneficence. Application was incomplete, however, for the available resources were limited, and were more urgently needed to provide the sinews of war. Following the downfall of the Robespierrists in Thermidor, the Convention and then the Directory moved back to a modified version of the pre-revolutionary arrangements.

While the Convention endeavored to create a general body of law to implement the constitution of 1793, it also took action on specific problems. As already mentioned, on July 11, 1794, hospitals were taken over by the state, and the government assumed responsibility for hospital indebtedness and maintenance. Hospital property was sold and the proceeds were used for the needs of the government. Many of the older institutions were turned into military hospitals, and new ones were built for this purpose. In the third report of the Committee on Mendicity, Papion *le jeune* had emphasized the need for single beds and ample ventilation, and had pointed to the example of other countries. On November 15, 1793, the Convention passed a decree that every hospital patient should have his own bed, and that beds should be separated from each other by a distance of three feet. Just how effective this decree was cannot be determined. Nonetheless, it is interesting that in a booklet published in the Year II and addressed to the Convention, Souquet, physician to the military hospital at Boulogne, calls attention to the facts that the wards are well ventilated, that the beds are not surrounded by curtains and are clean in every respect.[72]

V.

The thought and action of the Convention represent the most advanced point attained by the French Revolution in dealing with social assistance inclusive of medical care. This is of more than passing interest to an age which has developed its social services to a high degree and which prides itself on this achievement. It is in the programs and laws of the revolutionary governments that the first outlines of these developments may be discerned. The French revolutionaries deserve credit on various counts. They embodied the fundamental right of man to existence in the

[72] Souquet: *Essai sur l'histoire topographique physico-médicinale du district de Boulogne-sur-Mer, Department du Pas-de-Calais,* Boulogne, Dolet, l'an deuxième de la République Française, p. 148.

basic law of the land. They endeavored to set up a national system of social assistance, inclusive of health care. Their emphasis on home care wherever possible was salutory and progressive in the light of hospital conditions at the time. Furthermore, they called attention to the need for assistance, inclusive of medical care, in neglected areas and for neglected groups in the population. They endeavored to see the problem of assistance as a whole. Finally, they developed ideas on public policy which were to influence France profoundly during the first half of the nineteenth century, and through her other countries. Ideas of public service, public interest, and social utility provided the seed-bed in which germinated new views on the relations between health, medicine, and society.[73] The men of '89 and '93 could not forsee the consequences that would stem from their thought and action. The triumph of the machine and the concentration of capital were still in the future, but it was in terms of the situation created by these developments that the men of '48 endeavored to apply the ideas of their predecessors. In this attempt they carried them foreward to a more advanced level. Medicine, a social science—the idea of '48—must be seen as the first fruit of this historical process, a process which has continued in a variety of circumstances to our own day.

[73] J. Bélin: *La logique d'une idée-force. L'idée d'utilité sociale pendant la Révolution Française, 1789-1792,* Paris, 1939; Leroy, *op. cit.,* pp. 318-324.

POLITICAL ORDER AND HUMAN HEALTH IN JEFFERSONIAN THOUGHT *

The significance of health as a question of public policy was recognized and appreciated in eighteenth century Europe and America. Owing to varying political, economic, and social considerations, this awareness did not manifest itself everywhere to the same degree or in the same form. For example. it appeared most sharply in the concept of medical police, formulated within the framework of German absolutism and mercantilism. While there was no comparable systematic formulation of French and British thought and action on the question of social policy in relation to problems of health, it is possible to trace the various elements involved so as to have an ordered view of their origin and development.[1]

Here I shall deal with a related subject, that is, Jeffersonian views on the relations between political and social organization and states of health. As applied here, the term Jeffersonian is not limited to the views of Thomas Jefferson. It is used rather to describe the ideas of a group of men who were associated with Jefferson politically, scientifically, or socially, and who in varying degree shared his views. Among them may be mentioned Thomas Paine, Benjamin Rush, Joel Barlow, David Rittenhouse, and in his earlier years, Thomas Cooper. For the most part, however, this analysis will deal with Jefferson and Rush, as their thought offers the most sharply formulated views on the reciprocal relations of social and physical health.

Neither Jefferson nor Rush ever developed any systematic theory of the social relations of health. Nonetheless, their scattered ideas can be pieced together from a variety of sources to form a coherent whole. Jefferson's correspondence is the main source for his views, while Rush expressed his ideas throughout his numerous essays and books, as well as in his Commonplace Book. In considerable measure, the ideas of Jefferson, Rush, and the kindred spirits associated with them were not original, and in many instances were consciously borrowed to fill some immediate need.

* Read at the twenty-fourth annual meeting of the American Association of the History of Medicine, Baltimore, May 3, 1951.

[1] George Rosen: *The Idea of Social Medicine* (Chap. I, Mercantilism, Absolutism and Medical Police; II. Health and Social Policy in Britain and France from the Seventeenth Century to the End of the Ancien Régime) (unpublished manuscript).

This very fact, however, provided a definite frame of reference within which to operate, for they were immersed in the intellectual climate of the Enlightenment and therefore confidently adopted and applied certain clusters of ideas and patterns of thought very generally accepted as self-evident.

Design, Nature, Natural Law, Reason, and Happiness were key concepts in the thinking of the Enlightenment, and are employed with unhesitating regularity in Jeffersonian thought. It was accepted as a basic premise that the world had been established by the Creator according to a definite plan, within which there were ordered ways of behaving. These ordered ways were the laws of nature, which redounded to the glory of the Creator and the greater good of man. " What is natural law? " asked Volney. And in answer to his question replied that " It is the regular and constant order of events, by which God rules the universe." It followed ineluctably, therefore, that human nature and human institutions were subject to and resulted from the operation of these laws. Montesquieu pointed out that " Man is born in society and there he remains "; and Adam Ferguson echoed this in his comment: " If we are asked, therefore, where the state of nature is to be found? We may answer, it is here."

Underlying Jeffersonian political theory are these views, as well as the corollary, that the biological, social, psychological, and moral relations of man to his environment were so interlocked that they were all one. Indeed, the Creator had so designed the human body that it would flourish when it lived in harmony with its political and social environment, and conversely He had so framed the political order that human health was fostered by good social institutions. Both Jefferson and Rush are quite explicit on this point.

In his *Inquiry into the Natural History of Medicine among the Indians of North America,* which was read before the American Philosophical Society in 1774, Rush observed that disease, political institutions and economic organization were so interrelated that any general social change produced accompanying changes in health.

> The leprosy, elephantiasis, scurvy and venereal disease, appear to be different modifications of the same primary disorder. The same causes produce them in every age and country. They are diversified like plants by climate and nourishment. They all spring originally from a moist atmosphere and unwholesome diet; hence we read of their prevailing so much in the middle centuries, when the principal parts of Europe were overflowed with water, and the inhabitants lived entirely on fish and a few unwholesome vegetables. The abolition of the feudal system in

Europe, by introducing freedom, introduced at the same time agriculture; which by multiplying the fruits of the earth, lessened the consumption of animal food, and thus put a stop to these disorders. The elephantiasis is almost unknown in Europe. The leprosy is confined chiefly to the low countries of Africa. The plica polonica once so common in Poland, is to be found only in books of medicine. The small pox is no longer a fatal disorder, when the body is prepared for its reception by a vegetable regimen. Even the plague itself is losing its sting. It is hardly dreaded at this time in Turkey; and its very existence is preserved there by the doctrine of fatalism, which prevails among the inhabitants of that country. It may serve as a new and powerful motive against political slavery to observe, that it is connected with those diseases which most deform and debase the human body. It may likewise serve to enhance the blessings of liberty, to trace its effects, in eradicating such loathsome and destructive disorders.[2]

Despite its obvious historical and medical inadequacies, this passage has been quoted at length because it demonstrates explicitly the central Jeffersonian view of the connection betwen physical and social well-being. Nor is this an isolated instance. Later in the same essay, discussing the relation of health and civilization Rush observed that the complete enjoyment of health is as compatible with civilization, as the enjoyment of civil liberty.

We read of countries rich in everything that can form national happiness and national grandeur, the diseases of which are nearly as few and simple as those of the Indians. We hear of no diseases among the Jews, while they were under their democratical form of government, except such as were inflicted by a supernatural power. . . . The Empire of China, it is said, contains more inhabitants than the whole of Europe. The political institutions of that country have exempted its inhabitants from a large share of the diseases of other civilized nations. . . . But it is unnecessary to appeal to ancient or remote nations to prove, that health is not incompatible with civilization. The inhabitants of many parts of New England, particularly the province of Connecticut are strangers to artificial diseases.[3]

Twenty-five years later, in 1799, Rush published *Three Lectures on Animal Life* in which he reiterated his observations.

In no part of the human species is animal life in a more perfect state than in the inhabitants of Great Britain, and the United States of America. With all the natural stimuli that have been mentioned, they are constantly under the invigorating influence of liberty. There is an indissoluble union between moral, political and physical happiness; and if it be true, that elective and representative governments

---

[2] Benjamin Rush: An Inquiry into the Natural History of Medicine among the Indians of North America, and a comparative view of their diseases and remedies with those of civilized nations, *Medical Inquiries and Observations* . . . (second American edition). Philadelphia, Thomas Dobson, 1794, pp. 24-25.

[3] *Ibid.*, pp. 67-69.

are most favourable to individual as well as national prosperity, it follows of course, that they are most favourable to animal life. . . . Many facts prove, animal life to exist in a larger quantity and for a longer time, in the enlightened and happy state of Connecticut, in which republican liberty has existed above one hundred and fifty years, than in any other country upon the surface of the globe.[4]

Associated with or implicit in this central premise are certain logical inferences that the Jeffersonian thinkers did not hestiate to draw. Since the health of the body and the health of society are so intimately and positively related, it seemed an obvious inference that wherever the human species flourished and multiplied, there the political and social order was good and in accord with the laws of nature. The state of the population thus became a diagnostic criterion of a healthy society. According to Rush, " The population of a country is not to be accomplished by rewards and punishments. And it is happy for America, that the universal prevalence of the protestant religion, the checks lately given to negro slavery, the general unwillingness among us to acknowledge the usurpations of primogeniture, the universal practice of inoculation for the smallpox, and the absence of the plague, render the interposition of government for that purpose unnecessary." [5] Only a free and republican government could provide favorable conditions for population growth, while a monarchy which undertook to increase population by artificial means would inevitably fail.

At the same time, just because health and happiness were recognized as positive values, and accepted as symptoms of harmony with the order of nature, the existence of disease and physical disability even in America could not be overlooked. How could the ideas of order and design be reconciled with the individual and social loss resulting from disease and death? How justify the yellow fever epidemic which devastated Philadelphia and other American cities? In essence, this was a problem with which men had wrestled for thousands of years, and which many had attempted to solve. Earlier periods had in the main offered theological answers; the eighteenth century saw it as a problem of philosophy. Alexander Pope in his *Essay on Man* formulated the philosophical reply in its sharpest form.

[4] *The Selected Writings of Benjamin Rush,* edited by Dagobert D. Runes, New York, Philosophical Library, 1947, pp. 167-168.

[5] Rush, *Medical Inquiries and Observations* . . . ,second American edition), Philadelphia, 1794, pp. 74-75.

All Nature is but Art, unknown to thee;
All Chance, direction, which thou canst not see;
All discord, harmony not understood;
All partial evil, universal Good . . .

This is the Jeffersonian answer to the same crucial problem. Theirs is a reply essentially optimistic, perhaps even with Panglossian overtones.

In a letter to Rush dated September 23, 1800, Jefferson referred to outbreaks of yellow fever in Baltimore, Norfolk, and Providence, and offered this consoling thought. "When great evils happen," he wrote, "I am in the habit of looking out for what good may arise from them as consolations to us, and Providence has in fact so established the order of things, as that most evils are the means of producing some good. The yellow fever will discourage the growth of great cities in our nation, and I view great cities as pestilential to the morals, the health and the liberties of man."[6] On October 1, 1812, in a letter to Colonel William Duane, Jefferson returned to this problem. Discussing his physical condition, he indicated that he was still on the alert for the good which would compensate for the debility of old age. "As a compensation for faculties departed," he wrote, "nature gives me good health, and a perfect resignation to the laws of decay which she has prescribed to all forms and combinations of matter."[7]

Nor did Jefferson change his mind. In a letter to John Adams dated April 8, 1816, he expressed what may be considered his ultimate view of the matter. Measured optimism and a sense of design pervade Jefferson's remarks. While recognizing that happiness is never unalloyed, he still felt that in the long view all was for the best in this world. The justification of disease and pain would eventually come from those who studied this problem, the pathologists.

I think with you (he wrote to Adams), that it is a good world on the whole; that it has been framed on a principle of benevolence and more pleasure than pain dealt out to us. . . . . There are, I acknowledge, even in the happiest life, some terrible convulsions, heavy set-offs against the opposite page of the account. I have often wondered for what good end the sensations of grief could be intended. All our passions, within proper bounds, have an useful object. And the perfection of the moral character is, not in a stoical apathy, so hypocritically vaunted, and so untruly too, because impossible, but in a just equilibrium of all the passions. I wish the pathologists then would tell us what is the use of grief in the economy, and of what good it is the cause, proximate or remote.[8]

---

[6] *The Writings of Thomas Jefferson,* edited by Albert Ellery Bergh, Washington, D. C., 1905, vol. X, p. 173.

[7] *Ibid.*, vol. XIII, p. 187.

[8] *Ibid.,* vol. XIV, p. 467.

Rush shared the view that the creator's plan took both good and evil, health and disease into account. From his experience during epidemics, he concluded that fevers affected chiefly the poor, and consequently that the means to treat such diseases must be cheap and easy to apply. "From the affinity established by the Creator between evil and its antidotes, in other parts of his works," he observed, "I am disposed to believe no remedy will ever be effectual in any general disease, that is not cheap, and that cannot easily be made universal." [9]

This doctrine, that the world is a system which automatically works to produce good, was accepted by the Jeffersonians in association with the thesis of perfectibility. Faith in the growth of an order of peace, happiness, and health made it possible to accept the evils of life and yet remain an optimist. Belief in inevitable progress and perfectibility gives Jeffersonian thought a characteristically buoyant and confident cast. Poetically transfigured, this faith appears in the *Columbiad*, Joel Barlow's epic of the American Enlightenment.

> Sun of the moral world! effulgent source
> Of man's best wisdom and his steadiest force,
> Soul-searching Freedom! here assume thy stand
> And radiate hence to every distant land;
> Point out and prove how all the scenes of strife,
> The shock of states, the impassion'd broils of life,
> Spring from unequal sway; and how they fly
> Before the splendor of thy peaceful eye;
> Unfold at last the genuine social plan,
> The mind's full scope, the dignity of man,
> Bold nature bursting thro her long disguise
> And nations daring to be just and wise.

Clearly, then, government and the principles of political and social organization were matters of fundamental importance in relation to physical and mental health. According to Joseph Priestley, "The great instrument in the hand of divine providence, of this progress of society towards improvement, is *society* and consequently government." [10] To establish a healthy society, it was essential to determine and set up the right kind of government. This approach to the problem brings to light, however, a basic contradiction in Jeffersonian thought which was never resolved. With their faith in the common sense of mankind, the Jeffersonians

[9] Nathan G. Goodman: *Benjamin Rush, Physician and Citizen 1746-1813,* Philadelphia, University of Pennsylvania Press, 1934, p. 208.

[10] Basil Willey: *The Eighteenth Century Background,* London, Chatto and Windus, 1946, p. 195.

believed that free men could be trusted to discover the good society. At the same time, this voluntaristic approach to politics was coupled with determinism. Indeed, Jefferson's analysis of the nature and rôle of political parties was erected upon a basis of biological determinism. Republican theory accepted the origin and existence of political parties as inevitable in any human community. In attempting to account for this phenomenon Jefferson laid great stress on the biological basis of political activity. Indeed, if nothing else were known about Jeffersonian thought, one might be tempted to see in these views a biological theory of politics. Several years before becoming president, in a letter written to James Sullivan in 1779, Jefferson observed that " Where a constitution like ours, wears a mixed aspect of monarchy and republicanism, its citizens will naturally divide into two classes of sentiment, according as their tone of body or mind, their habits, connections and callings, induce them to wish to strengthen either the monarchical or the republican features of the constitution." [11] Similarly, in a letter to John Adams in 1813, Jefferson pointed out that political parties were both biological and social phenomena. In fact, he wrote, " the terms of whig and tory belong to natural as well as to civil history. They denote the temper and constitution of mind of different individuals. . . . To me, then, it appears that there have been differences of opinion and party differences, from the first establishment of governments to the present day, and on the same question which now divides our own country; that these will continue through all future time; that every one takes his side in favor of the many, or of the few, according to his constitution, and the circumstances in which he is placed. . . ." [12]

Inevitably, this point of view calls to mind the Gilbertian verse:

> Now Nature always does contrive . . .
> That every boy and every gal
> That's born into the world alive
> Is either a little Liberal
> Or else a little Conservative!

Nonetheless, this element of biological determinism in Jeffersonian thought must be taken seriously. Obviously, Jefferson was not a rigid biological determinist. He did take account of economic interests and social circumstances, yet these were closely linked with the biological element. Jefferson's thought on this subject was clearly influenced by the French Ideo-

[11] Jefferson, *Writings,* vol. IX, p. 377.
[12] *Ibid.,* vol. XIII, pp. 280, 283.

logists.[13] While visiting France before the Revolution, Jefferson met Cabanis, the leader of this school. When Cabanis published his work on the relations of body and mind in 1892, he sent a copy to Jefferson, who replied oñ July 12, 1803. How highly he regarded this work and its author is evident from this letter. He wrote:

> I lately received your friendly letter of 28 Vendem. an. II, with the two volumes on the relations between the physical and moral faculties of man. This has ever been a subject of great interest to the inquisitive mind, and it could not have got into better hands for discussion than yours. That thought may be a faculty of our material organization, has been believed in the gross; and though the "modus operandi" of nature, in this, as in most other cases, can never be developed and demonstrated to beings limited as we are, yet I feel confident you will have conducted us as far on the road as we can go, and have lodged us within reconnoitering distance of the citadel itself. . . .[14]

Jefferson was also a friend of Destutt de Tracy, whose commentary on Montesquieu he translated into English, and whose *Treatise on Political Economy* he arranged to have translated. His opinion of both Cabanis and de Tracy is clearly expressed in a letter of July 10, 1812, to Thomas Cooper. Discussing psychology and related topics, Jefferson commented that since "a course of anatomy lays the best foundation for understanding these subjects, Tracy should be preceded by a mature study of the most profound of all human compositions, Cabanis's 'Rapports du physique et du moral de l'homme.'" [15] Jeffersonian thought may thus be considered in part, at least, as an extension of Ideology to the American scene.

This linkage of biological and social organization was applied to a concrete case by Benjamin Rush in his *Account of the Influence of the Military and Political Events of the American Revolution upon the Human Body*.[16] Ostensibly this inquiry was intended to determine how conditions during the Revolution affected its friends or enemies. Actually, the findings were predetermined by Rush's conviction that individual and social health depended on correct political principles.

In general, good health fell to the lot of the patriots. "An uncommon cheerfulness prevailed everywhere among the friends of the Revolution.

[13] For Jefferson's relations with the Ideologic school, see Gilbert Chinard: *Jefferson et les idéologues d'après sa correspondance inédite avec Destutt de Tracy, Cabanis, J. B. Say et Auguste Comte,* Baltimore, Johns Hopkins Press, 1925.

[14] Jefferson, *Writings*, vol. X, p. 404.

[15] *Ibid.*, vol. XIII, p. 177.

[16] Benjamin Rush: *Medical Inquiries and Observations* (second American edition), Philadelphia, Thomas Dobson, 1794, vol. I, pp. 263-278.

Defeats, and even the loss of relations and property, were soon forgotten in the great objects of the war." [17] More specifically, Rush observed among other findings that hysterical women who favored the Revolution were cured of their condition. Furthermore, " marriages were more fruitful than in former years, and . . . a considerable number of unfruitful marriages became fruitful during the war." [18] Finally, many persons who had been sickly were restored to perfect health owing to change of occupation or location as a result of war conditions.

Sharply contrasted with the good health of the patriots was the mental and physical breakdown experienced by the Loyalists. In many instances, they tended to suffer from a hypochondriasis, which was popularly called the " Protection fever " and which Rush termed *Revolutiana*. It was called " protection fever " because it appeared to arise from the excessive concern of the Loyalists for the protection of their persons and possessions. This basic cause was accentuated by such other factors as loss of power and influence, the suspension of the Established Church, changes in manners and diet as a result of inflation, and lastly the legal and extra-legal oppression to which the Loyalists were subjected.

These effects upon the human body were produced through the medium of the mind. Thus the patriots themselves were not necessarily immune to such conditions, and Rush observed that following the peace in 1783, the Americans, unprepared for their new situation, were affected by an excess of liberty.

> The excess of the passion for liberty, inflamed by the successful issue of the war, produced, in many people, opinions and conduct which could not be removed by reason nor restrained by government. For a while, they threatened to render abortive the goodness of heaven to the United States, in delivering them from the evils of slavery and war. The extensive influence which these opinions had upon the understandings, passions and morals of many of the citizens of the United States, constituted a species of insanity, which I shall take the liberty of distinguishing by the name of *Anarchia*.[19]

In short, proper political stimuli, and a stable and ordered society were required for health. Jefferson was of the opinion that excess in society seized upon the mind and produced a kind of mental fever which might become incurable.[20] Mental health implied a society which would provide the proper stimuli and necessary conditions for well-being, and this the Jeffersonians saw in an agricultural economy. In Jefferson's

[17] *Ibid.*, p. 273. [18] *Ibid.*, pp. 273-274. [19] *Ibid.*, p. 277.
[20] Jefferson, *Writings*, vol. VIII, pp. 232, 344, vol. XIV, p. 381.

thinking this attitude was in large measure a result of his aversion for European social and political conditions. In Europe he saw the physical and moral oppression under which the great mass of the people labored. Wherever he looked he saw political injustice, social cruelty, poverty, and disease. By comparison, America was paradise. Jefferson found Europe "Much, very much inferior . . . to the tranquil, permanent felicity with which domestic society in America blesses most of its inhabitants; leaving them to follow steadily those pursuits which health and reason approve, and rendering truly delicious the intervals of those pursuits." [21] Rush concurred in these views, pointing out that "These advantages can only be secured to our country by agriculture. This is the true basis of national health, riches and populousness." [22] Consequently, the chief aim of the Jeffersonian statesman was to prevent the deterioration of agrarian virtue. In this task, he felt himself to be tending the vineyard of the Creator, for "Those who labor in the earth are the chosen people of God, if ever He had a chosen people, whose breasts he has made His peculiar deposit for substantial and genuine virtue." [23]

Urbanization and industrialization were to be avoided as far as possible if the United States was to remain an agricultural society. To the Jeffersonians urban civilization went hand in hand with poverty, disease, luxury, dissipation, political inequality, and social injustice. Jefferson agreed that cities "nourish some of the elegant arts," but insisted "the useful ones can thrive elsewhere, and less perfection in the others, with more health, virtue and freedom, would be my choice." [24] To Jefferson, cities meant an urban proletariat and this he rejected vigorously. In his opinion, "The mobs of great cities add just so much to the support of pure government, as sores do to the strength of the human body." [25] A letter to the economist Jean Baptiste Say, presents Jefferson's distrust of manufactures and cities in more measured tones. Discussing the question, Should the United States devote herself exclusively to agriculture?, he comments that in solving this problem, "we should allow its just weight to the moral and physical preference of the agricultural over the manufacturing man." [26]

This did not mean, however, that the Jeffersonians wished to do without

[21] *Ibid.*, vol. V, p. 153. See also *The Autobiography of Benjamin Rush*, edited by George W. Corner, Princeton, University Press, 1948, pp. 198-199.

[22] Rush, *Medical Inquiries* . . . I, p. 75.

[23] Jefferson, *Writings*, vol. II, p. 229.

[24] *Ibid.*, vol. X, p. 173.

[25] *Ibid.*, vol. II, p. 230.

[26] *Ibid.*, vol. XI, p. 3.

industry completely. Here, too, Rush made the point specifically in terms of health.

> Let us be cautious what kind of manufactures we admit among us. The rickets made their first appearance in the manufacturing towns in England. Dr. Fothergill informed me, that he had often observed, when a pupil, that the greatest part of the chronic patients in the London Hospital were Spittal-field weavers. I would not be understood, from these facts, to discourage those manufacturers which employ women and children: these suffer few inconveniences from a sedentary life; nor do I mean to offer the least restraint to those manufactories among men, which admit of free air, and the exercise of all their limbs. Perhaps a pure air and the abstraction of spirituous liquors might render sedentary employments less unhealthy in America, even among men, than in the populous towns of Great Britain.[27]

These views might be said to comprise the Jeffersonian conception of the agrarian ideal in relation to physical well-being. To complete the picture, however, we must examine the place of education and political institutions as instruments toward the achievement of their goal. Here, again, the unresolved ambiguity and duality of the Jeffersonian position is clearly revealed. To achieve the ideal agrarian society, an increasingly educated population was required which would produce natural leaders. Ignorant people, Jefferson insisted, cannot maintain their freedom, and he looked to the spread of education to enlighten men so that they would be able to decide issues for themselves. Other Jeffersonians like Rush agreed on the importance of education, but conceived its rôle in government in a more deterministic fashion. Rush leaned to a mechanical view of the educational process. "I consider it is possible," he observed, "to convert men into republican machines. This must be done, if we expect them to perform their parts properly, in the great machine of the government of the state. That republic is sophisticated with monarchy or aristocracy that does not revolve upon the wills of the people, and these must be fitted to each other by education before they can be made to produce regularity and unison in government." [28]

Jefferson's relation to education and the diffusion of knowledge may be symbolized in his connection with the American Philosophical Society,

[27] Rush, *Medical Inquiries* . . . I, p. 74.

[28] Benjamin Rush: *Essays, Literary, Moral and Philosophical,* Philadelphia, 1798, pp. 14-15. The reader will have noted that the emphases given by Jefferson and Rush are somewhat different even though basically they are in agreement. Apart from differences of personality this is due to the fact that they were influenced by different currents of European thought. While Jefferson reflected the French Enlightenment, Rush embodied the Scottish Enlightenment. In part at least this explains his combination of piety, humanitarianism, and desire to apply science to man.

which had been founded in 1742 through the cooperation of Benjamin Franklin, David Rittenhouse, and others. Jefferson was elected a member in 1780, and in 1797 president of the Society. It had been founded in the Baconian tradition to promote useful knowledge, and this view Jefferson shared. A new country with immense natural resources to develop needed a utilitarian viewpoint, and Jefferson strongly emphasized the usefulness of science.[29] Furthermore, in accepting the presidency of the Society he expressed his "ardent desire to see knowledge so disseminated through the mass of mankind that it may at least reach the extremes of society, beggars and kings." [30]

Beside increasing human knowledge, it was also necessary that the human mind be properly stimulated so that it would remain in a state of health. Stimuli deriving from politics and religion were most salutary in imparting strength to the intellectual faculties. The effects of such stimuli might be felt in several directions. Elections, as typical of representative government, were important in producing effects on the human mind. In his Commonplace Book, for instance, Rush noted that "Elections shake the public mind, improve the understanding, from influence of Passions on the understanding, promote longevity." [31] In addition, elections also increased intelligence.

> In monarchies the birth or death of a prince, the sickness of a king, and the events of a war, are the principal objects, that, by awakening the attention of a whole nation, infuse vigour into the public mind. But in republics, the same vigour is produced every two or three years by general elections. These important seasons, in which heaven renews one of the dividing lines between man, and the brute creation, interests every feeling of the heart. They stimulate the passions, which afterwards act upon the understanding, and impart to it a force, which prevents its relapsing into the repose of public apathy, during the intervals of a general suffrage. From a strict attention to the state of mind in this country, before the year 1774, and at the present time, I am satisfied, the ratio of intellect is as twenty are to one, and of knowledge, as an hundred are to one, in these states, compared with what they were before the American revolution.[32]

---

[29] Charles A. Browne: *Thomas Jefferson and the Scientific Trends of his Time.* Chronica Botanica, Volume 8, No. 3, Waltham, Mass. Chronica Botanica Co., 1944, pp. 387-391; *Proceedings of the American Philosophical Society . . . from the Manuscript Minutes of its Meetings from 1744 to 1838,* Philadelphia, 1884, p. 246 et passim.

[30] Edward Dumbauld: *Thomas Jefferson, American Tourist,* Norman, University of Oklahoma Press, 1946, p. 184.

[31] Rush, *Autobiography,* p. 199.

[32] Benjamin Rush: *Six Introductory Lectures to the Course of Lectures upon the Institutes and Practice of Medicine, delivered in the University of Pennsylvania,* Philadelphia, 1801, p. 111.

With this quotation we may bring to a fitting close our brief survey of Jeffersonian thought on the connections between health and social environment. By piecing together scattered expressions of opinion on specific subjects, it was possible to show that these were founded on certain basic principles. Philosophically, this aspect of Jeffersonian thought represents an important phase of the Enlightenment in America, and thus contained the basic ambiguities and unresolved contradictions of that great intellectual movement. In practice, the ideas expressed by the Jeffersonians would seem to have achieved little of immediate significance. Like its diametrical opposite, the concept of medical police, Jeffersonian thought was considering health and society in terms soon to be discarded. The new industrial society which was just appearing on the scene would have to be dealt with in other terms. Jeffersonian thought with its emphasis on agrarianism looked backward to a golden age. Its ideals were to be repudiated and its hopes disappointed. Nonetheless, this chapter in the history of American ideas and American medicine has a basic importance. As the pioneer endeavor in this country to explore the social relations of health and disease, it represents the earliest approach to an American theory of social medicine. Whether or not the Jeffersonians influenced with their ideas the generation that dealt with the social relations of health under new conditions in the nineteenth century is still to be determined. This, however, we can say. Jeffersonian ideas on the reciprocal connections between society and human health deserve recognition as a significant phase in the history of American medicine.

THE MEDICAL ASPECTS OF THE CONTROVERSY OVER FACTORY CONDITIONS IN NEW ENGLAND, 1840–1850 *

As in Europe, so in this country the factory had its origin in the textile industries, for it was here that machines first displaced hand processes. In the United States the factory system of manufacture obtained its initial foothold in New England. In 1814 Francis C. Lowell for the first time brought the various processes of spinning and weaving under one roof at Waltham, Massachusetts. As the new type of industrial organization spread, factory towns sprang up along the streams of New England and the Middle Atlantic states. Among these were Lowell, Lawrence, Holyoke, Fall River, and Paterson.

Among the problems of the new factories one of the most important was the need for recruiting a labor force. The factories needed workers, and the question of the day was: How to secure a sufficient number of wage workers, how to create a laboring class?

In his *Report on Manufactures* of 1791 Hamilton had already been cognizant of this problem. "The objections to the pursuit of manufactures in the United States," he wrote, "represent an impracticability of success arising from three causes; scarcity of hands, dearness of labor, want of capital." [1] But while admitting the scarcity, Hamilton also offered a solution. With the cold-blooded optimism characteristic of the early exponents of industrialism he had surveyed the possible sources of supply and had attracted attention to them. Among these was the employment of women and children. As he saw it, the employment of women and children could result only in positive human good. "It is worthy of particular remark," he wrote, "that, in general, women and children are rendered more useful, and the latter more early useful, by manufacturing establishments than they would otherwise be. Of the number of persons employed in the cotton manufactories of Great Britain, it is computed that four sevenths nearly are women and children,—of whom the greatest proportion are children, and many of them of a tender age." Not only would it benefit these workers, but also their fathers and husbands. In

* Paper read before the Johns Hopkins Medical History Club, April 5, 1943.

[1] Cited in Bogart, *Economic History of the American People*, 2 ed., New York, 1938, pp. 385-6.

Hamilton's opinion "The husbandman himself experiences a new source of profit and support from the increased industry of his wife and daughters, invited and stimulated by the demands of the neighboring manufactories."[2] In a measure these anticipations were realized as the invention and introduction of power machinery made it possible to utilize the labor of women and children. As one of the apostles of the new system of production expressed it, they could become the "little fingers . . . of the gigantic automatons of labor-saving machinery."[3]

The proportion of women and children employed in the new industrial establishments varied from district to district. To understand why this was so something must be said about the nature of factory organization. Two types can be distinguished in the textile industries, the Fall River type and the Waltham or Lowell type.[4]

The Fall River system of factory organization was similar to that prevailing in the English factories. Mule spindles were used and men spinners were employed with very young children as helpers. Unlike Great Britain, however, the labor force was recruited from among the local population, and the workers lived in their own homes or in company tenements.

The Waltham type, on the other hand, which was also adopted at Lowell, Lawrence and generally throughout Massachusetts and New Hampshire, relied more on automatic machinery, in particular the throstle spindle, a machine suited to women workers. Furthermore, centralized production was favored and the workers were housed in company boarding houses. As a result the cotton textile factories, particularly where the Waltham system prevailed, were conspicuous for the employment of women workers. In this study I shall deal chiefly with the controversy over conditions in factories where the Waltham system prevailed and will therefore pay little attention to conditions under the Fall River system.

Most of these women were quite young, in their late teens or early twenties. In part the employment of young women was a deliberate policy based on the use of the throstle, in part it was due to the high wages demanded by men workers who found the opportunities of commerce and agriculture more attractive. It should also be kept in mind

[2] Hamilton, *Report on Manufactures*, in G. S. Callender, *Selections from the Economic History of the United States 1755-1860*, Boston, 1909, pp. 550-1.

[3] Cited in Kirkland, *A History of American Economic Life*, New York, 1940, p. 333.

[4] Victor S. Clark, *History of Manufacture in The United States*, Vol. I, New York, 1929, pp. 397-398. See also Kirkland, *op. cit.*, pp. 332-341, and Bogart, *op. cit.*, pp. 429-431.

that with the decline of New England agriculture, and the migration of many young men to the more fertile lands and more roseate prospects of the West during the early decades of the nineteenth century, an over-proportion of the female population was created. Some of these women and girls were left without adequate means of support, while others were ready to welcome any opportunity of escaping the drudgery of farm life or domestic service. After surveying conditions in New England Harriet Martineau concluded: "There is reason to believe that there was much silent suffering from poverty before the institution of factories; that they afford a most welcome resource to some thousands of young women, unwilling to give themselves to domestic service, and precluded, by the customs of the country, from rural labour."[5]

Nevertheless, despite the potential availability of this labor force, certain prevalent impressions regarding the character of factory work had to be dispelled before it could be attracted to the factories. Investigations of conditions in the English factories had created an impression that factory work was degrading and immoral. In order to dissipate this idea, it was necessary to assure the farmers' daughters, whose labor was needed in the factories, of respectable surroundings and to control the conditions of both life and work. The product of this endeavor was the "Waltham system," which was later adopted at Lowell and most of the other textile centers north of Boston.

In order to break down the popular suspicion of factory work, the Waltham capitalists devised a system of paternalistic care which appears to have been modelled after the system organized by Robert Owen at New Lanark. Michel Chevalier, a French economist who visited the United States during the thirties described the conditions found in 1836 at Lowell, the most widely known of these first factory towns, in the following terms:

> The cotton manufacture alone employs six thousand persons in Lowell; of this number nearly five thousand are young women from 17 to 24 years of age, the daughters of farmers from the different New England States, and particularly from Massachusetts, New Hampshire and Vermont; they are here remote from their families, and under their own control. On seeing them pass through the streets in the morning and evening and at their meal-hours, neatly dressed; on finding their scarfs, and shawls, and green silk hoods which they wear as a shelter from the sun and dust . . . hanging up in the factories amidst the flowers and shrubs which they cultivate, I said to myself, this, then is not like Manchester. . . .
>
> The manufacturing companies exercise the most careful supervision over these girls. I have already said, that, twelve years ago, Lowell did not exist; when,

[5] Martineau, *Society in America* (1834-36), II, in Callender, *op. cit.*, p. 702.

therefore, the manufactories were set up, it also became necessary to provide lodgings for the operatives, and each company has built for this purpose a number of houses within its own limits, to be used exclusively as boarding houses for them. Here they are under the care of the mistress of the house, who is paid by the company at the rate of one dollar and a quarter a week for each boarder, that sum being stopped out of the weekly wages of the girls. These housekeepers, who are generally widows, are each responsible for the conduct of her boarders, and they are themselves subject to the control and supervision of the company, in the management of their little communities. Each company has its rules and regulations. . . .[6]

The rules to which Chevalier alludes required that the workers be neat, industrious, abstain from alcoholic liquors, attend religious services, and in general conduct themselves with an awareness of their moral and social obligations. Emphasis was laid on the maintenance of early hours. As an instance of these rules I wish to cite the first article of the regulations put out by the Lawrence company in 1833. It is as follows:

All persons employed by the Company must devote themselves assiduously to their duty during working-hours. They must be capable of doing the work which they undertake, or use all their efforts to this effect. They must on all occasions, both in their words and in their actions, show that they are penetrated by a laudable love of temperance and virtues, and animated by a sense of their moral and social obligations. The Agent of the Company shall endeavor to set to all a good example in this respect. Every individual who shall be notoriously dissolute, idle, dishonest, or intemperate, who shall be in the practice of absenting himself from divine service, or shall violate the Sabbath, or shall be addicted to gaming, shall be dismissed from the service of the Company.[7]

During the thirties there was a steady migration of women from the rural districts to the rapidly growing urban communities of Lowell, Lawrence and other factory towns. According to an estimate made in 1831, about two-thirds of all the employees in the cotton factories were women and girls.[8] As we have already mentioned, the companies provided boarding houses in which the workers were required to live under the strict supervision of the housekeepers who managed them. The same careful supervision was also exercised in the factory, where the women and girls were in charge of an overseer.

At first glance it would appear that here was an industrial idyl, and it is undoubtedly true that in its first blossoming conditions not usually found in factory towns were created at Lowell. Visitors to Lowell, such as Harriet Martineau, Chevalier, Poussin and others, were much impressed by the flower boxes in the factory windows, by the debating societies,

[6] Chevalier, *Society, Manners and Politics in the United States* (1836), in Callender, *op. cit.*, pp. 705-6.

[7] *Ibid.*, p. 706.

[8] Kirkland, *op. cit.*, p. 337.

by the groups that studied French and German, and by the generally modest and educated conduct of the female operatives. It must be remembered, however, that these factory workers did not yet form a permanent working class. They were recruited chiefly from the women of the farms and villages, who entered upon this work as a temporary measure. The average period of employment in the New England cotton factories was between four and five years.[9]

Nevertheless, all was not as serene as appeared on the surface. Even during the thirties when the industrial idyl had not yet completely faded, two strikes occurred at Lowell, one in 1834 and one in 1836. The first was against a reduction in wages, the second against an increase in the price of board which was equivalent to a reduction in wages.[10]

These strikes reflect the dynamic condition of the American labor movement during the late twenties and early thirties. From 1830 to 1837 the country was in the grip of one of the most extravagant eras of speculation and expansion in its history, and it was during this period that the early labor movement was most active. Labor organizations appeared in profusion, in answer to encroachments upon earnings and standards of living. It must be kept in mind that the American labor movement during its "awakening period" did not arise from factory conditions as in England.[11] In the United States at this time the factory system was still almost completely outside the labor movement. The first organizations appeared locally among the artisans and mechanics of the cities who still worked on a largely individual basis, but it was not long before such smaller units coalesced into central organizations to protect and promote the workers' common interests. Although they were primarily societies of craftsmen, the demands for better social and economic conditions put forth by these groups concerned also the factory operatives. In New England at least, factory workers were recognized as a distinct class, with problems and grievances different from those of the urban handicraft workers.[12]

In 1833 at the third convention of the New England Association of Farmers, Mechanics and other Workingmen the "condition of females and children in factories" attracted particular attention, and the Association asserted that this subject "ought to receive the sedulous care of

[9] Henry A. Miles, *Lowell, as it was, and as it is*, Lowell, 1845, p. 194.

[10] John R. Commons and associates, *History of Labour in the United States*, Vol. I, New York, 1918, p. 423.

[11] Professor Commons has called the period from 1820 to 1840 the "awakening period" of the American labor movement.

[12] Commons, *op. cit.*, p. 305.

the respective departments of government." In accordance with this policy a committee was appointed to study "the situation of the working women of this country." It seems not unlikely that this interest was due to the recent exposures of the evils of the factory system in this country by Seth Luther, the pioneer anti-child-labor crusader, who, by his own account, had "for years lived among cotton mills, worked in them, travelled among them." [13]

One year later the General Trades' Union of New York invited the trades' unions of the country to a national convention which met in New York during the last week of August 1834 and organized the National Trades' Union. In connection with a resolution that action be taken against the deplorable conditions under which children were employed in factories, Dr. Charles Douglass, president of the New England Association and editor of *The Artisan* bitterly denounced the entire factory system. The picture of the condition of the women workers of Lowell which he painted is the very opposite of that usually depicted. He pointed out that in the factories of that city there were about 4000 females of various ages "now dragging out a life of slavery and wretchedness." It is distressing, he said, "to behold these degraded females as they pass out of the factory—to watch their wan countenances—their woe-stricken appearance. These establishments are the present abode of wretchedness, disease and misery; and are inevitably calculated to perpetuate them—if not to destroy liberty itself!" Within the last few years, he pointed out, "the sons of our farmers, as soon as they are of sufficient age, have been induced to hasten off to the factory, where for a few pence more than they could get at home, they are taught to become the willing servants, the servile instruments of their employers' oppression and extortion!" To be sure, the daughter also earned a little more money, "but as surely loses health, if not her good character, her happiness!" [14]

The subject of female factory workers was again considered at the conventions of the National Trades' Union held in 1835 and 1836, at which Dr. Douglass was spokesman for the women and children employed in the Massachusetts cotton factories. A lengthy report on female labor was submitted to the 1836 convention in which the committee pronounced it a physical and moral injury to woman and a competitive menace to man.[15]

The panic of 1837 brought about a dissolution of the nascent trade union movement, but criticism of the effect of the conditions of labor on

[13] Commons, *op. cit.*, pp. 313, 319, 320.

[14] Cited by Commons, *op. cit.*, pp. 428-429.

[15] Commons, *op. cit.*, p. 436.

the health of women employed in the cotton mills did not abate. In fact it increased in vehemence. The long depression from 1837 to 1849 which followed the crisis of 1837 forced attention upon the conditions of labor. It was asserted that the factory rooms were hot, poorly ventilated, and the atmosphere in them saturated with moisture and cotton lint to such a degree that after a few years in the factory the workers went home to die.[16] In 1840 Orestes Brownson, then the radical editor of the *Boston Quarterly Review*, published an article on "The Laboring Classes" in which he depicted the effects of the factory system on the girls of New England. "The great mass," he wrote, "wear out their health, spirits and morals without becoming one whit better off than when they commenced labor. The bills of mortality in these factory villages are not striking, we admit, for the poor girls when they can toil no longer go home to die." [17]

These attacks could not go unanswered, and in 1841 Elisha Bartlett, M. D. of Lowell wrote *A Vindication of the Character and Condition of the Females Employed in the Lowell Mills*. Bartlett is best known perhaps as the "Rhode Island philosopher" celebrated by Sir William Osler, but as we shall soon see his philosophical acumen apparently did not extend to the medical aspects of social problems.[18] It was Bartlett's judgment that:

> The general and comparative good health of the girls employed in the mills here, and their freedom from serious disease, have long been subjects of common remarks among our most intelligent and experienced physicians. *The manufacturing population of this city is the healthiest portion of the population*, and there is no reason why this should not be the case. They are but little exposed to many of the strongest and most prolific causes of disease, and very many of the circumstances which surround and act upon them are of the most favorable hygienic character. They are regular in all their habits. They are early up in the morning, and early to bed at night. Their fare is plain, substantial, and good, and their labor is sufficiently active, and sufficiently light to avoid the evils arising from the two extremes of indolence and over-exertion. They are but little exposed to the sudden vicissitudes, and to the excessive heats and colds of the seasons, and they are very generally free from anxious and depressing cares.[19]

---

[16] Kirkland, *op. cit.*, p. 350.

[17] Cited by Commons, *op. cit.*, p. 495. For Brownson see Helen S. Mims, Early American Democratic Theory and Orestes Brownson, *Science and Society*, Vol. III, 1939, pp. 166-198.

[18] W. Osler, "Elisha Bartlett, a Rhode Island Philosopher," in *An Alabama Student, and Other Biographical Essays*, New York, 1909.

[19] Elisha Bartlett, *A Vindication of the Character and Condition of the Females Employed in the Lowell Mills*, Lowell, 1841, p. 13.

In his essay on the philosophy of medicine Bartlett emphasizes that science depends above all on the observation and collection of facts, but it would seem that this dictum was not meant to apply to a problem such as the effect of conditions of labor on the health of workers. For Bartlett's opinion is based upon facts gathered in a rather curious manner. He inquired of 2611 girls at work whether they enjoyed better health than before working in the mills, whether their health was as good, or whether it was not as good as before. Of this group 170 (6.51 percent) replied that their health was better than before, 1563 (59.87 percent) that it was as good, and 878 (33.62 percent) that it was not as good as it had been.[20] Secondly, he queried the overseers regarding the health of the operatives. As an instance of the information obtained we may cite the overseer of one spinning room in which fifty girls were employed, who described his charges as follows: "'Looks well,' 25; 'rosy,' 9; 'fat and looks well,' 4; 'looks healthy,' 2; 'very healthy looking,' 2; 'fat and rosy,' 2; 'fat and pale,' 3; 'thin,' 2; 'pale,' 4." This can hardly be described as a scientific analysis, but perhaps Bartlett's approach to the question may be illuminated in some degree by the fact that after the incorporation of Lowell as a city in March 1836, he had become its first mayor.[21]

Facts and opinions such as those of Elisha Bartlett made no impression on the factory workers of Lowell. For instance, a Lowell petition of 1842 requested the passage of a ten-hour law on the ground that "it would, in the first place, *serve to lengthen the lives of those employed*, by giving them a greater opportunity to breathe the pure air of heaven, rather than the *heated* air of the mills. In the second place, *they would have more time for mental and moral cultivation*, which no one can deny is necessary for them in future life."[22] The movement for shorter hours during the forties had developed out of the social unrest which followed the panic of 1837 and the collapse of the unionism of the thirties. The chief demand of this movement was for the legislative enactment of a ten-hour working day. Agitation for the ten-hour day was most intense in Massachusetts, the chief factory state of the nation. From 1842 to 1845 efforts were made to exert pressure on the legislature by petitioning the General Court of Massachusetts. In 1844 the Mechanics Association of Fall River issued a call for a convention which would devise plans for further action towards limiting the hours of labor. In justifying the convention, it was pointed out that "the system of labor . . . requiring of the mechanic and laborer of New England from twelve to fifteen

[20] *Ibid.*, p. 11. [21] Miles, *op. cit.*, p. 41. [22] Kirkland, *op. cit.*, p. 353.

hours of labor per diem is more than the physical constitution of man can bear, generally speaking, and preserve a healthy state. . . ."[23] It is of interest in this connection that a Doctor Nelson was active in this movement and helped to formulate the policy of the organization. In October 1844 this convention met in Boston and organized the New England Working Men's Association.

Almost contemporaneously with the formation of the Association, in January 1845, the women operatives of Lowell, led by Sarah G. Bagley, organized the Lowell Female Labour Reform Association. The purpose of the organization was to work for the ten-hour day, on the ground that "such unmitigated labor is to the highest degree destructive to the health . . . and serves to injure the constitutions of future generations."[24] The Lowell Association joined forces with the New England Working Men's Association in sponsoring the ten-hour day. The effectiveness of these groups may be seen from the fact that in 1845 petitions signed by 2,139 persons were presented to the legislature, and in 1846 petitions with 10,000 signers.[25] As a result of this insistent pressure the Massachusetts legislature in 1845 appointed a committee to investigate the factory system, in particular the subject of hours in factories.

The report presented by the committee was unfavorable to the workers, as it claimed to have found no need for legislative action. In support of this stand the report cited among other evidence the testimony of certain Lowell physicians: "It is the opinion of Dr. Kimball, an eminent Physician of Lowell, with whom the committee had an interview, that there is less sickness among the persons at work in the mills than there is among those who do not work in the mills; and that there is less sickness now than there was several years ago, when the number was much less than at present. This we understand to be, also, the opinion of the City Physician, Dr. Wells."[26] The Dr. Kimball mentioned in the report was physician to the Lowell Hospital, established in 1839 by the mill owners as a hospital for sick operatives.

This evidence as well as the previously mentioned opinion of Elisha Bartlett were used to paint a pleasanter picture of factory conditions in a little book entitled *Lowell, as it was, and as it is,* published by the Reverend Henry A. Miles in 1845. Miles presents a survey of the history and development of Lowell until 1845, and describes the city in that year. Among the subjects with which he deals is the "comfort and health of

[23] Commons, *op. cit.*, p. 537.

[24] Cited by Commons, *op. cit.*, p. 539.

[25] Kirkland, *op. cit.*, pp. 354-355.

[26] Quoted by Miles, *op. cit.*, pp. 122-123.

the operatives."[27] Indeed, in the preface he emphasizes that "the great questions relating to Lowell are those which concern the health and character of its laboring classes. It is believed that more full and precise information on these points is given in the following pages, than has ever before been published." At the very outset of his discussion Miles declares: "The mills themselves are kept of a uniform temperature, being heated in cold weather either by steam, or by hot air furnaces. The rooms are lofty, are well ventilated, and are kept as free from dust as is possible, while the machinery is carefully boxed, or otherwise secured against accidents." He then goes on to point out that "on no point are such conflicting statements put forth as on that of the health of the operatives. It is extremely difficult to arrive at the exact facts of the case." Nevertheless Miles tries to show that work in the mills does not impair the health of the workers. For this purpose he cites the results of a poll which he had undertaken in the mills, a comparison of mortality in Lowell with that in other places, the testimony of the Lowell physicians which has been presented, and finally, the opinions of the boarding house keepers as to the health of their charges.

Miles had prepared a questionnaire which he sent to the superintendent of each mill. Among the questions asked were the following: "How many [girls] say that they enjoy better health than before working in the mill? How many as good health? How many not so good?" The replies to the questionnaire contained the responses of 1424 girls. Of these 154 (10.82 percent) reported themselves in better health, 827 (58.08 percent) replied that their health had not changed, and 443 (31.10 percent) said their health was not as good as it had been. It must be kept in mind that these answers were not made directly to Miles, but to the overseers or superintendents who transmitted the information to him.

For further support Miles draws a comparison between the rates of mortality for Lowell and for other cities such as Providence, Salem, and Worcester. He concludes that the Lowell rate is lower than that of the other towns, and consequently the population is healthier. But he takes no account of a pertinent fact pointed out by Lemuel Shattuck in the following year (1846).[28] Shattuck drew attention to the fact that the age composition of Lowell, owing to its history, was unlike that of other towns. As might be expected of a community which was only a little over two decades old, the population consisted preponderantly of younger

[27] Miles, *op. cit.*, pp. 116-127. See also pp. 146-161.

[28] Lemuel Shattuck, *Report to the Committee of the City Council appointed to obtain the Census of Boston for the Year 1845 . . .*, Boston, 1846, pp. 165-167.

people, who had migrated from the surrounding countryside. In 1840 the 15-40 age group made up 65.44 percent, and in 1845 62.35 percent of the population. Furthermore, as Miles himself points out, a considerable portion of this population was unstable, remaining at the factories for 4 to 5 years and then returning home. Consequently, any statistical comparison such as that made by Miles has little validity.

Finally, he refers to the demand for a shorter working day and in this connection cites the previously quoted opinions of the Lowell doctors. He concludes his discussion of the entire question with the following statement: "A walk through our mills must convince one, by the generally healthy and robust appearance of the girls, that their condition is not inferior in this respect, to other working classes of their sex."

In 1846, a year after the publication of Miles's book, Dr. John O. Green joined the fray when he addressed the annual meeting of the Massachusetts Medical Society on the subject of "The Factory System, in its Hygienic Relations." [29] Dr. Green first pointed out the significance of the new industrial system and then went on to describe and to compare factory conditions in England and in America, paying particular attention to Lowell "as the type and exemplification of . . . the Factory System of New England. . . ." [30] After enumerating the advantages of temperance, sobriety, regular hours of rest, moderate labor, comfortable dwellings, and well ventilated workrooms enjoyed by the Lowell operatives, he proceeded to discuss whether factory work is injurious to health. "While we maintain," he said, "that many of the conditions of health are as little violated by manufacturing industry, as by an immense proportion of other pursuits, we still believe that factory labor, is, on some accounts, injurious. How, indeed, can it be otherwise, when regarded as a whole? Individuals thus employed, do not spend in the open air, on an average, more than an hour or an hour and a half in the twenty-four: and work is resumed almost the moment the meal is swallowed, allowing scarcely any rest for the commencement of a healthy digestion. Causes like these must and do depress, more or less, the vital powers, and induce certainly, perhaps slowly, a lower state of the general health than would exist with the opposite state of things." [31]

Green admitted that long hours were injurious to health, and agreed that they ought to be shortened. Nevertheless he hastened to dissociate himself from the proponents of the ten-hour day. "Among the most

[29] John O. Green, *The Factory System in its Hygienic Relations*, . . . Boston, 1846.
[30] Green, *op. cit.*, p. 12.
[31] *Ibid.*, p. 20.

prominent perhaps of the adverse influences, as must occur to every one," he said, "is the too long confinement by the protracted hours of labor, amounting in the case of the mills at Lowell, to an average per day, throughout the year, of twelve hours and eighteen minutes. It is in no spirit of sympathy with a certain class who are seeking to turn the public attention to this matter, that we would declare ourselves in favor of abridging these hours. On the contrary, nothing can be more ill-judged than these attempts to create distrust and ill-will between the employers and employed, between whom, every thing should be designed to cherish the utmost kindness and consideration." [32]

Having delivered himself of these pious sentiments Dr. Green mentions briefly the medical conditions that European doctors had observed among textile workers, but says nothing about the Lowell operatives. Instead he appends several statistical tables indicating the deaths in Lowell from 1830 to 1845. While these figures are admittedly not very accurate, yet they do reveal a very high mortality from pulmonary disease.[33]

While these opinions were being expressed and circulated, the battle for shorter hours continued. In 1847 the Lowell corporations bowed to public opinion and reduced the working day to 11 hours and 58 minutes, but the demand for the ten-hour day did not abate. Finally in 1849 a new committee was appointed by the legislature to "inquire and report . . . whether any, and what legislation ought to be adopted for the limitation of the hours of work of the laboring people." [34] This time the committee brought in a majority and a minority report. The majority believed such legislation to be inexpedient. The minority, however, favored a reduction of the working day and an eleven-hour bill embodying this proposal was introduced. Although the bill passed the house, it was defeated in the senate. Of interest to us is the fact that the minority report was based for the most part on evidence presented by Dr. Josiah Curtis of Lowell in 1849 before the American Medical Association.[35]

In 1848 at the annual convention of the American Medical Association a committee on public hygiene had been appointed. Among the members was Dr. Curtis. The purpose of the committee was to make a sanitary survey of the principal cities of the United States. When the Association

[32] *Ibid.*, pp. 20-21.

[33] *Ibid.*, pp. 28, 31.

[34] Commons, *op. cit.*, p. 541.

[35] J. Curtis, "Public Hygiene of Massachusetts; but more particularly of the Cities of Boston and Lowell," *Transactions of the American Medical Association*, II, 1849, pp. 487-554.

met again in 1849 the committee presented its first report, and this was followed by twelve special reports describing sanitary conditions in various cities. Among these was a report by Dr. Curtis on public hygiene in Massachusetts in which he devoted particular attention to Boston and Lowell.

I shall not enter into a detailed description of the information contained in Curtis's report, but shall deal only with his discussion of the effect of factory work on health in Lowell. The report attempted an impartial appraisal of this question. Curtis pointed out that the population was an unstable one. "In the first place," he says, "we perceive the instability of our operative population. While there are a very few who have remained some twelve or fifteen years or more, the average length of time of remaining on the Merrimack corporation for the last nine years, has been only nine months. It is believed, that the entire population of other corporations changes a little oftener than this. Some go from one corporation to another in the city, to do the same or some other kind of work; some to other manufacturing places; some, either temporarily or permanently, return to their country homes; and some—are married." Furthermore, he continues, "we are not able to say how many leave on account of ill health, nor how many of these become ill while connected with the mills, nor how many of these can trace the cause of declining health to influences concomitant with their employment."[36] In this connection Curtis presents the statistical material compiled by Bartlett and Miles, but does not comment on it.

Curtis agrees with the previously mentioned authors that the work of the factory operatives is "light, but constant. Their hours of labour, and rest, and meals are regular, and this is highly conducive to health." But he was unable to agree with the opinion that "the rooms in which they work are kept of a uniform temperature, and are lofty and well ventilated."[37] To disprove this notion Curtis calculated the amount of air required by each person in a certain mill and then found that even the best Lowell mills did not approach his standards. In a footnote he added: "There is not a State's Prison, or House of Correction, in New England, where the hours of labour are so long, the hours for meals so short, or the ventilation so much neglected, as in all the cotton-mills with which I am acquainted."[38] He concluded that while "many points demand attention, yet, to imperfect ventilation, or rather to an absence of venti-

[36] Curtis, *op. cit.*, p. 513.

[37] Green, *op. cit.*, p. 18, see also Miles, *op. cit.*, p. 116.

[38] Curtis, *op. cit.*, p. 531 (footnote).

lation, more than to any other one cause, can we trace the origin of impaired health." [39]

In his report Curtis also discussed the various hospitals and dispensaries of Boston, and Lowell, among them the Lowell Hospital which has already been mentioned. Here he presents further evidence bearing on the question of the health of the factory workers. The physician to the Lowell Hospital had recently read a paper before the Middlesex District Medical Society in which he had presented statistics showing the high incidence of typhoid fever among the patients of the Hospital, all of whom were factory workers. From this paper Curtis presents the following extract. "From the statements here furnished," the physician said, "it appears quite obvious that typhoid fever is not only a very constant, but also the most important, disease among the operative population. It gives no evidence of the proportion it bears to the same disease, as it occurs with the rest of our adult population. Nevertheless, I think it must have been impressed upon the conviction of every physician of several years' standing in our city, that our operatives, as a class, have suffered from it to a much greater degree than the citizens at large. If such is the fact, it becomes a matter of interest to inquire why it is so; and then, again, to ascertain if it is an evil which admits of a remedy, and if so, what it is. My own opinion, however, is that *imperfect ventilation,* in our cotton-mills particularly, may have a very important bearing upon the question of causes of fever among our operative population . . . Air thus confined for the space of several months, in rooms occupied by some fifty persons, for twelve hours every day, except Sundays, must, sooner or later, make an impression upon the constitution, thus indirectly, at least, become the means of inducing disease." [40]

Curtis does not mention the name of the physician to the Lowell Hospital, but this information is provided by a *Report of the Lowell Hospital* which appeared several months after the completion of Curtis's survey.[41] The author of the *Report* is Gilman Kimball, M. D., physician and surgeon to the hospital. It is probable that the *Report* is an extended version of the paper to which Curtis referred, as it contains almost verbatim the passage just quoted. Furthermore, it is of interest to note that this is apparently the same Dr. Kimball who in 1845 had stated that the factory workers had less sickness than the rest of the population of Lowell. Kimball's report does not add much to the information already

[39] *Ibid.*, p. 519.
[40] *Ibid.*, p. 529.
[41] Gilman Kimball, *Report of the Lowell Hospital, from 1840 to 1849,* Lowell, 1849.

presented, but it is of interest as the first printed report of what may be regarded as the first industrial hospital in this country.

With this our account of the New England factory controversy of the forties may be concluded. I have no doubt that further investigation of the medical and non-medical literature of this period will produce a great deal more information than is contained in this rather sketchy account. For the present, however, I think that the material presented here will suffice. It shows the rôles played by physicians and health problems in social criticism and social change, and presents one facet of a very much larger subject, namely, the history of industrial medicine in this country.

THE HOSPITAL
Historical Sociology of a Community Institution

Introduction

Illness creates dependency. The sick need not only medical treatment but also personal care and shelter. Throughout history societies have accepted such need as a responsibility of community life, and have created various institutions to provide the necessary services. One of these institutions, the hospital, is today a cornerstone of any modern system of health care.

Arrangements to provide for the needs of the sick have always been intimately linked with the varying economic, political, social, and cultural conditions that govern the life of man. Whether man lived in a city or on the land, whether he suffered scarcity or enjoyed abundance, how he saw his fellow men and how they looked upon him, the religion he practiced and the values he prized, the learning, arts, and sciences that gave shape to his society—all have affected the development of the hospital, the form it has achieved, and the services it offered. To be understood, the hospital has to be seen, therefore, as an organ of society, sharing its characteristics, changing as the society of which it is a part is transformed, and carrying into the future evidence of its past.

A historical sociology of the hospital in this sense requires a delineation of political and economic conditions, social structure, value systems, cultural organization, and social change in relation to the health conditions and needs of populations at various historical periods. However, a task of this kind far exceeds the limits of this chapter, and will not be undertaken here. Instead, I have selected a number of hospital types that can be distinguished in different historical periods, and in each case described and discussed how the hospital was conceived, organized, financed, and operated, how it was related to its societal context, and how it changed or gave way to other kinds of institutions.

The Medieval Hospital

The concept of a need for social assistance in case of sickness or other misfortune was highly developed during the Middle Ages. This was as true of the Moslems and Jews as of the Christians, and was most evident in the creation of hospitals. Religious and social considerations were preeminent in the development of these facilities.

To be sure, separate institutions for the care of the sick existed even earlier. Temples were probably the earliest institutions concerned with such care, as in the case of the cult of Asclepius. Separate medical institutions for the care and shelter of the sick first appear in Rome,[1] but the guiding motives in their development were clearly military or economic for the most part, and obviously related to the structure and purposes of Roman society. Other values underlie the creation of hospitals by Christian communities during the later Empire and the medieval period. The teaching of Paul, "and now abideth faith, hope and charity, these three; but the greatest of these is charity," sets forth one of the basic values that motivated the rise of such institutions. The Christian had a duty to his sick and suffering fellows, and the practical expression of this charitable idea became evident after Constantine accepted Christianity and recognized it as a state religion. Bishops had an obligation to receive strangers or the needy into their homes, or to see that they were cared for by the community in other ways. The Council of Nicaea (A.D. 325) instructed the bishops to establish a hospital in every city that had a cathedral, and at the end of the fourth century the Council of Carthage (A.D. 398) urged them to maintain a hospice (*hospitiolum*) not far from the church. The model for these Christian institutions was very probably the Jewish hospice, which already existed in the Talmudic and pre-Christian period.

The motive of charity was reinforced by another Christian value—that Grace and salvation might be achieved by giving alms. Thus, the so-called second letter of St. Clement, which dates from the second or third century, informed the congregation of Corinth that "almsgiving relieves the burden of sin."[2] Moreover, through sickness and suffering man became a participant in the Grace of God. To care for the sick was not only a Christian duty but also beneficial for the salvation of the soul. Through association with the sick, and by providing for them, the healthy could participate in their grace. Had not Christ said: "I was sick and you visited me. Whatever you have done unto one of these, the least of my brethren, you have done it unto me"? This motive is found throughout the entire medieval period.

From the fourth century on, institutions were founded to care for the sick and those in need. An early example is the hospital established by St. Basil at Caesarea in Cappadocia (369–372).[3]This institution comprised several sections, and cared for travelers, the indigent, the infirm, and the sick. Even those suffering from contagious ailments such as leprosy were admitted. The entire staff, including physicians, resided in the hospital. The land with which the Emperor Valens had endowed the church of Caesarea was its principal source of revenue. The example provided by St. Basil was followed in 398 by St. John Chrysostom when he became Patriarch of Constantinople. A number of similar hospitals were constructed in the capital. The administration of each of these establishments was entrusted to two priests. Institutions of the same kind also came into being at Alexandria and elsewhere in the Eastern Empire.

While these early institutions combined social and medical functions, hostels, hospitals, and other charitable establishments were set up separately. Fabiola, a Roman matron who had aided in founding a hospice at Ostia, also created an infirmary (*nosocomium*) in Rome, and according to St. Jerome "gathered into it sufferers from the streets, giving their poor bodies worn with sickness and hunger all a nurse's care." An awareness of the distinction between the hospital in a strict sense and other facilities designed for the care of groups with different needs is evidenced by the various terms used to designate them.[4] *Xenodochia* were hostels or hospices for pilgrims, travelers, and all those who needed a lodging when in a strange town. *Nosocomia* designated hospitals, that is, institutions for the care of the sick. *Gerocomia* were establishments for the aged; *lobotrophia* provided asylum for the disabled or for lepers; *orphanotrophia* were orphanages, and *brephotrophia* designated foundling homes.

A number of different officials administered these institutions. In imperial decrees, the director of such a facility is designated as *administrator, antistes,* or *praepositus.* When referring to the chief administrator of a specific type of institution, terms such as *noscomos* or *xenodochos* were employed. Such titles as *oeconomos* or *circuitor* designated the superintendent of an institution.

The degree to which the hospital in the East Roman or Byzantine Empire tended to achieve a clear-cut institutional character is most sharply revealed by the organization of the important hospital attached to the Monastery of the Savior Pantocrator at Constantinople, Our knowledge of this and similar institutions is derived from their *typica,* or charters of foundation. The monastery and its associated welfare facilities were established by John II Comnenos in 1112, and seem to have been completed by 1136.[5]

The hospital had an outpatient department and five sections, each for a different class of ailments. A surgical ward of ten beds was provided for patients with fractures and wounds. A second ward of eight beds was assigned to patients with acute infectious diseases, particularly ailments of the eyes and the intestinal tract. Twelve beds in another ward were reserved for women. Then there were two wards of ten beds each for simpler cases. Furthermore, each ward had an extra bed for emergency cases. However, in addition to these there were six more beds, each with a mattress that had a central hole for patients so seriously ill that they could not move.

The medical staff was quite large. Each ward had no less than two physicians, three assistants, and several orderlies. The women's ward had a woman physician in addition to the two male physicians. These women physicians probably developed from midwives, and it is quite likely that obstetrics was practiced on the women's ward.[6] Two chief surgeons headed the surgical service of the hospital, and provided care for female patients when required. In addition, the surgical service included a specialist for hernia operations. Furthermore two physicians, two surgeons, and eight assistants provided care for ambulatory patients in the dispensary. In difficult cases the chief physicians were called upon for consultation. The entire medical staff was divided into two groups, each serving alternately for a period of a month. Physicians on service were expected to visit patients at least once daily and twice a day in summer. Physicians also had night duty. The hospital was administered by two physicians, the *primmikerioi*. Under their direction two chief physicians supervised the medical staff.

Both the Moslems who overran large parts of the Eastern Empire and the Europeans who came into contact with it for religious, commercial, or political reasons were impressed and influenced by its hospitals and other welfare institutions. As first the Moslems used existing institutions; then they built new ones. In the ninth century, during the reign of the Caliph Harun al-Rashid, a hospital was founded at Baghdad. Another hospital was built there in the next century by the Caliph al-Muktadir. A third hospital founded at Baghdad in 970 had a staff of twenty-five physicians and was used for the teaching of medical students. All in all, there are records of some thirty-four hospitals in countries under Islamic rule. These hospitals were generally well organized, and reflect the high state of development attained by medicine in Moslem lands. At Cairo, for example, the hospital founded in 1283 had separate sections for patients with febrile illnesses, for the wounded, and for those with eye diseases, as well as special rooms for women. Medical care was provided by a staff of physicians under a director, and three male and female nurses or aides. The similarity to the type of institution exemplified by the Pantocrator is unmistakable.

The hospital as concept and as institution developed much more slowly in the West. In view of the close linkage to the Church, it is not surprising that the most significant early contribution to the establishment of hospitals came from medieval monasticism. The manner in which the monks cared for their own sick became a model for the laity. The monasteries had an *infirmitorium,* where the sick monks were taken for treatment, a pharmacy, and frequently also a garden with medicinal plants. In addition to caring for members of the monastic community, the monasteries also provided for pilgrims and travelers. The beginnings of this practice cannot be precisely established, but it is quite likely that they go back to the early Middle Ages.

Benedict of Nursia, the founder of Western monasticism, dealt with these matters explicitly in the code of religious life that he created on Monte Cassino about A.D. 535. In Chapter 36 of his *Rule,* Benedict specified that "a cell be set apart by itself for the sick brethren, and one who is God-fearing, diligent and careful, be appointed to serve them." Another chapter deals with guests who are to be received like Christ Himself. Moreover, special care should be "taken in the reception of the poor and of strangers." For this purpose a guesthouse is to be established.[7] Other monastic orders had similar rules. The Franciscans were told to care for the sick in the same manner that they themselves would wish to be treated in case of illness.

As monastic houses were established, these injunctions were carried out, and the simple cell set aside for a sick monk in many instances became a large institution. Thus, an architectural plan of the Abbey of St. Gall, in Switzerland, in 820 contains a hospital, with rooms for seriously ill patients (*cubiculum valde infirmorum*), for a chief physician (*mansio medici ipsius*), and for other physicians (*domus medicorum*). Nearby is the pharmacy (*armarium pigmentorium*), and behind the physician's quarters lies the herb garden with sixteen plots for various plants.[8]

The visitor to Tintern Abbey, in Monmouthshire, founded in 1131 for monks of the Cistercian order, will find a similar establishment. The infirmary of the abbey housed both the sick and the aged monks, and comprised a large hall, a cloister, and a kitchen. Attached to the hall at one end is a room with a drain that was probably the latrine. A passage connects the infirmary hall with the church.[9] Similar arrangements can be found in various parts of Europe.

Further important impulses toward the creation of hospitals came from ecclesiastical as well as secular sources. At the Council of Aachen, in 816, it was decided that a refuge for the poor (*receptaculum, hospitale pauperum*) would be established by bishops and abbots.[10] In the course of the following two to three hundred years, establishments for the poor, the sick, and for strangers were founded at bishops' sees and in connection with cathedral chapters and religious communities. Meffert has clearly demonstrated this development for Bavaria.[11] In Germany, hospitals were first founded in the seventh century in the Rhineland-Westphalia area, and not earlier than the ninth century in the northern section.[12]

The hospital also spread because it became a central institution around which great hospital and nursing orders established themselves. Thus, hospitals were founded along the routes taken by the Crusaders, and several knightly orders organized during the holy wars assumed the mission of establishing and maintaining hospitals. The best known of these orders, the Knights of St. John or the Hospitalers, for example, founded hospitals as far apart as Malta and Germany. Another trend developed with the founding of the Holy Ghost Hospital at Montpellier by Guido, a pious layman. Sanctioned in 1198 by Pope Innocent III, the Order of the Holy Ghost established and maintained similar hospitals throughout Europe.

As time went on, many different kinds of benefactors founded hospitals. Kings, queens, high ecclesiastics, noble lords, wealthy merchants, guilds, fraternities, and municipalities—all endowed houses for the care of the sick, the poor, the infirm, the aged, and for numerous other purposes. The first hospital in England was founded in 937 by Athelstan, favorite grandson of Alfred the Great, at York, and was dedicated to St. Peter. Later, in 1155, after a great and destructive fire, it was reestablished by King Stephen and dedicated to St. Leonard. It became a vast establishment which in 1370 maintained over two hundred sick and otherwise infirm inmates. Still surviving today is the vaulted undercroft that was the basement story of a large infirmary hall.[13]

Another extant relic in York is the undercroft or hospital in the Merchant Adventurers' Hall. Built between 1357–1368, the hall housed the guild of York mercers and merchants. The guild was a dual organization comprising (1) a fraternity concerned with religious and social matters and (2) a mystery concerned with trade and commercial affairs. In 1371 the fraternity created a hospital. Two years later, the Archbishop of York undertook the reorganization of the hospital, and Johannes de Roncliff, a benefactor of the guild, became its patron. Thirteen poor and feeble people, apparently impoverished mercers, under the charge of a resident master, were to inhabit the hospital. Attached to the hospital was a chapel in charge of a chaplain. The hospital was called the Hospital of the Blessed Mary and the Holy Trinity. With the Reformation, the religious aspects of the hospital disappeared, but the pensioners remained. Indeed, pensioners continued to live in the accommodations on the street floor of the hall until the end of 1900. Thereafter they were boarded out with relatives or others.[14]

York simply illustrates a significant trend. The guilds took an important and active part in founding hospitals as well as other establishments for medical care and social assistance. Funds were created for the relief of their sick and disabled members. Wealthy guilds built their own hospitals; others paid regular fees to a cloister hospital that assumed responsibility for the accommodation and care of their members.

By the end of the fifteenth century, as a result of the developments described above, Europe was covered with a network of hospitals. For example, in England alone, by the middle of the fourteenth century, there were more than six hundred institutions of this kind, ranging in size from numerous small foundations caring for a dozen or so persons to the great establishments like St. Peter's and St. Leonard's of York.[15] Developments on the Continent were similar. According to the chronicler Giovanni Villani, Florence in 1300, with a population of some ninety thousand inhabitants, had thirty hospitals and welfare establishments capable of providing medical aid and shelter to more than a thousand sick and needy people. They were staffed by more than three hundred monks or other nursing personnel. During the later fifteenth century, under Lorenzo the Magnificent, there were some forty hospitals of various kinds. Paris at the beginning of the fourteenth century is reported to have had about forty hospitals and as many leper houses.

The hospitals varied considerably in purpose, and there were variations in the way they functioned. The medieval hospital was not only a center for medical care but a philanthropic and spiritual institution as well. Provision was made at various times and in different places for lepers, orphans, pregnant women, the aged and invalid, and strangers, as well as for those suffering from illness. Smaller establishments frequently dealt with a limited group or specific problem, while large institutions handled a wide range of health and welfare problems. Actually, this was a logical consequence of the premises on which the whole system developed, namely, the religious obligation to provide care and support for the sick, the poor, and the disabled. Those admitted to a hospital were to be received and cared for in a spirit of Christian charity. Tierney in discussing medieval poor law notes that the church lawyers of the period seldom discussed in detail the kind of administrative problems that have most perplexed writers on institutional poor relief in more recent times. There is very little, for instance, on criteria of admission to hospitals, or on the relative values of outdoor relief and institutional care in different types of cases. There was certainly no idea of a "workhouse test."[16]

While the hospital was created as a philanthropic institution and an agency of poor relief, it was simultaneously also a religious and spiritual institution. Spiritual care, prayer, and religious provision for the dying were predominant in every Christian hospital. Even when hospitals were taken over from the ecclesiastical authorities by municipalities in the later Middle Ages, they were not secularized.[17] Essentially, the hospital was a religious house in which the nursing personnel had united as a vocational community under a religious rule.[18] Spenser in *The Faerie Queene* sums up succinctly this side of the institution:

> Eftsoones unto an holy Hospitall
> That was foreby the way, she did him bring:
> In which seven Bead-men, that had vowed all
> Their life to service of high heavens King,
> Did spend their daies in doing godly thing.
> Their gates to all were open evermore,
> That by the wearie way were traveiling;
> And one sate wayting ever them before,
> To call in commers-by that needy were and pore.[19]

The medieval hospital generally had clergy attached to it; frequently it was also a church, and religious services were conducted in it for the edification of the faithful. In short, the hospital was a *locus religiosus* from an ecclesiastical viewpoint, and legally a *pia causa*. As such it enjoyed certain privileges and rights. Most frequently the hospital was tax-exempt; thus, the Hôtel-Dieu of Angers was able to sell its wine to taverns without paying any taxes to the government. The right of burial (*jus funerandi*) was also granted to hospitals, as was the right of asylum.

The financing of the medieval hospital reflected its origins and purpose. Medieval charity was a consequence of one of the strongest and most widespread feelings of the period, the desire for salvation and sanctification. An effective means for the achievement of this aim and to avoid suffering and pain in the next world was the performance of good works, including charity toward the poor and needy. Countless endowments, almshouses, hospitals, and other charitable institutions bear witness to the strength of this religio-social principle. Endowment, legacies, donations, lands and buildings provided the financial basis for the medieval hospital. The revenues of the Hôtel-Dieu of Beauvais in 1450 may serve as an example (Table 1).

TABLE 1

Revenues of Hôtel-Dieu of Beauvais, 1450

Revenues (in specie)	*Livres*
Quitrents, leases, farms	144
Legacies, donations, offerings, and so forth (including 11 livres from the sale of beds, clothes, and the like)	27
Seigneurial rights	2
Revenues (in kind)	
Quitrents, tithes, and so forth	33
Direct exploitation	
Wine	297
Wheat	170
Grains	56
Animals	35
Wood	2
	593
Grand Total	*766*

A number of hospitals at the death of a member of the parish took the bed and linen of the deceased. Judicial fines were sometimes given to hospitals by royal or seigneurial order. In 1395, for example, the Parlement of Paris laid a fine of 10,000 livres on the Jews living there, of which 500 livres were to go to the Hôtel-Dieu of Paris, the remainder for the construction of a bridge that would essentially serve the needs of the same institution.

The concept of good works as a means to salvation tends to emphasize the role of the donor in giving charity. It is the giving that is important—this is the essential good work. However, the founder, sponsor, or patron of a charitable institution had certain rights in it that were determined by law. All such institutions operated under a constitution granted by the local diocesan bishop. By 1414, the Archbishop of Canterbury had formulated a general framework for this purpose, namely, "The Statutes of St. James, according to the use of the Church of England."[20] Founders or patrons could determine what kinds of persons were to be admitted to the institution; they appointed the administrator (warden, master, keeper) and had a right to make a visitation whenever they desired to inspect the premises, the observance of the rule, the accounts, and other aspects of the operation of the institution. Moreover, they could set rules of behavior and punish those who broke them.[21] Indeed, even when municipal or national governments took over the administration of hospitals and other charitable institutions, the rights and intentions of the original founders were taken into account.[22] As Tierney points out, canonistic writers on hospital law were largely concerned with the regulation of the property rights of the institution and the definition of its legal status in relation to the local parish and diocesan authorities.[23]

But while a bishop could act to prevent maladministration of charitable bequests in his diocese, before the fourteenth century there was no general regulation of hospitals and related institutions. The individualistic, private characters of these caritative foundations made possible the appearance of various abuses, especially during the later Middle Ages. Hospital funds were misappropriated; in various instances hospitals were turned into ecclesiastical benefices to provide an income for some cleric; and toward the end of the Middle Ages hospitals frequently became boarding homes for the aged or for able-bodied individuals. In 1321, for example, Bishop Johann von Strassburg ordered the master of the Andreasspital at Offenburg to receive only the infirm and invalid poor and not to admit any idle, healthy individuals who could support themselves outside the institution. Excepted were persons who had sufficient means to support themselves and would therefore not disadvantage the sick.[24] Similarly, in 1414, an English statute for the institution of hospital reforms is justified on the basis that "many hospitals . . . be now for the most part decayed, and the goods and profits of the same, by divers persons, spiritual and temporal, withdrawn and spent to the use of others, whereby many men and women have died in great misery for default of aid, livelihood and succor."[25]

Ecclesiastical authorities were aware of various abuses that had become notorious, and in 1311 Pope Clement V promulgated the decretal *Quia contingit,* later incorporated in the *Extravagantes Joannis XXII.*[26] This decretal required all administrators of hospitals to swear to administer honestly property entrusted to them, and to prepare for the bishop an annual statement of hospital accounts. Moreover, the administrator did not have to be a cleric; that is, the hospital was not to be considered an ecclesiastical benefice, and its resources were to be devoted wholly to the charitable end for which it was created. Bishops were required to look into the administration of all hospitals in their dioceses, and to correct abuses.

The Medieval Hospital in Transition

Despite such efforts, however, the decline in the medieval hospital system continued. The authorities, both ecclesiastical and civil, neglected to take action where abuses existed and to enforce reforms; founders or their descendants failed to curb the malfeasance of administrators; and a number of other influences and elements, economic, social, and political, came into play to create a new situation.[27] For one thing, from the thirteenth century on, the hospital came increasingly under secular jurisdiction. As cities in Europe prospered and the bourgeoisie grew wealthy and powerful, municipal authorities tended to take over or to supplement the activities of the Church. In part, this was politically motivated, a desire of the civil authorities to be independent of clerical domination or to render the ecclesiastical power subordinate. Yet, this does not mean that the clergy were entirely eliminated. Monks and nuns continued to provide nursing care as they had done before. Administratively, the municipal authorities were responsible for the hospital facilities, but the Church might participate in some way. At Amiens, in the fifteenth century, for example, the master of the Hôtel-Dieu was elected by the municipality, but installed in his office by the bishop. At Louvain from 1473 to 1476, the ecclesiastical authorities played a part in removing two unsatisfactory administrators from the town hospital.[28]

Second, the hospitals and related establishments were increasingly inadequate to deal with new situations in which problems of health and welfare were considered from a new viewpoint. From the medieval standpoint, the poor, the sick, and the infirm might almost be considered necessary for the salvation of the donor of charity. They did the almsgiver a service, and had they not been present they might have had to be created. However, such an attitude tended to encourage begging and the acceptance of the beggar as a necessary part of human society. Little or no consideration was given to bettering the condition of the poor and the sick. During the late Middle Ages, and especially following the Reformation, the whole approach to this problem changed.[29]

Though the causes of poverty changed but little from the thirteenth century to the sixteenth, economic and social circumstances altered their significance and intensified their impact. As a result, the condition of the poor, which was bad in the earlier period, had become increasingly severe by the early sixteenth century. Increased unemployment, higher prices, enclosure of peasant lands and related factors brought into being the problem of vagrancy, which was constant throughout the fourteenth and fifteenth centuries. Vagrancy appeared in the Netherlands and Germany even earlier than in England, and then assumed increasingly large proportions. In their endeavors to piece out a livelihood, many vagrants pretended to be crippled or diseased, so as to be able to beg with impunity and to obtain admission to a hospital. There is little doubt that the large number of poor and sick wanderers overtaxed the facilities available in various countries. Whether these vagrants were sick or not, there was a great deal of economic and social distress by the sixteenth century, and the problem was what to do about it. As Simon Fish put the case in 1529 in his famous *Supplicacyon for the Beggers*: "But whate remedy to releve us your poore sike lame and sore bedemen? To make many hospitals for the relief of the poore people? Nay truely. The moo the worse, for ever the fatte of the hole foundacion hangeth on the prestes berdes."[30] Fish proposed a solution: that the clergy be expropriated and the hospitals and related facilities be taken in hand by the king.

In fact, this was the course followed, a course influenced essentially by the Reformation and the rise of the absolutist state. While the intervention of the civil authorities in matters of welfare and health before the sixteenth century has been noted, the notion that poor relief, including medical care, was a community and not a church responsibility was definitely established during the Reformation period. Those who wished to bring some order into the area of welfare and health, whether Vives in Bruges or Zwingli in Zürich, were guided by the same principles and were oriented to the same goals: elimination of all beggary, organization of effective agencies of public assistance, and unification of all facilities and resources (hospitals, domiciliary relief, and the like) in the hands of municipal or national authorities.

However, throughout the period the hospital changed little in its character. It remained a combination of an institution for the care of the sick, an old-age home, an almshouse, and an orphanage, possibly a guesthouse. Many aspects of medieval hospital administration were retained.

For example, religious services continued to be held in many places, not only in Catholic countries. Sweden's first general legislation on hospital administration of 1571 laid down specific instructions that at least once a day, at a given time, prayers were to be said collectively for peace on earth, for the welfare of the authorities, and for all concerned with the management of the hospital.[31]

Hospital administration of the period is clearly described in an account of the organization of the London hospitals in the middle of the sixteenth century.[32] Over-all administration was in the hands of a board of governors comprising sixty-six members. Of these, fourteen were aldermen and fifty-two "grave commoners, citizens and freemen of the said citie." Furthermore, the latter group included at least four scriveners, or notaries. The board of governors was headed by two aldermen termed governors general; the other twelve aldermen and the fifty-two commoners were divided into four subcommittees, each of which supervised one of the four London hospitals. Each subcommittee had at least sixteen members; one of these, an alderman, acted as president, and another, a commoner, served as treasurer. Members of the board of governors were elected at an annual meeting held on St. Matthew's day at Christ's Hospital or one of the others. A majority of the board was required, and each new member was elected for a two-year term. In a special situation a longer term was permitted.

The administration of each hospital was in the hands of a staff consisting of two groups. Officials concerned with the business management and administration of the institution were called governors, and comprised the following: a controller general and a surveyor general who were responsible for all the affairs of the hospital and represented it at meetings of the governors of the London hospitals; a president who was the actual director or administrator of the hospital; a treasurer who looked after the financial affairs and internal property; three almoners who supervised the inmates, their diet, activities, hygiene, as well as the personnel who looked after such matters (matron, nurses, steward, and others); two "scruteners" who were responsible for gifts, legacies, and bequests given to the hospital, and in general for fund raising in our terms; a renter who collected rents on all properties and holdings of the hospital; and two surveyors who were responsible for managing the real and other property of the hospital.

In addition to the above officials, or governors, the hospital staff, or officers, consisted of the following personnel, whose titles essentially describe their jobs. The clerk acted as secretary and bookkeeper. Those concerned with housekeeping functions included the matron, the steward, the cook, the butler, the porter, and the beadle. The matron was responsible for all women and children in the institution, as well as for the nurses and keepers of the wards. In addition, she was a housekeeper who looked after laundry, bedding, and the like. Food supply and maintenance were the major responsibilities of the steward, while the butler dealt with the baker and the brewer who supplied the hospital with bread and beer. A separate official maintained liaison with the churchwardens and the local parish collectors who had to bring in money to the hospital and with the poor who needed care and assistance. A surgeon and a barber were connected with the hospital and provided the necessary professional and technical attention.[33]

The medical staff and its activities are essential to the hospital as we conceive it today. As has already been indicated, this was not the case in the medieval hospital in Europe. During the early Middle Ages the presence of monastic physicians in religious houses makes it probable that the sick received some medical care.[34] From the fourteenth century on, however, physicians were increasingly associated with hospitals to provide care for patients. Thus, in Frankfurt am Main the municipal surgeon appointed in 1377 was required to treat surgical patients at the Holy Ghost Hospital. Similarly, the municipal physician appointed in 1381 agreed to attend gratis all persons employed by the municipality and to care for patients in the hospital.[35]

In Nürnberg a specific hospital physician was first appointed in 1486 at the new Holy Ghost Hospital with private funds.[36] By the beginning of the sixteenth century, this example began to be followed by other communities. This was done in Strassburg around 1515 on the ground that medical attention might help some patients and would eventually cost less than if no medical care was provided. It had been noted that patients who received no medical care remained longer in the hospital, and even though some died, the expenses to the institution were higher.[37]

Karl Sudhoff suggested that the association of the physician with the hospital and the provision of medical care in it became permanent when the inunction cure of syphilitics required public funds and when results showed that this treatment was successful.[38] As we have indicated, however, this trend began earlier, and was influenced by other factors as well. The so-called "Reformation of the Emperor Sigmund" (*Reformatio Sigismundi*), a work prepared in or about 1439, which contains proposals for the reform of medical care in the German cities, indicates that this was a problem that caused considerable concern.[39] The author insisted on the need for a municipal physician in every town, and emphasized that the medical profession should attend the poor gratis. This work was widely circulated during the fifteenth century and may have influenced governments to provide care by physicians on a more regular basis.

As it emerged from the medieval period the hospital was essentially an instrument of society to ameliorate suffering, to diminish poverty, to eradicate mendicity, and to help maintain public order. It had also come under different management in many places, under the jurisdiction of the royal power, of a municipality, or of some voluntary charitable organization. The same period also saw the beginning of an association with the medical profession, but the physician was not yet a part of the hospital, and remained independent. However, this association did provide the basis for another trend that from the seventeenth century on would lead the medical profession increasingly to use the hospital for the study of disease and for its own practical education. The view that hospitals should be places for the treatment of the sick and at the same time centers for the study and teaching of medicine was to have extraordinarily fruitful consequences in succeeding centuries. Holland led the way in this development; bedside teaching was established at Leyden in 1626. The same idea was also advanced in England by Francis Bacon, Samuel Hartlib, William Petty, and John Bellers.[40] Later, in the eighteenth century under the leadership of Hermann Boerhaave, this idea was developed at Leyden and put into practice so that other medical centers were influenced, notably Edinburgh.

New Conditions Produce New Hospitals

The eighteenth and early nineteenth centuries saw a growth of hospitals in Great Britain, on the European continent, and in America that exemplified and was formed by major political and social currents, especially mercantilism and enlightened despotism, private initiative and cooperative action, and the concept of a national health policy. Taking as a point of departure the mercantilist position in relation to health, a few far-seeing men had been led in the seventeenth century to adumbrate the idea of health as a significant element of national policy. Problems of health were considered chiefly in connection with the aim of maintaining and augmenting a healthy population, and thus in terms of their significance for the political and economic strength of the state. On a theoretical plane, this idea had been developed in varying degree in different countries. However, owing to the lack of knowledge and administrative machinery, it had nowhere been possible to develop and to implement a health policy on a national basis. While this goal was not actually achieved until the later nineteenth century, significant changes occurred during the eighteenth and earlier nineteenth centuries that did affect the hospital.

During the period under consideration, health problems in Great Britain were handled overwhelmingly by local authorities. Local government was carried on by the counties and the parishes into which the counties were divided. These administrative units provided the frame of reference for thought and action in matters of community health. Furthermore, the Elizabethan Poor Law (1601) had laid upon the parish the duty of providing relief for the indigent, and in time this came to include medical care. Each parish was responsible for the maintenance of its own poor, and consequently was concerned to reduce this burden as far as possible. It was believed that this could be accomplished by arranging to employ the poor in workhouses. While the enthusiastic belief in the efficacy of workhouses to deal with poverty was never realized, many of the plans and programs developed for this purpose also turned attention to health problems. As a result there was an increasing recognition in Great Britain of the need for medical assistance to certain groups of the population.[41]

It was this period, particularly the years from 1714 to 1760, that witnessed the creation in London and the provinces of dispensaries and general hospitals, as well as hospitals for special groups. The hospital and dispensary movement found its impetus chiefly in private initiative and contributions, although there was some governmental assistance in the form of legislative action. To be sure, private benefactions had never been absent in the support of the older London hospitals. In fact, as Jordan has recently shown, the sums contributed by private persons between 1480 and 1660 were large.[42] Moreover, fund-raising appeals to the public and the establishment of charities were not unknown before the eighteenth century.[43] The development of private initiative coupled with cooperative action, which is so characteristic of Britain in the eighteenth century, is to a very considerable degree related to the character of activity by local government. While the parish officers had to assume considerable responsibilities, generally they had neither the training nor desire to perform their functions. In many ways, this very aspect of the governmental system gave increasingly greater scope to private initiative, making it necessary and possible to deal pragmatically with new problems as they presented themselves. Indeed, throughout this period parliamentary action was generally undertaken on the basis of previously initiated local programs and projects.

The first institutions to provide medical care for the sick poor appeared in London. The metropolis was growing, wages were high, and workers were attracted to the city. Many of them, however, unable to establish the needed residence requirement, were ineligible for parochial relief when sick. The Act of Settlement of 1662 gave the parish authorities the right to remove within forty days any newcomer unable to rent a dwelling worth £10 if they believed that such a person was likely to be a burden to the parish.[44] Furthermore, the two older hospitals, St. Bartholomew's and St. Thomas's, were overcrowded and unable to care for all those in need. Recognizing the problem, a group of London laymen and physicians in 1719 organized the Charitable Society in Westminster to provide for such sick persons as were unable to obtain proper care. This was the beginning of the Westminster Hospital, which was soon followed by the establishment of other institutions: Guy's (1724), St. George's (1733), London Hospital (1740). About the middle of the century special hospitals were created. The Middlesex Hospital was founded in 1746 for smallpox patients and to encourage inoculation. The same year also saw the establishment of the Lock Hospital for patients with venereal diseases. St. Luke's, for the reception of mentally ill persons, was established in 1751.

From 1760 to 1800 the growth of hospitals in London slowed down, but thereafter the process of development was resumed. During the first four decades of the nineteenth century, fourteen hospitals were founded in London. While some were general hospitals, it is noteworthy that most of them were special hospitals. Thus, the London Fever Hospital was founded in 1802, the Royal London Ophthalmic Hospital in 1804, the Royal Chest Hospital in 1814, the Royal Ear Hospital in 1816, and the Royal National Orthopedic Hospital in 1838.

The influence of these trends was soon felt and paralleled outside London. The movement began to spread rapidly to Bristol (1737), York (1740), Exeter (1741), and Liverpool (1745). By 1760 there were 16 provincial hospitals of which 14 were general in character. There were 38 by 1780, and 114 by 1840. Similar forces were at work in Scotland and Ireland, and by the end of the eighteenth century hospitals were to be found in most of the cities and larger towns of Great Britain.[45]

But even while hospitals were being founded, it was realized that these institutions would have to be supplemented by some other kind of establishment. To fill this need the dispensary was developed. The dispensary idea may be traced to the seventeenth century, but it was not until 1769 that a more permanent establishment of this type came into being. This was the Dispensary for the Infant Poor, opened by Dr. George Armstrong at a house in Red Lion Square, Holborn, London. The opening of Armstrong's dispensary was followed in 1770 by the founding of the General Dispensary by John Coakley Lettsom, a Quaker physician, and a group of associates. Following the example set by Lettsom, dispensaries sprang up in London and the provinces. From 1770 through 1792, fifteen were founded in London, and from 1775 through 1798, thirteen in the provinces.[46]

The causes of this expansive growth were varied, but they may be considered in two major categories: medical and scientific, and socioeconomic. The great scientific outburst of the sixteenth and seventeenth centuries laid the foundation for the application of science to medical care, and increasingly knowledge of the structure of the human body was provided through dissection and observation by Vesalius, his contemporaries, and his successors. Obstetrics and surgery were already able to benefit from this knowlege in the eighteenth century. Equally basic, though on a more complex level, was Harvey's discovery of the circulation of the blood, which provided a firm basis for consideration of the body as a functional system. Observation and classification also made possible the more precise recognition of diseases. In creating institutions where it was possible to apply this knowledge, the hospital and dispensary movement gave a concrete form to the social philosophy of Bacon, Petty, and others who saw in science a means for improving human health and welfare.

However, the mere accretion of medical ideas and knowledge cannot of itself assure application. Social environment and intellectual milieu must provide favorable conditions and patterns of behavior in terms of which knowledge can be put to use. Precisely this, however, characterized England during the eighteenth century, particularly during the latter part of the period. The tempo and character of economic life had been changing in England before the middle of the eighteenth century, but by comparison the industrial and agricultural changes during the latter half of the century were both rapid and radical. These profound alterations in the economic life of the country necessarily disturbed its social structure and gave rise to a new attitude of mind toward problems of community life. Representing essentially the views of the middle classes, this distinctive ethos was characterized by two dominant facets: an insistence on order, efficiency, and social discipline, and a concern with the conditions of men. Appreciation of the social factors and consequences of ill health led merchants, physicians, clergymen, and other public-spirited citizens to undertake ameliorative efforts. It is significant that the hospital and dispensary movement, the infant-welfare movement, and other similar activities originated in urban centers, first in London, then in other cities and towns. Wealth, commerce, and industry were largely centered there, and at the same time it was much easier for the middle class, many of whose members were Dissenters, to make themselves felt. They fostered the growing social conscience, but it was a humanitarianism coupled with a firm belief in the sober and practical virtues of efficiency, simplicity, and cheapness.[47]

The English colonies in America followed the general pattern set by the mother country, but with a considerable lag. The first successful effort to establish a general hospital occurred in Philadelphia, in the middle of the eighteenth century, with the opening of the Pennsylvania Hospital in 1751. The causes that led to its founding were well stated by Benjamin Franklin in 1754:

> About the end of the year 1750 [he wrote] some persons, who had frequent opportunities of observing the distress of such distemper'd poor as from time to time came to Philadelphia, for the advice and assistance of the physicians and surgeons of that city; how difficult it was for them to procure suitable lodgings, and other conveniences proper for their respective cases, and how expensive the providing good and careful nurses, and other attendants for want whereof, many must suffer greatly, and some probably perish that might other wise have been restored to health and comfort, and become useful to themselves, their families, and the publick for many years after; and considering moreover, that even the poor inhabitants of this city, tho' they had homes, yet were therein but badly accommodated in sickness, and could not be so well and so easily taken care of in their separate habitations, as they might be in one convenient house, under one inspection, and in the hands of the skilful practitioners; and several of the inhabitants of the province, who unhappily became disordered in their senses, wander'd about, to the terror of their neighbours, there being no place (except the House of Correction) in which they might be confined, and subjected to proper management for their recovery, and that House was by no means fitted for such purposes; did charitably consult together, and confer with their friends and acquaintances, on the best means of relieving the distressed, under those circumstances; and an Infirmary, or hospital, in the manner of several lately established in Great Britain [was proposed and approved].[48]

Franklin also pointed out that the hospital could serve an educational purpose by training physicians. Moreover, the idea that in terms of social economy it may be cheaper to provide medical care in an efficient and accessible way so that sick persons can be restored, if possible, to a useful place in society, which had been noted in the early sixteenth century, now appears as an integral motivating value of the eighteenth-century hospital movement.

The hospitals founded in Great Britain and in America during the eighteenth century and the early nineteenth century were not governmental undertakings. They were the outcome of voluntary efforts by private citizens, and were financed by subscription and bequest. It is clear that the voluntary hospital was not an outgrowth of experience with the social and economic changes brought about by the Industrial Revolution in the nineteenth century, but preceded them. Moreover, the voluntary hospital had a purpose that was primarily social rather than medical. It was intended to serve the sick poor "whose home conditions were deficient in the accommodation their distress needed."[49] However, the sick poor who had to go to a hospital because they could not obtain care at home were faced with two possibilities: they might be admitted by a voluntary general hospital; if not, the almshouse or the workhouse was their lot. The choice was determined by hospital policy. Patients with chronic, incurable, or terminal conditions were not accepted by the voluntary hospitals. For example, in 1808 attention was drawn to the circumstance that certain medical practitoners tended to refer to the Dundee Royal Infirmary patients far advanced in illness who had no prospect of recovery. These people were not regarded as "proper objects" of the infirmary, which was "never intended as an almshouse or poorhouse." Furthermore, with a limited number of beds such a practice would tend to exclude those who might truly benefit from the care provided by the institution. Finally, "what opinion would the public form of the skill of the medical attendants in the house, if upon looking at the annual reports it should appear that the cases of death were to those of recovery as three to one?"[50] This situation continued to exist throughout the nineteenth century. Louisa Twining commented some seventy years later that there were "a large number of persons afflicted with incurable disease who are not proper objects for admission into general hospitals." Furthermore, the workhouses were "hospitals for those who are incurable, and who are turned out of our best London hospitals."[51]

On this basis there developed in Great Britain, and in a modified form in the United States and Canada, a pattern of hospital services that persisted until well into the twentieth century and whose influence is still evident in hospital organization in the United States. Hospitals were simply institutions maintained through public funds or private charity, where the indigent poor could be cared for more economically than in their own homes. Voluntary hospitals tended to take acute cases, the short-stay patients, while the chronic cases, the incurable, the insane, and those suffering from communicable diseases went to public institutions.

This pattern explains in part the number of hospitals, hospital beds, and hospital patients in the United States and Britain in the nineteenth century. As late as 1873 there were only 149 hospitals and related institutions in the United States, and of those one-third were for the mentally ill. Fifty years later there were 6,762. During the same period the number of beds increased from 35,453 to 770,375. Similarly, in 1851, in all of England and Wales the census enumerators recorded only 7,619 patients as resident in hospitals. In 1871 there were 19,585 patients in general and special voluntary hospitals, but over 50,000 patients in workhouse infirmaries.[52]

The public hospitals of this period, and to a lesser extent the voluntary general institutions, left much to be desired. Owing to prevailing concepts of administrative economy, wards were overcrowded, hygienic conditions were poor, and nursing was primitive. Small wonder when as late as 1877, W. Gill Wylie, a prominent physician, asserted that hospitals did more harm than good by removing the "healthful stimulus of necessity" that was essential to recovery. In his opinion, hospitals should be limited "to those who have no homes and to those who cannot be assisted at their homes."[53] However, Wylie did emphasize the importance of hospitals for medical education, a view that was stated even more strongly by John Green, another physician concerned with hospital construction and operation. Hospitals, he said, "are essentially charitable institutions, and the welfare of the patients must ever hold the first place in the minds of their founders. Nevertheless, we must not lose sight of the fact that they are also our great schools of clinical observation and instruction; and have thus, perhaps, rendered their most important service to mankind."[54]

Hospital organization and staffing of the nineteenth century were simple. The Charity Hospital in New Orleans was jointly administered at first by the state and the city through a board of administrators, and later by a state board. The operating personnel of the hospital consisted in 1823 of an attending physician, an apothecary who also served for a time as a house surgeon and purveyor, an assistant apothecary, a ward master, a porter, and ten nurses, including slaves belonging to the institution. Later, the board annually elected four physicians, one visiting surgeon, and a house surgeon to provide professional attendance. In 1843 the number of attending physicians was increased to eight, the surgeons to two, and elections to these posts were made semiannual. About six medical students served as interns and performed tasks ordered by the attending physicians.[55]

The Modern Hospital Appears

Application of the knowledge derived from bacteriology and laboratory studies in clinical medicine led in the twentieth century to an increase in the number of medical and technical personnel required by the hospital. A striking illustration of this development was offered in 1938 by Alphonse R. Dochez in a comparative picture of the complex changes in hospital medical practice during the first three decades of this century. He did this by contrasting the histories of two patients with similar types of heart disease; one was recorded in 1908, the other at the same hospital in 1938. The total written record of the first patient occupies two and one-half pages, and the observations represent the combined efforts of two physicians, the attending and the house officer, and of one specialist, a pathologist-bacteriologist. The record of the second patient, who was still in the hospital when Dochez made this comparison, comprised twenty-nine pages and represented the combined observations of three visiting physicians, two residents, three house officers, ten specialists, and fourteen technicians, a total of thirty-two individuals.[56] Naturally, such an elaborate study as that of the latter patient is not made of everyone admitted to a hospital, but the organization necessary for such studies is continuously maintained, not only for patients with heart disease but also for others.

Obviously the change described by Dochez could not have occurred without specific alterations in the hospitals and in the communities they served. Thus, it had long been recognized that different categories of patients should be separated. In 1865, for instance, a report to the administration of the Paris hospitals advised a reorganization of the maternity service, that patients be separated into appropriate groups, and the building of special pavilions for those with communicable diseases.[57] However, this reorganization was not undertaken until 1880. This was also the period in which operating rooms were constructed that took account of the principles of asepsis and were specifically designed for the purpose. Hospital laboratories were also introduced in the eighties and nineties. The first laboratory in a municipal hospital in Paris was created in 1893.[58] Lankenau Hospital in Philadelphia established the first bacteriological and chemical laboratory in that city in 1889, and the first hospital X-ray laboratory in 1896.[59]

It was also during this period that nursing was reformed and training schools for nurses were introduced. This along with the increasing recognition of the medical value of bedside care led to changes in hospital administration. The introduction of trained nurses involved conflicts with the physicians, the older nurses, and the administration. As Abel-Smith has so succinctly put it: "If the new matron was to undertake what she considered to be her duties, she had to carve out an empire of her own. She had to take over some of the responsibilities of the medical staff and some of the responsibilities of the lay administration. In addition she had to centralize the administration of nursing affairs," thereby lowering the status of the other nurses.[60] Moreover, not only for the matron but also for the nurses under her direction there existed the problems of role definition, status, and the other sociological elements involved in such innovations. Doctors were afraid that nurses would undermine their authority, and no one had yet drawn a line between general nursing that was a responsibility of the matron and her staff and medical treatment for which the physicians were responsible. Eventually, of course, a *modus vivendi* was developed, and, especially in the English voluntary hospitals, nursing became essentially an independent department, of which the head had a position of authority between the medical staff and the lay administration. Similar changes in the English workhouse infirmaries occurred much more slowly, essentially because of the deterrent philosophy that was the basis of the whole system of poor-law administration.[61]

The suspicion and hostility encountered by the trained nurses when they first entered the hospital were not peculiar to this group. Such attitudes and the conflicts they engender have been the fate of other new groups also. This happened to the first social workers in hospitals and for the same reasons. Richard C. Cabot found such a situation at the Massachusetts General Hospital. In 1909 he wrote:

> Unless there is at least one doctor who really knows what the social worker is trying to do, the scheme fails. If he thinks of her merely as a nurse and asks of her only such help as a nurse can render, she will either fall short of his expectations . . . or finally she will exceed his expectations and his horizon—which will make him think her "uppish" or interfering or visionary. Unless a doctor has already acquired the "social point of view" to the extent of seeing that his treatment of dispensary patients is slovenly, without some knowledge of their homes, their finances, their thoughts and worries,—he will think that the social worker is teaching him how to do his work whenever she does what he didn't and couldn't do before. Naturally he will resent this indignantly . . . he will not care to be advised by any "woman charity worker."[62]

In this manner the hospital in the more developed countries of the world was taking unto itself the various elements that were eventually to create the institution that we know today as the workshop of the physician and the eventual community health center. At the same time other factors also made their impact felt. One of these was urbanization; the other was population growth. During the later nineteenth century more and more hospitals were constructed.

In New York City twelve hospitals came into existence from 1850 to 1860, at a time when Brooklyn was not yet a part of the greater city. The decades of the seventies and eighties were prolific in the creation of new hospitals. Many of the special hospitals were created during this period. This growth of special institutions was due in part to the development of specialism, but even more so to the limitations of the voluntary general hospital. The latter had no facilities for the new specialties as they appeared, nor could they undertake any pioneering initiative because of financial limitations.

Furthermore, public attitudes toward hospitals changed. As early as 1802, the municipal authorities of Paris converted the Hospice de Jésus into a hospital known as the Maison Dubois to which paying patients were admitted,[63] and in New York City, St. Vincent's Hospital, built in 1850, was the first to provide private accommodations. None the less, the rich for a long time continued to receive medical care, including surgery, at home, and the poor feared admission to the hospital as a death sentence, a way station to a pauper funeral. By the middle of the second decade of the twentieth century, the situation had changed completely. Around the turn of the century the adoption of asepsis had so lowered operative mortality that the public began to accept hospitals as agencies of social good. It was realized that various forms of ill-health could be treated more effectively in the hospital than in the home. This trend was further strengthened and intensified by the development of roentgenology, of laboratory techniques for diagnosis, and of a variety of costly therapeutic modalities. At the same time the value of the hospital as an educational institution for physicians, students, and nurses was increasingly recognized. As a result, by the beginning of the twentieth century hospitals were admitting increasing numbers of paying patients in private rooms and other accommodations set apart from those for the indigent.[64]

With increasing complexity of medical care and increased acceptance of hospital service, there developed a need for adjunct services in addition to the usual medical and nursing care. These have involved social work, nutrition, and more complex record and business procedures. As hospitals had to accommodate more complex functions, additional personnel, facilities and equipment, their organization has also grown increasingly complex and their operation more costly. These consequences, interacting with or affected by developments outside the hospital, have in turn led to new phenomena and situations, namely, the appearance of hospital administration as a profession, the growth of voluntary prepayment plans for hospital expenses, an increased awareness and greater attention to the quality of hospital service and medical care, and a more prominent role of government, at all levels, in the hospital field, especially in the financing and construction of hospitals.[65]

The consequence of these developments has been to give the hospital a central role in modern medical care, to make it responsible for complex and wide-ranging tasks, but at the same time to produce painful tensions and conflicts most evident in the voluntary general hospital.

The source of this situation is to be found in the characteristic administrative structure the voluntary hospital inherited from its eighteenth century origins in Great Britain and the United States.[66] Each voluntary hospital was an independent institution managed by its own trustees or governors, and staffed by physicians and surgeons who donated their services gratis. In return the medical staff were enabled to use suitable and interesting cases for teaching and research. Later, as the public began to accept the advantages of hospitalization, physicians began to use the hospital for their private patients. At the same time, the physician had no administrative or financial responsibility to the hospital. Moreover, as scientific medicine emerged and became institutionalized in the hospital, the physician became essential for its operation, while the institution became more and more indispensable for the practice of good medicine. This administrative duality was possible as long as most of the patients were indigent, as long as the hospital tended to remain a self-contained, relatively simple organization, and as long as the physician could use the hospital and still retain his position as an independent entrepreneur.

However, as the hospital increased in size and complexity, as the development of medicine required the use of costly equipment, as changing social and economic conditions altered the financing of medical care and created new patterns of hospital utilization, the organizational relationships within the hospital have been disturbed and have become unstable. It is no longer a question of trustees, administrator, and medical staff alone. Another set of people, the organized consumers, have to be considered and satisfied if possible. In short, having become a large-scale organization, the hospital requires a more explicit organizational division of labor and more efficient, responsible management. For the physician this means accommodation to institutionalized teamwork, a prospect that is highly distasteful to many. The degree of control will vary with the hospital, but the prospect is that increased administrative rationality will characterize the developing hospital and that the practice of the physician will be under the continuing scrutiny of others, not only his professional colleagues, who will appraise his activities. Indeed, the very nature of large-scale organization raises problems of administrative efficiency and rationality, productivity, and accountability of all personnel, including physicians.

Conclusion

At various periods in history the need to care for the sick and the disabled, the needy and the dependent has crystallized sufficiently in terms of attitude and practice that one may speak of institutional models characteristic of certain societies. In this sense, the history of the hospital may be seen in terms of certain types that have predominated in given historical periods. The medieval hospital in all its varied forms was essentially an ecclesiastical institution, not primarily concerned with medical care. This institutional type was eventually replaced in the sixteenth century by another kind of hospital whose goals were not religious, but primarily social. To achieve this, the medieval hospital was to a large extent secularized, placed under governmental control, and its activities accepted as a community responsibility. In its organization and operation, however, the early modern hospital still retained various features of its predecessor, one being that medical care was not its primary function. That is, the hospital as it existed from the sixteenth century into the nineteenth century was intended primarily to help in the maintenance of social order while providing for the sick and the needy. During this period, however, various forces and developments external to the hospital eventually transformed it into what is now characteristic of economically developed countries. This hospital, the product of the industrial and scientific revolutions, may be called the health-workshop or medical-factory type. Here medical care is the primary goal of the institution, and its provision is governed chiefly by scientific-technological norms and the requirements of organizational rationality and economy. Yet this hospital type still has features derived from its past that are not always congruent with its ostensible goals and norms. For this reason, the better we understand how "within living memory an age-old institution has been transformed from a hostel for sick-poor into a medical center for everyone,"[67] the clearer will we as scientists be able to see the hospital, and the more effectively can we as practitioners contribute to its evolution.

REFERENCES

1. Cyril Bailey, ed., *The Legacy of Rome* (London: Oxford University Press, 1951), pp. 292-296.
2. "The So-called Second Letter of St. Clement," trans. Francis X. Glimm, *The Apostolic Fathers,* The Fathers of the Church Series (New York: Cima Publishing Co., 1947), p. 76.
3. E. Jeanselme and L. Oeconomos, "Les Oeuvres d'Assistance et les Hôpitaux Byzantins au siècle des Comnènes," *1er Congrès de l'Histoire de l'Art de Guérir (août, 1920)* (1921), pp. 239-256.
4. *Ibid.*, p. 240.
5. Georg Schreiber, *Gemeinschaften des Mittelalters. Recht und Verfassung. Kult und Frömmigkeit,* Gesammelte Abhandlungen, Bd. I (Regensberg Münster, 1948), pp. 3-80 (p. 10); Steven Runciman, *Byzantine Civilization* (New York: Meridian Books, 1956), p. 190.
6. Schreiber, *op. cit.*, pp. 45-46.
7. *The Rule of St. Benedict,* ed., with an English translation and explanatory notes by D. Oswald Hunter Blair, 3rd ed. (Fort Augustus, Scotland, Abbey Press, 1914), pp. 101-103, 133-137.
8. F. Keller, *Bauriss des Klosters St. Gallen vom Jahre 820, im Faksimile herausgegeben und erläutert* (Zurich, 1844). Cited by Alfons Fischer, *Geschichte des deutschen Gesundheitswesens,* 2 vols. (Berlin: F. A. Herbig, 1933), Vol. 1, p. 49.
9. These comments are based on a personal inspection of the site in 1960. See also O. E. Craster, *Tintern Abbey, Monmouthshire,* Ministry of Works Official Guide-Book (London: H.M.S.O., 1956), pp. 17-19; also plan between pp. 11-12.
10. Wilhelm Liese, *Geschichte der Caritas,* 2 Bde. (Freiburg im Breisgau, 1922), Vol. I, p. 143.
11. Franz Meffert, *Caritas und Krankenwesen* (Freiburg, 1927), p. 147.
12. Liese, *op. cit.*, Vol. II, p. 118; E. A. Meinert, *Die Hospitäler Holsteins im Mittelalter,* Kiel Dissertation (1949).
13. J. M. Hobson, *Some Early and Later Houses of Pity* (London: George Routledge and Sons, 1926), pp. 14-15.
14. Maud Sellers, *The Merchant Adventurers of York,* Printed for the Company of Merchant Adventurers of the City of York (Ben Johnson & Co., Ltd., 1946, reprinted 1956). Comments based also on visit to building in 1960.
15. For a list of the English hospitals, see D. Knowles and R. N. Hadcock, *Medieval Religious Houses* (London: Longmans, Green & Co., Ltd., 1953), pp. 250-324.
16. Brian Tierney, *Medieval Poor Law: A Sketch of Canonical Theory and Its Application in England* (Berkeley: University of California Press, 1959), p. 87.
17. Siegfried Reicke, *Das deutsche Spital und sein Recht im Mittelalter,* Kirchenrechtliche Abhandlungen (Stuttgart, 1932), p. 198.
18. For different religious rules of various French hospitals in the twelfth, thirteenth, and fourteenth centuries, see Léon Le Grand, *Statuts d'Hôtels-Dieu et de Léproseries. Recueil de textes du XIIe au XIVe Siècle* (Paris: Alphonse Picard et Fils, 1901); also Dorothy-Louise Mackay, *Les Hôpitaux et la Charité à Paris au XIIIe Siècle* (Paris: Honoré Champion, 1932), pp. 34-50.
19. *The Faerie Queene,* Book I, Canto X, 36.

20. Rotha Mary Clay, *The Medieval Hospitals in England* (London: Methuen & Co., 1909), pp. 120-126.
21. *Ibid.*, p. 138; Liese, *op. cit.*, Vol. I, p. 173.
22. F. R. Salter, ed., *Some Early Tracts on Poor Relief* (London: Methuen & Co., 1926), pp. 10-11, 117.
23. Tierney, *op. cit.*, p. 87.
24. W. Haid: "Über den kirchlichen Charakter der Spitäler, besonders in der Erzdiözese Freiburg," *Freiburger Diozesanarchiv*, Bd. 2 (1866), p. 136, 2.2, p. 305, Document No. 7; cited by Fischer, *op. cit.*, Vol. I, p. 137.
25. Clay, *op. cit.*, p. 212.
26. Tierney, *op. cit.*, p. 86.
27. W. J. Ashley, *An Introduction to English Economic History and Theory*, 2 vols. (New York: G. P. Putnam's Sons, 1893), Vol. II, p. 319.
28. Martha Goldberg, *Das Armen- und Krankenwesen des mittelalterlichen Strassburg, Freiburg Dissertation* (Strassburg, 1909), p. 2; E. Becker, "Geschichte der Medizin in Hildesheim," *Archiv für klinische Medizin*, 38 (1899), p. 317; Reicke, *op. cit.*, pp. 93-97; Liese, *op. cit.*, Vol. I, pp. 231 ff.; A. de Calonne, *La Vie municipale au XVe siècle dans le nord de France* (Paris: Didier et Cie, 1880), p. 126.
29. Charlotte Koch, *Wandlungen der Wohlfahrtspflege im Zeitalter der Aufklärung*, Erlangen Dissertation (Erlangen, 1933), pp. 11-29.
30. Simon Fish, "A Supplicacyon for the Beggers" (1529), in *A Miscellany of Tracts and Pamphlets*, ed. A. C. Ward (London: Oxford University Press, 1927), pp. 1-17 (p. 16).
31. Claude Lillingston, "Sweden's Hospital Administration in the Sixteenth Century," *British Medical Journal* (December 10, 1955), p. 1445.
32. *The Order of the Hospitals of K. Henry the VIII and K. Edward the VI, viz. St. Bartholomew's. Christ's. Bridewell. St. Thomas's.* By the Maior, Cominaltie, and Citizens of London, Governours of the Possessions, Revenues and Goods of the sayd Hospitalls, 1557.
33. The organization as described in the preceding reference lists a surgeon and a barber, but does not discuss their duties or their specific position as members of the hospital staff.
34. E. A. Hammond, "Physicians in Medieval English Religious Houses," *Bulletin of the History of Medicine* 32 (1958), pp. 105–120.
35. G. L. Kriegk, *Deutsches Bürgertum im Mittelalter*, 2 vols. (Frankfurt am Main, 1868-1871, Vol. I, pp. 8, 53, 524.
36. Ernst Mummenhoff, "Die öffentliche Gesundheits- und Krankenpflege im alten Nürnberg," in *Festschrift zur Eröffnung des neuen Krankenhauses der Stadt Nürnberg*, herausgegeben von den Städtischen Collegien (Nürnberg, 1898), p. 53.
37. O. Winckelmann, *Das Fürsorgewesen der Stadt Strassburg vor und nach der Reformation bis zum Ausgang des 16. Jahrhunderts*, Quellen und Forschungen zur Reformationsgeschichte (Leipzig, 1922), Vol. V, p. 25; Fischer, *op. cit.*, Vol. I, p. 140.
38. K. Sudhoff, "Ein Wendepunkt im Spitalwesen des Mittelalters," Bericht über einen am 24 Sept., 1913, gehaltenen Vortrag, *Münchener medizinische Wochenschrift* (1913), p. 2482.
39. *Die Reformation Kaiser Sigmunds, Eine Schrift des 15. Jahrhunderts zur Kirchen und Reichsreform*, herausgegeben von Karl Beer, Beiheft zu den Deutschen Reichstagsakten herausgegeben durch die Historische Kommission bei der Bayerischen Akademie der Wissenschaften (Stuttgart, 1933), pp. 124-126; Karl Beer: "Was ein deutscher Reformer vor einem halben Jahrtausend vom Ärztestand erwartete," *Gesnerus*, 11 (1954), pp. 24-36; Lothar Graf zu Dohna, *Reformatio Sigismundi. Beiträge zum Verständnis einer Reformschrift des fünfzehnten Jahrhunderts* (Göttingen, 1960).
40. George Rosen, "Medical Care and Social Policy in Seventeenth Century England,"

Bulletin of the New York Academy of Medicine, 29 (1953), pp. 420-437.

41. Dorothy Marshall, *The English Poor in the 18th Century* (London: George Routledge & Sons, 1926), pp. 127-128; Karl de Schweinitz, *England's Road to Social Security* (Philadelphia: University of Pennsylvania Press, 1943), pp. 53-55; H. R. Fox Bourne, *The Life of John Locke,* 2 vols. (New York: Harper & Brothers, 1876), Vol. II, pp. 376-392; A. Ruth Fry, *John Bellers, 1654–1725: Quaker, Economist and Social Reformer* (London: Cassell & Co., 1935), pp. 5-28; George Rosen, "An Eighteenth Century Plan for a National Health Service," *Bulletin of the History of Medicine,* 16. (1944) pp. 429-436; Bernard Mandeville, *The Fable of the Bees: or Private vices, publick benefits. With an essay on charity and charity schools . . .,* 5th ed. (London: J. Tonson, 1728), pp. 341-366.
42. W. K. Jordan, *The Charities of London, 1480–1660: The Aspirations and the Achievements of the Urban Society* (London: George Allen and Unwin, 1960), pp. 186-196.
43. *Bute Broadsides* (Houghton Library, Harvard University), Vol. 1, pp. 44, 53, 65, 76-77, 164-166.
44. Dorothy Marshall, *English People in the Eighteenth Century* (London: Longmans, Green & Co., 1956), pp. 186 ff.
45. B. Kirkman Gray, *A History of English Philanthropy* (London: P. S. King & Son, 1905), pp. 126-131; S. Wilks and G. T. Bettany, *A Biographical History of Guy's Hospital* (London, 1892), pp. 52-53, 56-73; Thomas Ferguson, *The Dawn of Scottish Social Welfare* (Edinburgh: Thomas Nelson & Sons, 1948), pp. 255-284; K. H. Connell, *The Population of Ireland 1750–1845* (Oxford: Clarendon Press, 1950), pp. 198-207; M. C. Buer, *Health, Wealth and Population in the Early Days of the Industrial Revolution* (London: George Routledge & Sons, 1926), pp. 257-258.
46. Ernest Caulfield, *The Infant Welfare Movement in the Eighteenth Century* (New York: Paul B. Hoeber, 1931), pp. 55-58, 146-176; Gray, *op. cit.,* pp. 132-134; A. M. Carr-Saunders and P. A. Wilson, *The Professions* (Oxford: Clarendon Press, 1933), pp. 72-73; Harvey Cushing, "Dr. Garth. The Kit-Kat Poet," *Bulletin Johns Hopkins Hospital* 17 (1906), pp. 1-17; G. F. Still, *The History of Pediatrics* (London: Oxford University Press, 1931), pp. 417-421; J. J. Abraham, *Lettsom, His Life, Times, Friends and Descendants* (London: William Heinemann, Ltd., 1933), pp. 109–110; T. J. Pettigrew, *Memoirs of the life and writings of the late John Coakley Lettsom . . .,* 3 vols. (London, 1817), Vol. I, pp. 36-38; J. C. Trent, "John Coakley Lettsom," *Bulletin of the History of Medicine,* 22 (1948), pp. 528-542.
47. *Reports of the Society for Bettering the Conditions and Increasing the Comforts of the Poor* (London, 1802), Vol. III, p. 2; Dorothy Marshall, *English People in the Eighteenth Century* (New York: Longmans & Co., 1956), pp. 147-157.
48. Benjamin Franklin, *Some Account of the Pennsylvania Hospital,* ed. I. Bernard Cohen (Baltimore: Johns Hopkins Press, 1954), p. 3; see also p. 19-22.
49. Henry J. C. Gibson, *Dundee Royal Infirmary with a Short Account of More Recent Years* (Dundee: William Kidd & Sons, 1948), p. 11.
50. *Ibid.,* pp. 12-13.
51. Louisa Twining, *Recollections of Workhouse Visiting and Management during Twenty five Years* (London, 1880), p. 37; *idem, A Letter to the President of the Poor Law Board on Workhouse Infirmaries* (London, 1866), pp. 26-27.
52. Michael M. Davis, *Clinics, Hospitals and Health Centers* (New York: Harper & Brothers, 1927), pp. 4-5; Brian Abel-Smith, *A History of the Nursing Profession* (New York: W. Heineman, 1960), pp. 2, 4.
53. W. Gill Wylie, *Hospitals: Their History, Organization, and Construction* (New York: D. Appleton & Co., 1877), pp. 60, 67.
54. John Green, *City Hospitals* (Boston: Little Brown & Co., 1861), p. 14.
55. Elizabeth Wisner, *Public Welfare Administration in Louisiana* (Chicago: University of

Chicago Press, 1930), pp. 37-38.
56. Alphonse R. Dochez, "President's Address," *Transactions of the American Clinical and Climatological Association,* 54 (1939), pp. 19-23.
57. Pierre Vallery-Radot, *Un Siècle d'Histoire hospitalière de Louis-Philippe jusqu'à nos jours* (1837–1949) (Paris, 1948), pp. 27–28.
58. *Ibid.*, pp. 31-32.
59. Herman M. Somers and Anne R. Somers, *Doctors, Patients and Health Insurance* (Washington, D.C.: Brookings Institution, 1961), p. 63.
60. Abel-Smith, *op. cit.*, p. 25.
61. *Idem,* Chaps. 2–3.
62. Richard C. Cabot, *Social Service and the Art of Healing* (New York: Dodd, Mead & Co., 1931), pp. 180-182; see also E. Moberly Bell, *The Story of Hospital Almoners; The Birth of a Profession* (1961), pp. 27-30.
63. René Sand, *The Advance to Social Medicine* (New York: John de Graff, Inc., 1952), p. 86.
64. Davis, *op. cit.*, pp. 13-14; Somers and Somers, *op. cit.*, pp. 64-65.
65. George Rosen, "Hospital," *Encyclopedia Americana* (1959), Vol. XIV, pp. 432-433.
66. George Bugbee, "The Physician in the Hospital Organization," *New England Journal of Medicine* (1959), pp. 896-901.
67. Michael M. Davis, *Medical Care for Tomorrow* (New York: Harper & Brothers, 1955), p. 111.

This study was financed by a grant (M-3171) from the National Institute of Mental Health, U. S. Public Health Service. The paper is an expansion of one read at the 1960 meetings of the American Sociological Association.

THE FIRST NEIGHBORHOOD HEALTH CENTER MOVEMENT
Its Rise and Fall

Introduction

Among aspects of urban life in modern times which have been regarded as conducive to social dis-ease and decay, the connection between poverty and ill-health has long been recognized as a major focus of community concern and action. Awareness of the widespread prevalence of disease among the poor and of the inadequacy of the health care available to them has at various times motivated efforts to improve their health by providing more effective medical care. Historically, such concern has expressed itself in the creation of programs and facilities ranging from the dispensaries of the 18th century to the current neighborhood health centers.

Indeed, the latter grew out of a recognition that existing arrangements and programs in the United States were not satisfactorily meeting the complex health needs of the poor.[1] As a result, the neighborhood health center had been developed to remedy this situation by providing "a one-door facility, in which virtually all ambulatory health services are available; close coordination with other community resources; professional staff of high quality; and intensive participation by and involvement of the population to be served."[2] In these terms the current wave of neighborhood health centers has been viewed by some as having brought forth a new institutional form. Yet neither the concept of providing health services on a local basis, nor the creation of facilities to deliver such care, nor the stated objectives of the neighborhood center are essentially new. The concept of a community health center providing service on a neighborhood basis, and its embodiment in organizational forms provided the core for a widespread movement which developed in the United States during the second and third decades of this century, reached its peak during the 30s, and then declined. Since the circumstances out of which this movement grew, the objectives at which it aimed, and the organizational forms it assumed are not unlike those characteristic of the neighborhood health center movement, an examination of the earlier movement may perhaps throw some light on the future possibilities of current trends.

Urbanism, Immigration, and Health

The roots of the health center movement, which began around 1910, are to be found in the changes which occurred in American society during the preceding decades. From 1860 to 1910 the urban portion of the population rose from 19 to 45 per cent of the total, due in large measure to a flood of immigrants which poured into the cities and industrial towns where workers were in demand.[3] From about 1880 the majority of the immigrants came from southern and eastern Europe where they had left the backward, wretched circumstances of countryside and hamlet to seek a better life in the New World.[4] Some were skilled workers and craftsmen, a category which was largest among Jewish immigrants, of whom thousands entered the needle trades. A certain number of Italian immigrants also possessed skills adaptable to urban conditions, and some, particularly women, took jobs in the garment industry. Others entered service occupations or set up as shopkeepers or peddlers. As early as 1890, for example, most fruit peddlers and bootblacks in New York City were Italian, and not much later Italians were already heavily represented among waiters, barbers and shoemakers. Most immigrants, however, were unskilled and had to accept poorly paid jobs performing heavy manual work. But even those who were skilled worked excessively long hours for low wages under unhealthful conditions. Frequently they worked for their compatriots, often converting their dwellings into sweatshops.

Separated from the native Americans by language and custom, the immigrants crowded together in segregated neighborhoods where mutual aid and understanding were available. These neighborhoods were a geographic expression of the immigrants' endeavor to maintain their identity by living within a cultural environment in which they had roots, and from which they might make contact with and learn about the unfamiliar American world in which they found themselves. To the native American, however, the areas where these impoverished aliens congregated were loathsome, sickening slums whose denizens challenged and threatened the fabric of his social and psychological order. As early as 1883 Henry George, anticipating the end of the public domain viewed the flooding immigrant tide with alarm and asked "What in a few years are we to do for a dumping ground? Will it make our difficulties the less that our human garbage can vote?"[5] George was not alone in his opinion, which was echoed with numerous variations in succeeding decades. Robert A. Woods, a leading Boston social worker of the period, recoiled from the "unspeakable degraded standard of life" of the immigrants, while his collaborator Joseph Lee was amazed that this "human rubbish" produced a "number of physically, mentally and morally efficient citizens."[6]

The revulsion and dismay expressed in such statements are related to two reactions to the immigrants which clashed in principle but in practice tended to blend in various, sometimes ambiguous ways. One was a reaction to the differing life-styles and values of the immigrants, comprising feelings of contempt, distrust and fear, as well as a sense that the alien masses were inferior and a menace. General anti-foreign attitudes, views of foreigners as unruly and dangerous were refracted through specific ethnic or national stereotypes to which unfavorable characteristics and qualities were attributed.[7] This attitude found its more unsophisticated expression in the tendency to single out "wops," "sheenies," "polacks," "bohunks" or some other group as inherently criminal, avaricious or subversive.

But even those Americans who were sympathetic to the foreign-born were not completely exempt from the influence of the current stereotypes. In the early 1900s, the distinguished physician, Richard Cabot, examining his reactions to foreign-born patients at the Massachusetts General Hospital, noted that "the chances are ten to one that I shall look out of my eyes and see, *not* Abraham Cohen, but *a Jew* . . . I do not see *this* man at all. I merge him in the hazy background of the average Jew. But," he went on, "if I am a little less blind than usual today . . . I may notice something in the way his hand lies on his knee, something that is queer, unexpected. That hand . . . it's a muscular hand, it's a prehensile hand; and whoever saw a Salem Street Jew with a muscular hand before . . . I saw *him.* Yet he was no more real than the thousands of others whom I had seen and forgotten, forgotten—because I never saw *them,* but only their ghostly outline, their generic type, the racial background out of which they emerged."[8]

Cabot's self-analysis is an aspect of the other reaction to the immigrants, an aspect of an endeavor to come into close enough contact with them to learn about them as people, to begin to understand the stresses and strains to which they were exposed in an alien environment. This tendency appeared most prominently with the establishment of social settlements in the 1890s in the poorest sections of Chicago, New York and other cities. Since these sections, the slums, were also overwhelmingly the foreign quarters, most of those with whom settlement dwellers worked were immigrants. The settlement workers soon became aware of the deep gulf which separated the poor immigrants from the larger society in which they lived, but to which they did not belong. Recognizing the need for social integration of the newer immigration with the older America, they set themselves the task, as Lillian Wald put it, of "fusing these people who come to us from the Old World Civilization into . . . a real brotherhood among men."[9]

For the most part, the settlements approached this task in practical, concrete terms. Recognizing that the influences to which the immigrants were subjected, and the treatment which they received after arrival, resulted in exploitation and neglect, they endeavored to prevent or repair the damage by turning to social action and dealing with specific problems such as economic exploitation, overcrowded and decrepit housing, destitution, broken homes, crime, alcoholism, prostitution and ill-health. The settlement dwellers worked largely on a local basis, directing their efforts and programs specifically at immigrant needs, at the needs of an oppressed minority. In so doing, they planted the seeds of a national social welfare program but their immediate concern was the neighborhood. This positive interest in the welfare of the immigrant poor went hand-in-hand with a desire to work with them, as well as for them, and also with a growing awareness that by accepting the cultural heritage and enhancing their self-respect, the slum dwellers were more likely to become involved in solving or ameliorating the problems of their group and their neighborhood.[10]

The great importance of health problems within this complex context was well-recognized. In 1909, Edward T. Devine,[11] a leading social worker, noted not only that "Ill health is perhaps the most constant of the attendants of poverty," but he went on to emphasize that "An inquiry into the physical condition of the members of the families that ask for aid . . . clearly indicates that whether it be the first cause or merely a complication from the effect of other causes, physical disability is at any rate a very serious disabling condition at the time of application in three-fourths . . . of all the families that come under the care of the Charity Organization Society, who are probably in no degree exceptional among families in need of charitable aid."[12]

Activities in New York and Chicago also are indicative of the importance attached to health work among the poor immigrants. In 1893, Lillian D. Wald and Mary Brewster opened the Nurses' Settlement on Henry Street in New York in order to bring the benefits of public health nursing to an entire neighborhood. The Henry Street Settlement developed an organized community service intended to prevent disease, as well as to help the sick. As its program grew, involvement in studies of health and social welfare extended the influence of Henry Street far beyond the locality.[13]

Also in 1893, four years after Jane Addams opened Hull House, a public dispensary was organized at the settlement in Chicago. It was open every day from three to four in the afternoon and from seven to eight in the evening. There was also a physician in residence at Hull House, and another doctor who lived nearby helped out. A nurse from the Visiting Nurses' Association was stationed at the settlement, and received her orders there. In addition, various studies and programs were undertaken to improve health conditions in the neighborhood where the settlement was located. These involved improvement of housing and garbage collection, combating cocaine addiction among minors, regulation of midwifery, studies of tuberculosis in relation to overcrowding, and of typhoid fever and poor sanitation.[14]

Thus, throughout the last decades of the 19th century and the early years of this century, the growing cities of the United States were increasingly confronted by the problems of poverty, crime, disease and other attendant ills of the slums, problems most often associated with immigration.[15] The inescapable fact of these urban problems, plus a growing conviction of the need for social change led to a broad movement of reform dedicated to the eradication of demonstrable social ills and the realization of conditions for a better life through planned social action. From this standpoint campaigns were mounted to deal with a wide range of problems: poverty and dependency, tenement house reform, sweatshops, prostitution, juvenile delinquency, and others among which ill health was prominent as a cause or a consequence.[16]

Coordinating Health Work

While these changes were taking place, the work of Pasteur, Koch and their contemporaries had been answering some of the pertinent questions concerning the causation and prevention of communicable diseases, and this knowledge was being applied in public health programs. As a result, by the end of the first decade of this century, there was a solid basis for the control of a number of infectious diseases and throughout succeeding decades advances along this line continued.[17] Alongside these trends, a shift was beginning to take place in the concept and orientation of community health action, a shift of attention from the environment to the individual. As health authorities and others became aware of noxious influences, other than those emanating from the physical environment, as activities in connection with maternal and child health, industrial hygiene, tuberculosis, venereal disease and mental ill-health developed, public health expanded. As new areas of concern became a part of public health, new programs developed and new personnel were trained to execute them.[18] Increasing expansion of the scope of community health work created problems for official and voluntary health agencies. As more and more special programs, operated by separate personnel and often through special agencies, came into being, it also became increasingly clear that better ways of organizing and administering health work were needed.[19] It was recognized that there was a need for the coordination of hitherto separated agencies, facilities and services, many of which were concerned with the same population. Even within a single agency (such as a large urban health department), duplication of effort and lack of coordination among its constituent units were found both wasteful, inefficient and irritating to the people who needed the services. In 1914, S. S. Goldwater, the Health Commissioner of New York City, observed that "Various brueaus send their representatives into the same districts, often into the same house, which results in undue expenditure of time and energy and in annoyance to the individual citizens."[20] A similar point of view was expressed by Charles F. Wilinsky in Boston. . . . "Gaps in the programs," he said, "duplication and consequent waste, frequent inefficiencies and misunderstandings, could not help but lead to the conclusion that there was a great need for better coordination and correlation, more efficient organization, and more harmonious understanding between those agencies concerned with the public health and with the amelioration of human suffering." He went on to add "that the fault of public health administration in large cities particularly was due to the fact that it was too far removed from the people it attempted to served."[21]

Wilinsky's last remark touches on another factor which reinforced the tendency to develop local health work, namely, recognition that effective application of health programs, especially among the poor and the foreign-born, required an approach to the people on their own ground, in their neighborhood. By locating a service in the section where they lived, one avoided the necessity of drawing these people away from familiar streets and landmarks. Strangeness and distance, as well as language barriers and long waiting periods, were serious limiting factors in the use of health facilities such as dispensaries and hospitals.[22] As Michael M. Davis pointed out, long waits were particularly important for mothers, "when children must either be brought along or left at home in the care of a busy neighbor, or of children too young to take the responsibility."[23] Moreover, "the mother in her home, seldom, if ever, getting out to gatherings of any sort, is the hardest member of the immigrant group to reach, and often the slowest to give up her racial habits; yet in her position as homekeeper she has most to do with the health of her family. Taking our health work into her neighborhood is the surest way to get acquainted with her."[24]

Nevertheless, even such a localization of health and social services was not enough as long as the prospective users, the consumers, confronted a multiplicity of uncoordinated agencies in a situation where they were Alices in a Wonderland of confusing community resources. About the time of the First World War, in East Harlem, in New York City, for example, there were many clinics, dispensaries, and district offices of welfare agencies, but the ordinary citizen had only the vaguest idea of what they did, what services they provided. Nor did he have any more precise notion of the service he needed. "He might be in trouble of some kind," wrote Homer Folks, "his health failing, or one of the children backward at school, or running afoul of the police, or the family just could not make ends meet. He needed assistance badly, somewhere, from somebody, but just what sort of help, or where to go to find it, or whether it could be had, were vague uncertainties . . . Possibly he remembered having seen a sign somewhere in the locality or someone had told him that somebody had said that someone had been helped from an office on the north side of 116th Street near First Avenue. If of an optimistic and pioneering type, he bravely started on a voyage of discovery of what we call the social resources of the community.

"If his courage were strong, and his health not too bad, the needy person might persevere and by making the rounds, calling, on one office and clinic after another, and being referred from one agency to another, he might finally arrive at the place where he should have gone in the first instance for real help for his particular trouble." The consequences of this situation were frequently deplorable; ". . . the fact of not knowing just what was needed, nor just where to go, resulted on the part of the less enterprising, in not going anywhere. And, going nowhere and doing nothing meant that things went from bad to worse."[25]

An implicit consequence of this statement is that health and welfare agencies should, as far as possible, be brought together, perhaps under one roof. As settlement workers had already recognized, the problems for which poor people needed help were usually neither simple nor single and had no easy solutions. More often than not their health and social problems were closely linked, so that those endeavoring to solve them had to establish the closet possible collaboration. This point was explicitly underscored by Robert A. Woods. "The local health center," he wrote, "gathers under one head a group of services which in greater or lesser degree have been undertaken in the past by the settlement. In all their technical phases the settlement clearly and unquestionably must be ready to pass them over to the health center. It is, however, equally clear — and this the promoters of the health centers do not always appreciate — that all the values of acquaintance and influence which the settlement has in its various organizations — must continue to be of indispensable importance to any sort of comprehensive local health campaign."[26] With this comment Woods touched upon another important dimension, the sociopsychological. Unless geographic localization and administrative coordination were complemented by social organization of the neighborhood with active participation of the population served, the fullest benefits of localized services would not be achieved. What was needed was a democratic educational process involving local people on an organized basis.

This aspect was most fully developed by Wilbur C. Phillips and his wife Elsie Cole Phillips.[27] The initial source for his idea of a community health plan was his experience as secretary of the New York Milk Committee established in 1907 by the Association for Improving the Condition of the Poor.[28] The objective of the Committee was to reduce infant mortality in New York City by improving its milk supply, and seeing that babies received clean milk. Phillips undertook to achieve this aim by establishing infant milk depots throughout the city. This in itself was not new; the philanthropist Nathan Strauss had begun to establish a system of milk stations in 1893.[29] However, Phillips soon recognized that distribution of milk was not enough. Stimulated by the work of Pierre Budin, professor of obstetrics at Paris who, in 1892, established a system of infant consultation centers, and based on his own experience, by 1909, Phillips had developed a concept of the milk depot as a "centre of influence for child life" where babies could receive medical examinations, where mothers could be taught how to keep their babies well, and from which would "radiate the influences of education and social betterment."[30]

The First Health Centers, 1910–1919

In 1911, this idea was expanded by Phillips in a Polish district of Milwaukee into a demonstration center for maternal and child care on a broad democratic basis using a so-called "block plan."[31] After resigning from the New York Milk Committee in 1910, he left for Milwaukee where implementation of his idea appeared feasible. Milwaukee had a high infant mortality, and seemed ready to deal with such problems in terms of basic social change, since it had recently elected a Socialist administration to office, the first large American city to do so. Phillips was then a member of the Socialist Party, having joined because as he says, "I knew at that time no other way of registering my opinion that poverty could and should be abolished — and that it could not be abolished through charity. But first, as the Socialists preached, came education — getting wider and wider numbers of people to understand the root causes of poverty and the way to remove them."[32]

In May, 1911, at the instigation of Phillips, a non-partisan Child Welfare Commission was appointed of which he became secretary. Its objective was to investigate the causes of infant mortality, and to formulate and carry out a plan of child welfare work from the standpoint of the entire community. By the end of the year the studies had been completed and a child health program based on a system of preventive health centers was proposed. This program was to be carried out by the municipality through its health department which would direct the work of social organizaiton, promotion and education that was regarded as absolutely essential for the development of the child health program, and which the Phillipses had been doing. As a demonstration, they set up a child health station in a Polish area, comprising 33 city blocks with a population of 16,000 people and between 350 to 400 mothers and babies. The medical staff to provide the preventive consultations was selected by the physicians of the district, who also agreed on a fixed fee of $2.00 to be paid each doctor for his period at the clinic. Cooperation of midwives and other local people was obtained. An unprecedented degree of support was obtained from the mothers by the creation of block committees headed by a block worker for each of the blocks in the demonstration area. This was the germ of the social unit idea which Phillips was then to try and implement in Cincinnati.

This was in the spring of 1912, but by June of that year, Wilbur Phillips and his wife were on their way to New York. Their activities had been upset by a change in the municipal administration. The Child Welfare Commission was terminated, and the child health program was limited to its purely medical aspects as part of a health department activity. But the idea of an "Educational Health Center" had been formulated, an idea which was to provide the basis for the Social Unit Organization, which in 1917 took form under Phillips' leadership in the Mohawk-

Brighton district of Cincinnati. This was undertaken as a demonstration of the National Social Unit Organization created by Phillips in 1916, with headquarters in New York City. The purpose of this group was "to promote the type of democratic community organization through which the citizenship as a whole can participate directly in the control of community affairs, while at the same time making constant use of the highest technical skill available."[33]

After some deliberation, the Mohawk-Brighton district of Cincinnati was chosen for the purpose of carrying out a "social unit" community experiment on a large scale, and funds were made available by the national organization for a period of three years, with a certain proportion of the budget to be raised in Cincinnati. This city was chosen in large measure because Courtenay Dinwiddie, secretary of the Cincinnati Anti-Tuberculosis League (realizing the importance of community organization) worked hard to have the demonstration there. The League had developed plans in 1917 for a neighborhood health center through which its aims might be attained, and now felt that the Social Unit Plan was capable of achieving even more than their initial goals.

The demonstration was carried out in a neighborhood of some 15,000 inhabitants, of whom between 5 and 10 per cent were recent immigrants.[34] The area was divided into thirty-one "blocks" of approximately 500 people each, and in each block, the residents over 18 years of age elected a council. This council elected a block worker who represented the residents of the block on the Citizens' Council of the Unit. Her duties were to visit the families in her section, keep them in touch with the Unit, and to bring specific problems they had to the proper department of the organization. The block worker was paid four dollars a week for the time lost from her household activities. Just as the Citizens' Council represented the people of the district, an Occupational Council secured the interest and cooperation of the various occupational and professional groups in the district, while the doctors, nurses, and social workers had their groups for the consideration of problems involved in their work. The Occupational Council was a neighborhood planning body working with other groups in the city. No new activities were undertaken until they had been endorsed by the people of the district through their representatives on the various councils. Most of the health and welfare agencies in Cincinnati, not only the Anti-Tuberculosis League, but also the Associated Charities, the Better Housing League and the Humane Society, cooperated with the Social Unit Organization.

The Cincinnati Social Unit demonstration was an experiment in applied democracy with health as its focal point. The health activities carried on included antepartum care, well child care for infants and pre-school children, anti-tuberculosis work, dental examination of school children, nursing service, medical care during the influenza epidemic of 1918, and periodic examination of adults. In short, beginning with health as a field of activity, Phillips and his co-workers endeavored to develop a consciously self-governing local unit in the midst of a large city. This enterprise was one of the most seminal experiments in social organization for health in the United States. It offered a vision of a community in which citizens working together as members of a vitally cooperating group sought the common welfare rationally and intelligently. It also raised profound political and social questions which are still unresolved. Can such a vision be realized in the heart of a large urban center? Can its inhabitants become truly conscious of mutual interests and be, in some degree, self-governing? Do such aims require a stable population, and how can such stability be maintained?

The Cincinnati experiment answered some but not all the questions. Opposition to it developed from the Director of Public Welfare, the newly elected Mayor, a local medical society and various conservatives who charged that the Social Unit demonstration was a Red plot, a not uncommon occurrence in the supercharged patriotic atmosphere at the end of the First World War. Although an investigation of the charges showed that they were unfounded, and a referendum within the Mohawk-Brighton district revealed a strong sentiment for the demonstration, the municipal administration withdrew its support, the funds that had been pledged were not forthcoming, and by 1920 the Social Unit demonstration was over. Without political and economic leverage, the inhabitants of the district could hardly make their wants felt. Phillips had not adequately established a financial basis nor had there been adequate time to create a political power base. The demonstration raised questions but provided only partial or ambiguous answers.

Meanwhile, efforts had been made elsewhere to provide health services to a definite population on a local basis. In 1912, William C. White, a physician and medical director of the Tuberculosis League of Pittsburgh, tried such an approach to tuberculosis control. As his model, he took the district system of the public schools. "In the educational field," he said, "there has gradually developed a knowledge of the equipment necessary for a given population, and this equipment has been apportioned so as to be readily accessible to those whom it is to serve. The management of these units is centered in a legally constituted governing body which also controls the expenditure of funds collected by taxation. The same form of control is applicable to tuberculosis and other health problems."[35] However, White's scheme lasted only six months. That year also saw an effort in Philadelphia by Samuel M. Hamill, a physician, to apply the same idea to child health work creating a basis for a growing program. Broader and more enduring efforts were also undertaken in New York, Boston and Buffalo.

In 1913, the New York Milk Committee established a health center on the lower West Side of Manhattan to serve a district populated largely by Syrians and Irish-Americans, where housing was poor and medical resources were limited.[36] The Bowling Green Neighborhood Association composed of local residents and outside specialists was formed to administer the center which provided chiefly antepartum and infant care. Neighborhood associations composed of voluntary groups of citizens were not new in New York City and many of them had worked with the Health Department in one way or another.[37]

S. S. Goldwater, Health Commissioner of New York, was aware of these developments and in September, 1914 formulated a plan to apply the principle of localization to health administration in order to see how far the work of the Department could "be improved by the substitution of a system of local or district administration for the present purely functional administrations."[38] To answer this question an experimental health district was established by January, 1915 on the lower East Side of Manhattan in an area populated almost entirely by Jews.[39] The district comprised a highly congested area of twenty-one blocks housing 25,000 people. The staff comprised a part-time district health officer in full charge of local administration, a part-time medical inspector who was responsible for medical inspection of preschool and school children as well as the infants' milk station, three nurses and one nurses' assistant, a food inspector and a sanitary inspector, both part-time. The basic principles underlying district work were coordination of health department functions, local administration in terms of local needs, and establishment of a community spirit. In accordance with the latter point, the health officer of the district was a Jewish physician who understood the people, their language, backgrounds and characteristics.

The experiment proved so satisfactory that on May 1, 1916 it was extended by Haven Emerson, (Health Commissioner from 1915 – 1917), to Queens, where four health districts were opened (Long Island City, Flushing, Ridgewood and Jamaica). In 1916, there was also created within the Health Department a Division of Health Districts under the

Deputy Commissioner of Health, and in 1917 the district health officers were placed on a full-time basis.[40] Unfortunately, at this time, there was a change in the city government, and the new administration slipped smoothly back into the established rut of the *status quo ante*. Among other actions, it halted the plans to extend district health administration to other parts of the city, and it was not until more than twelve years later that district health centers were established on a more solid basis in New York. Nevertheless, experience had been gained for such a program, and some advantages to be derived from decentralized public health administration were demonstrated. For example, as a consequence of the coordination of services, it was possible to serve families more efficiently, with all services rendered to a family provided by a single nurse. This led to the introduction of a Family Record Card which contained a continuous history of the family as far as Health Department services were concerned. However this abortive attempt to apply the principle of local administration to health work in New York City brought forth a problem which was to plague the revived district system in 1930s, namely, the division of responsibility and the relationships between the district health officers and the chiefs of the central functional bureaus of the Department.

During this period, health departments and private health and welfare agencies in a number of American cities and towns undertook to coordinate their activities on a localized basis and to develop neighborhood health centers and programs. In 1916, on the initiative of Charles F. Wilinsky, Deputy Health Commissioner of Boston, (who has been referred to above), the Blossom Street Health Unit was opened in the West End, one of the most congested sections of the city.[41] The objective was to provide a local center from which agencies engaged in health and welfare work could serve a geographically defined population. Among the agencies included in the center were the Consumptives Hospital Department, the Instructive District Nursing Association, the Milk and Baby Hygiene Association, the visiting physican of the Boston Dispensary, and the Hebrew Federated Charities. Later additions were clinics for dental care and mental health counseling. Eventually, Boston had eight centers, each serving a population of 50,000. This expansion was assisted by a bequest by George Robert White of six million dollars to the city of Boston for this purpose.

Similar developments occurred in other large cities. Beginning with one experimental station in 1914, Buffalo developed a citywide system of district services. By 1920 there were seven districts of 26,000 to 91,000 population (average about 75,000) with a center in each. The system represented a cooperative arrangement between the Department of Health and the Department of Hospitals and Dispensaries. Arrangements and proceedings were also worked out to govern relationships with private medical and social agencies. Basically this system was intended for the poor people of the city, and the districts were correlated with the existing tracts covered by the Charity Organization Society.[42]

Health Centers Spread

As C.-E. A. Winslow noted in 1919, "The most striking and typical development of the public health movement of the present day is the health center."[43] The First World War had emphasized the possibilities of coordinated effort in achieving results, as well as the importance of health, and these lessons were not lost on community leaders. When the War ended, health centers and demonstrations financed by foundations, voluntary health agencies, or other social welfare organizations, as well as by local governments were established in many parts of the United States. A decision by the American Red Cross at the end of the War to further the establishment of health centers gave additional impetus to this trend.[44] Local chapters undertook to create health centers, and more generally such facilities became the fashion in community health work.

The scope of this development is evident from the following figures obtained by the Red Cross during the latter part of 1919 in a survey of existing and planned health centers.[45] The report showed that as of January 1, 1920 there were 72 centers in 49 communities, of which seven cities had more than one center. In addition to the existing centers, 33 centers were being proposed or planned in 28 other communities. An analysis of the existing and proposed centers showed that at the time of the report, 33 were administered entirely by public authorities, 27 were under private control, and 16 were under combined public and private control. The Red Cross was involved in 19 instances. There was considerable variation in the work and aims of the existing health centers. In 40 communities with health centers in operation, 37 contained clinics of some type, 34 carried on visiting nursing, 29 did child welfare work, and 27 did antituberculosis work. Twenty-two had venereal disease clinics, 14 had dental clinics, and 11 had eye, ear, nose and throat clinics. Only 10 had laboratories, and nine had milk stations.

The succeeding decades witnessed a further development of health centers and districting of health services. In 1930, a subcommittee on health centers collected information for the White House Conference on Child Health and Protection. It obtained data for 1,511 major and minor health centers throughout the United States. Eighty per cent had been established since 1910. Of the total number, 725 were operated by private agencies, 729 by county or municipal health departments, and a small number by the Red Cross, hospitals, tuberculosis associations, case-work agencies and the like. In nearly half these centers, the principal support came from public funds, while supplementary aid came through community chests, or from private funds.

As is not infrequently the case when a professional development or trend is in "fashion," the name by which it is designated acquires an aura of approval, and is used to describe activities and enterprises that differ widely, so that they may share some of the aura. This was also the fate of the health center concept, and is in part responsible for its decline. As one observer put it in 1921, "We find it used as a name for child welfare stations, tuberculosis dispensaries, venereal disease clinics, out-patient departments of hospitals, settlement houses, and substations of local health departments."[46] The Red Cross concept of a health center was that of an institution which could be locally operated with a minimum of outside direction and with an emphasis on its function as an educational, informational facility. "Functionally, the health center is an institution through which the community may get in touch with all health promoting agencies and with the health problems of local and of national importance."[47] Administratively, however, the Red Cross view was that the health center should be under the combined guidance and control of all the local health agencies.

Michael M. Davis, writing in 1927, defined the health center more definitely and related it more specifically to health care, both preventive and curative. "Observation of a large number of health centers," he said, "leads to an indication of two factors which all those studied appeared to present: first, the selection of a definite district, or of a population unit, with the aim of serving all therein who need the services offered; second, coordination of services within this area, embracing both the facilities furnished by the health center itself and those provided by other agencies. A definition might therefore be stated as follows: A health center is an organization which provides, promotes and coordinates needed medical service and related social service for a specified district."[48] Davis also emphasized that there were still many unanswered questions concerning policy, objectives, organization, administration and evaluation of health centers. For example, he asked, "How far is organization of the people of a district themselves a practical means of promoting the services at the center, and of advancing health education throughout the district? Experience shows great value in a loose local organization of agencies interested in medical or health work,in education, especially public and parochial schools, and neighborhood and recreational bodies. On the other hand, the attempt to organize the people of a district into a local council, with or without block workers, has generally yielded little result in proportion to the effort expended. The reasons for this difficulty lie deep in the characteristics of American neighborhood life, whether among native or foreign-born."[49]

Meanwhile, significant district health programs were created and developed in a number of American communities. It is obviously impossible to discuss those developments in detail, but several selected examples can indicate some of their characteristics. In New York City a program of district health administration was developed after 1929, and a group of health centers was opened beginning with one in rented quarters in central Harlem. Actually, this program grew out of two demonstrations in the 1920s. The East Harlem Health Center was initiated in 1920 by the New York County chapter of the Red Cross, and was opened in November, 1921. The demonstration was planned as a three-year project involving the cooperation of the Health Department and 21 voluntary agencies, and was described as a "department store of health and welfare"[50] where clients could find under one roof almost all the health and welfare services needed. Throughout the decade the Health Center continued to develop, and eventually became one of the municipal district health units. While East Harlem was the first general health center, the Bellevue-Yorkville Health Demonstration, organized in 1924 and opened to the public in 1926, led eventually to the adoption by New York City of the principle of district health administration.[51] Financed by the Milbank Memorial Fund and the Health Department, the Demonstration was carried on for ten years in cooperation with a very large number of participating official and voluntary agencies.[52] With the example of two health centers in operation, and under pressure from leaders in the private health and welfare field, the Health Department developed a citywide plan of district administration, with a health center building in each district serving as a local headquarter for both private health and welfare agencies and for the field activities of the Department. In 1934, under the administration of Fiorello H. La Guardia, the city embarked on a program of districting which has had its ups and down over the years — but is still in existence at present. Owing to changing policies and intramural conflicts the potential of this system was never fully realized.

Plans initially started by William H. Welch in Baltimore in the twenties eventuated in 1932 in the establishment of the Eastern Health District as a cooperative endeavor of the Baltimore City Health Department, the Johns Hopkins School of Hygiene and Public Health, as well as several voluntary agencies. This district has made possible the intensive study of public health problems and has provided a field laboratory for the testing of new administrative procedures and for the training of personnel. A second district was organized in 1935.

The district health center, coordinating hitherto separated clinics and services, was inaugurated to replace centralized control of particular services. Generally, the health center has been a branch or unit of a local health department or some other official health agency. Except for such diseases as tuberculosis, venereal diseases and a few other conditions considered as public health problems, most medical care concerned with diagnosis and therapy remained outside the sphere of activity of health centers, which emphasized prevention. Far-sighted leaders in the health field realized that the health center concept might be employed to improve the organization and provision of medical care, issues which had come to the forefront of public attention at the same time as the health center. The Social Unit experiment in Cincinnati had touched on this problem, as did J. L. Pomeroy, the County Health Officer of Los Angeles, in his ambitious program undertaken in 1919.[53] In his centers, Pomeroy originally included clinics staffed by physicians, nurses and social workers to provide preventive and curative services on an ambulatory basis. The clinics were available to the poor whose eligibility was established by a means test. Due largely to the complaints of physicians that medical care was being given to patients who should go to private practitioners, by 1935 this work had, for the most part been turned over to the Welfare Department and the county general hospital. This attempt foundered on the slogan that undeserving individuals were abusing the service intended only for the indigent, a theme which has been played with variations for about one hundred years.[54]

The most imaginative approach was made by Hermann Biggs in 1920 when he endeavored to deal with health service for rural areas in New York State.[55] As Commissioner of Health, he proposed the establishment of local health centers to include one or more of the following elements: hospital, clinics (for tuberculosis, venereal diseases, prenatal and child care, mental illness, dental care, and general medical care), laboratories, public health nursing, and district health administration. Such centers could be established in any county with the approval of the State Health Commissioner. The proposal was permissive and not mandatory in any of its details. In addition to coordinating public health services, these centers were intended "to encourage and provide facilities for an annual medical examination to detect physical defects and disease;" and "to provide for the residents of rural districts, for industrial workers and all others in need of such service, scientific medical and surgical treatment, hospital and dispensary facilities and nursing care at a cost within their means or, if necessary, free." State aid in the form of 50 per cent cash grants for buildings, a cash allowance for the treatment of patients unable to pay, together with certain allowances toward maintenance, were to be furnished to all communities fulfilling the requirements of the State Health Department. While a large number of community organizations supported these proposals, the Sage-Machold Bill which embodied this health center program, was defeated in the New York Legislature. The whole concept was ahead of public opinion, and especially of opinion in the medical profession.

Biggs had realized that the next step in the development of community health services required a coalescence of preventive and curative medicine. Since 1920, this seminal concept has evolved in several directions. Among these the idea of comprehensive group practice coupled with prepayment, as exemplified by the Kaiser-Permanente Foundation and the Health Insurance Plan of Greater New York, has been demonstrated as practicable. Another approach was promoted by Joseph W. Mountin, of the U. S. Public Health Service, based on his belief that hospitals and health departments must eventually combine or coordinate their facilities and resources to provide a comprehensive health service for the communities they serve. As part of such a plan, he proposed to correlate the health center with the general hospital in the community.

After 1946, following the passage of the Hill-Burton Act, there was a renewal of the earlier interest in the role of the health center. A proponent of the idea who tied it to regionalization was John B. Grant of the Rockefeller Foundation. In fact, in 1949, he pointed out that the health center of the future had not yet been established.[56] Nevertheless, such centers did not really take hold after the 1940s.

Why Did the Health Center Movement Decline?

The concept of a local health center had developed largely in response to the circumstances and the needs of the urban poor, particularly the immigrants. From the time of the First World War, however, these elements were changing, especially during the decades of the twenties and the thirties. Consequently, the time setting in which the movement for local health centers emerged and became institutionalized is important for understanding its further development.

The cessation of immigration during the war years and the restrictive legislation of 1921 and 1924 were undoubtedly important factors in changing the circumstances of the foreign-born. As the flow of new immigrants was cut down to a trickle, the foreign-born and even more so their children adapted to American life under the influence of economic and educational factors.[57] As they moved up the economic ladder, there was an increasing tendency to move out of the areas of initial settlement and toward the periphery of the community. Between 1920 and 1930 there appeared to be a growing trend toward less clustering of the foreign-born in ethnic neighborhoods. Movements within the cities and towards suburbs scattered members of these groups in areas that were mixed. Many of those involved in this process were younger persons of the second generation, largely native-born, with a greater earning capacity than their parents or older families with few children below working age. Hand-in-hand with these changes went higher levels of schooling among the children of the foreign-born and a wider use of English by their parents, changes clearly reflected in the foreign language press of the period.

As this potential clientele for local health centers changed its character, it turned more and more to the use of private health care. This tendency was reinforced by the limited nature of the services provided in most local health centers. Thus, there was practically no integration of preventive and curative services. As Michael Davis saw in 1921, "curative work furnishes the best approach to preventive" service."In the field of preventive medical and health work," he said, "there is particular need for emphasizing . . . that the study of people must run parallel to the study of technique. As a corollary to this, curative work must be connected with preventive work, so that the service which the people seek of their own initiative can be supplemented by the service which we believe the larger interests of all require."[58] Therapeutic services were provided only to a limited degree, for the most part to patients with tuberculosis and venereal disease. At the same time medical practice was changing. Immunization, antepartum care and well child care were incorporated into the work of the private practitioner, and this was to happen later with the treatment of tuberculosis and venereal disease when the antibiotics became available.

The depression of the 1930s retarded these tendencies, but they were reinforced indirectly as the attention of many concerned with the provision of medical care and its costs turned to the problem of organizing the financing of such care on a compulsory or voluntary basis. The improvement of economic conditions toward the end of the decade coincident with the outbreak of World War II made it financially possible for more people to seek private medical care, especially when labor-management negotiations provided varying forms of health insurance. Thus, the local health centers tended to lose one part of the rationale for their creation.

The same period also saw the erosion of another part of the theoretical underpinning of the health center movement. Need for coordination of health and welfare services had been adduced as a reason for bringing them together under one roof or at least in close contiguity. However, the role of social agencies changed greatly during the depression as government, particularly on the Federal level, assumed a larger and more active part in welfare, specifically in its financial aspects. At the same time social work was beginning to move away from an interest in social problems and reform. Case work became the dominant facet of social work, and in turn social work focused on the individual, on his personal strengths and weaknesses, and on individual psychological mechanisms, with psychoanalysis providing a theoretical rationale for this orientation.[59] Along this line of development, social agencies withdrew from health centers to other locations where they could centralize their therapeutic services and utilize them more efficiently.

In addition to the factors discussed above, there were a number of others that hindered the development of health centers and led to the decline of the movement. Thus, despite the often expressed aim of involving the local population in the neighborhood health program, this goal was hardly realized and remained more of a pious intention. Although Bellevue-Yorkville in New York City may have been envisaged as an experiment to crystallize community consciousness around health as a center, the demonstration was actually run by a group of voluntary health and welfare agencies, financed by a foundation in collaboration with the municipal health department.[60] In the New Haven Health Center Demonstration (1920–1923), efforts to develop active participation by local people were admittedly unsuccessful, mainly because the necessary rapport was not established with the largely Italian population.[61]

Another negative factor was the resistance by political forces in the broadest sense. The ability of government (municipal or state) to hinder or to facilitate the creation and development of health center programs is evident from the examples of Milwaukee, Cincinnati, and New York. Antagonism of professional groups such as physicians or welfare agencies were significant in some cases. Administrative infighting within the municipal health department was a factor in weakening the New York City health center program, and such a factor may have been operative elsewhere. Finally, one should note that the health center movement participated in the general pattern of development of public health during this period. In the late 1930s public health was beginning to approach the end of a period of development that had begun around the first decade of the century. World War II was an interlude in this transition which is still in process. By that time, however, the health center movement had run out of steam.

Questions?

Analysis of the earlier health center movement raises certain questions about the current neighborhood health centers. These too have come into being to provide for the needs of the urban poor, of people who have migrated to the city and who live under circumstances highly adverse to health. These centers clearly fill an immediate need, and no doubt fulfill their purpose better than did the earlier centers.[62] Today they are located in impoverished areas. But what should happen if and when the economic status of the population changes? One aim of the centers is job training, which implies a change in economic condition. Is it not possible that improved economic circumstances may lead to a shift of population, and thus to a loss of health center clientele? Or is there an unexpressed assumption that the poor will always be with us and a separate system is needed for them? Furthermore, should neighborhood centers remain purely local, or should they become part of a larger system of health care toward which we appear to be moving? Should they become part of a national health insurance system and of a larger health-care delivery system? Obviously, such questions have no immediate answer, but they do arise from a consideration of the earlier local health center movement.

REFERENCES

1. Sar A. Levitan: The Great Society's Poor Law. A New Approach to Poverty, Baltimore, Johns Hopkins Press, 1969, pp. 191–197.
2. Lisbeth Bamberger: Health Care and Poverty: What Are the Dimensions of the Problem

from the Community's Point of View? Bull. N.Y. Acad. Med., 42:1140, 1966.
3. U. S. Bureau of Census: Historical Statistics of the United States, Colonial Times to 1957, Washington, D.C., Government Printing Office, 1960.
4. For the following see Moses Rischin: The Promised City: New York's Jews, 1870 – 1914, Cambridge, Harvard University Press, 1962; Hutchins Hapgood: The Spirit of the Ghetto, Cambridge, Belknap-Harvard University Press, 1967; Giuseppe Prezzolini: I Trappiantati, Milano, Longanesi, 1963, pp. 401 – 430; Phyllis H. Williams: South Italian Folkways in Europe and America, New Haven, Yale University Press, 1938; Robert E. Park and Herbert A. Miller: Old World Traits Transplanted, New York, Harper & Bros., 1921. The literature on this theme is large and the above references are simply illustrative.
5. Henry George: Social Problems, New York, 1886, pp. 40–46, 161–162.
6. Barbara M. Solomon: Ancestors and Immigrants. A Changing New England Tradition, Cambridge, Mass., Harvard University Press, 1956. Quotation is from the edition published by John Wiley & Sons, 1965, pp. 140–141.
7. John Higham: Strangers in the Land. Patterns of American Nativism, 1860-1925, (1955), New York, Atheneum, 1963, pp. 88–94.
8. Richard C. Cabot: Social Service and the Art of Healing. (1909), New York, Dodd, Mead & Co., 1931, pp. 4–7.
9. R. L. Duffus: Lillian Wald: Neighbor and Crusader, New York, 1939, p. 147.
10. Jane Addams: Hull House: An Effort Toward Social Democracy, Forum 14:226, 1892; Jane Addams et al.: Philanthropy and Social Progress: Seven Essays, New York, 1893, pp. 2–3, 15–16, 35–38. Lillian D. Wald: The House on Henry Street, New York, 1915, pp. 66, 184, 290, 310; Frank J. Bruno: Trends in Social Work . . . 1874–1946, New York, 1948.
11. Edward Thomas Devine (1867 – 1948) was General Secretary of the Charity Organization Society in New York City, 1896 – 1912, and Secretary until 1917; Director of the New York School of Philanthropy, 1904 – 1907, 1912 – 1917, and from 1905 to 1919 Professor of Social Economy at Columbia University.
12. ——— Misery and Its Causes, New York, Macmillan Company, 1910, p. 55. See the section on ill health in this book, pp. 53–112.
13. Lillian D. Wald: The House on Henry Street, New York, Henry Holt and Co., 1915, Ibid.: Windows on Henry Street, Boston, Little, Brown and Co., 1934.
14. Hull House Maps and Papers. A Presentation of Nationalities and Wages in a Congested District of Chicago, together with Comments and Essays on Problems Growing Out of the Social Conditions by Residents of Hull House, New York and Boston, Thomas Y. Crowell, 1895, p. 228; Jane Addams: Twenty Years at Hull House, New York, Macmillan, 1910, pp. 342–358.
15. Kate H. Claghorn: The Foreign Immigrant in New York City. In United States Industrial Commission: Reports on Immigration (Washington, D.C.), 15:449ff, 1901; see also Harper's Weekly, January 12, 1895, p. 42, 60–62, and June 22, 1895, pp. 586–587.
16. George Rosen: A History of Public Health, New York, MD Publications, 1958, pp. 344–349.
17. Ibid., pp. 319–343.
18. Health and National Efficiency. Modern Medicine 1:2–3, 1919; H. W. Hill: The New Public Health, Ibid.: 1:57–58, 1919.
19. Michael M. Davis: Immigrant Health and the Community, New York, Harper and Brothers, 1921, pp. 406–407.
20. Annual Report of the Department of Health of the City of New York for the Calendar Year 1914, New York City 1915, p. 25. The House that Health Built. A Report of the First Three Years' Work of the East Harlem Health Center Demonstration, prepared under the Direction of Kenneth D. Widdemer, New York City, 1925, p. 4.
21. The Health Units of Boston, 1924–1933, City of Boston Printing Department, 1933, quoted in I. V. Hiscock: The Development of Neighborhood Health Services in the United States, Milbank Memorial Quarterly, 13:30–51, 1935 (p. 35).
22. Davis, op. cit., p. 299.

23. Ibid., p. 329.
24. Ibid., p. 299.
25. Homer Folks, Preface, House that Health Built (fn. 20), p. 3.
26. Robert A. Woods: The Neighborhood in Nation-Building, Boston and New York, Houghton Mifflin Co., 1923, p. 279.
27. Wilbur C. Phillips: Adventuring For Democracy, New York, Social Unit Press, 1940. Unfortunately, Phillips rarely dates the events he describes so that the evolution of his activities and ideas has had to be reconstructed from other sources indicated below.
28. Charles E. North: Milk and Its Relation to Public Health, in A Half Century of Public Health, edited by Mazyck P. Ravenel, New York, American Public Health Association, 1921, pp. 279–280; William H. Allen: Health Needs and Civic Action, in The Public Health Movement, Philadelphia, American Academy of Political and Social Science, 1911, pp. 3–12 (see p. 7).
29. Rosen, op. cit., pp. 354–355.
30. Wilbur C. Phillips: The Achievements and Future Possibilities of the New York Milk Committee, Proceedings of the Child Conference for Research and Welfare, 1909, Clark University, Worcester, Mass., July 6–10, 1909, New York, G. E. Stechert & Co., 1910, pp. 189–192.
31. Wilbur C. Phillips: The Trend of Medico-Social Effort in Child Welfare Work, American Journal of Public Health 2: 875 – 882, 1912 (see pp. 881 – 882); idem, Adventures in Democracy, pp. 46–47, 55–56, 63–114.
32. Ibid., Adventures in Democracy, pp. 59–60.
33. A. C. Burnham: The Community Health Problem, New York, Macmillan Co., 1920, p. 108.
34. N. A. Nelson: Neighborhood Organization vs Tuberculosis, Modern Medicine 1:515–521, 1919; Courtenay Dinwiddie and A. G. Kreidler: A Community Self-Organized for Preventive Health Work, Modern Medicine 1:26–31, 1919. Wilbur C. Phillips: Democracy and the Unit Plan, Proceedings of the National Conference of Social Work, Atlantic City, New Jersey, June 1–8, 1919, National Conference of Social Work, 1920, p. 562.
35. William C. White: The Official Responsibility of the State in the Tuberculosis Problem, J.A.M.A., 65:512–514, 1915.
36. Davis, op. cit., p. 381.
37. Shirley W. Wynne: Neighborhood Health Development inthe City of New York, Milbank Memorial Fund Quarterly Bulletin, 9:37–45, 1931.
38. Annual Report of the Department of Health of the City of New York for the Calendar Year 1914, New York City, 1915, p. 25.
39. Davis, op. cit., pp. 381 – 384. According to Herbert Kaufman: The New York City Health Centers (Inter-University Case Program #9), Indianapolis, Bobbs-Merrill Co., 1959, the population was 35,000.
40. Annual Report of the Department of Health of the City of New York for the Calendar Year 1916, New York City, 1917, pp. 23, 31; Annual Report of the Department of Health of the City of New York for the Calendar Year 1917, (n.p., n.d.), pp. 12 – 13; Ira V. Hiscock: The Development of Neighborhood Health Services in the United States, Milbank Memorial Fund Quarterly, 13:30–51, 1935, pp. 38–39.
41. Charles F. Wilinsky: The Blossom Street Health Unit, The Nation's Health 6:397–398, 1924; ibid: The Health Center, American Journal of Public Health 17: 677–682, 1927.
42. Michael M. Davis: Clinics, Hospitals and Health Centers, New York, Harper & Brothers, 1927, pp. 354–355; Hiscock, op. cit., p. 48.
43. [C.-E. A. Winslow] The Health Center Movement, Modern Medicine 1:327, 1919.
44. Burnham, op. cit., pp. 99 – 100; E. A. Peterson and W. H. Brown; The American Red Cross and Health, the Nation's Health 3:73–80, 1921.
45. James A. Tobey: The Health Center Movement in the United States, Modern Hospital 14:212–214, 1920.
46. Peterson and Brown, op. cit., p. 79.

47. E. A. Peterson: What Is a Health Center? The Nation's Health 3:272–274, 1921.
48. Michael M. Davis: Goal-Post and Yardsticks in Health Center Work, A.J.P.H. 17:433-440, 1927 (p. 434).
49. Ibid., p. 439.
50. House that Health Built (see fn. #9), p. 4. A Decade of District Health Center Pioneering, A Report of Ten Years Work of the East Harlem Center, New York City, 1932, p. 23; George R. Bedinger: Cooperative Health Plan in New York County, the Nation's Health 3:486–489, 1921.
51. C.-E. A Winslow and Savel Zimand: Health Under the "El," New York and London, Harper & Brothers, 1937.
52. The exact number seems uncertain, but was probably close to 70. According to Hiscock there were 85, according to Kaufman about 65.
53. J. L. Pomeroy: County Health Administration in Los Angeles, A.J.P.H., 11:796–800, 1921; ibid.: Health Center Development in Los Angeles County, J.A.M.A., 93: 1546–1550, 1929.
54. George Rosen: The Impact of the Hospital on the Patient, the Physician and the Community, Hospital Administration 9:15–33, 1964.
55. Milton Terris: Hermann Biggs' Contribution to the Modern Concept of Health Centers, Bull. Hist. Med. 20:87 – 412, 1964; B. R. Rickards: What New York State has done in Health Centers, A.J.P.H. 11:214–216, 1921.
56. John B. Grant: Health Care for the Community. Selected Papers edited by Conrad Seipp, Baltimore, Johns Hopkins Press, 163, pp. 5–6, 21–24, and passim.
57. Recent Social Trends in the United States. Report of the President's Research Committee on Social Trends, New York McGraw-Hill, 1933, pp. 469, 560, 563 – 564, 582; John C. Gebhart: The Health of a Neighborhood. A Social Study of the Mulberry District, New York Association for Improving the Condition of the Poor, 1924, pp. 5–7.
58. Davis, Immigrant Health and Community, p. 419.
59. George Rosen: Madness in Society. Chapters in the Historical Sociology of Mental Illness, Chicago, Ill., University of Chicago Press, 1968, pp. 310–312.
60. Winslow and Zimand, Health Under the "El," pp. 11–13, 38–48.
61. Philip S. Platt: Report on New Haven Health Center Demonstration July 1920–June 1923, (n.p., n.d.), pp. 21–23, 98.
62. Gerald Sparer: Evaluation of OEO Neighborhood Health Centers, A.J.P.H. 61:931 – 942, 1971.

Library of Congress Cataloging in Publication Data

Rosen, George, 1910–
From medical police to social medicine.

1. Social medicine—Addresses, essays, lectures.
2. Medical care—History—Addresses, essays, lectures.
I. Title. [DNLM: 1. Delivery of health care.
2. Social medicine—History. WA11 R813f]
RA418.R67 362.1′09 74-10819
ISBN 0–88202–015–3
ISBN 0–88202–016–1 (pbk.)